The Diabetic Foot

Editor

ANDREW J.M. BOULTON

MEDICAL CLINICS
OF NORTH AMERICA

www.medical.theclinics.com

September 2013 • Volume 97 • Number 5

ELSEVIER

1600 John F. Kennedy Boulevard • Suite 1800 • Philadelphia, Pennsylvania, 19103-2899

http://www.theclinics.com

MEDICAL CLINICS OF NORTH AMERICA Volume 97, Number 5
September 2013 ISSN 0025-7125, ISBN-13: 978-1-4557-7598-9

Editor: Pamela Hetherington

Medical Clinics of North America (ISSN 0025-7125) is published bimonthly by Elsevier Inc., 360 Park Avenue South, New York, NY 10010-1710. Months of publication are January, March, May, July, September, and November. Business and editorial offices: 1600 John F. Kennedy Boulevard, Suite 1800, Philadelphia, PA 19103-2899. Periodicals postage paid at New York, NY, and additional mailing offices. Subscription prices are USD $241.00 per year (US individuals), $441.00 per year (US institutions), $121.00 per year (US Students), $307.00 per year (Canadian individuals), $572.00 per year (Canadian institutions), $190.00 per year (Canadian and foreign students), $372.00 per year (foreign individuals), and $572.00 per year (foreign institutions). To receive student/resident rate, orders must be accompanied by name of affiliated institution, date of term, and the signature of program/residency coordinator on institution letterhead. Orders will be billed at individual rate until proof of status is received. Foreign air speed delivery is included in all Clinics' subscription prices. All prices are subject to change without notice. **POSTMASTER:** Send address changes to *Medical Clinics of North America*, Elsevier Health Sciences Division, Subscription Customer Service, 3251 Riverport Lane, Maryland Heights, MO 63043. **Customer Service: Telephone: 1-800-654-2452** (U.S. and Canada); **1-314-447-8871** (outside U.S. and Canada). **Fax: 314-447-8029. E-mail: journalscustomerserviceusa@elsevier.com** (for print support); **journalsonlinesupport-usa@elsevier.com** (for online support).

Reprints. For copies of 100 or more of articles in this publication, please contact the Commercial Reprints Department, Elsevier Inc., 360 Park Avenue South, New York, NY 10010-1710. Tel.: 212-633-3874; Fax: 212-633-3820; E-mail: reprints@elsevier.com.

Medical Clinics of North America is also published in Spanish by McGraw-Hill Interamericana Editores S. A., P.O. Box 5-237, 06500 Mexico, D.F., Mexico.

Medical Clinics of North America is covered in *MEDLINE/PubMed (Index Medicus), Current Contents, ASCA, Excerpta Medica, Science Citation Index,* and *ISI/BIOMED.*

Printed and bound by CPI Group (UK) Ltd, Croydon, CR0 4YY

Transferred to digital print 2013

PROGRAM OBJECTIVE
The goal of the *Medical Clinics of North America* is to keep practicing physicians up to date with current clinical practice by providing timely articles reviewing the state of the art in patient care.

TARGET AUDIENCE
All practicing physicians and other healthcare professionals.

LEARNING OBJECTIVES
Upon completion of this activity, participants will be able to:
1. Review topical and biological therapies for diabetic foot ulcers as well as hyperbaric oxygen therapy as adjunctive treatment of diabetic foot ulcers.
2. Discuss peripheral arterial disease and bypass surgery in the diabetic lower limb.
3. Recognize, manage, and diagnose osteomyelitis in the diabetic foot.

ACCREDITATION
The Elsevier Office of Continuing Medical Education (EOCME) is accredited by the Accreditation Council for Continuing Medical Education (ACCME) to provide continuing medical education for physicians.

The EOCME designates this enduring material for a maximum of 15 *AMA PRA Category 1 Credit*(s) ™. Physicians should claim only the credit commensurate with the extent of their participation in the activity.

All other health care professionals requesting continuing education credit for this enduring material will be issued a certificate of participation.

DISCLOSURE OF CONFLICTS OF INTEREST
The EOCME assesses conflict of interest with its instructors, faculty, planners, and other individuals who are in a position to control the content of CME activities. All relevant conflicts of interest that are identified are thoroughly vetted by EOCME for fair balance, scientific objectivity, and patient care recommendations. EOCME is committed to providing its learners with CME activities that promote improvements or quality in healthcare and not a specific proprietary business or a commercial interest.

The planning committee, staff, authors and editors listed below have identified no financial relationships or relationships to products or devices they or their spouse/life partner have with commercial interest related to the content of this CME activity:
Mostafa A. Albayati, BSc, MBBS, DMCC; David G. Armstrong, DPM, MD, PhD; Andrew JM Boulton, MD, DSc (Hon), FACP, FRCP; Santha Priya Boorasamy; Javier La Fontaine, MS, DPM; Robert Frykberg, DPM, MPH; Frances L. Game, FRCP; Pamela Hetherington; Brynne Hunter; Adam L. Isaac, DPM; William Jeffcoate, MRCP; Edward B. Jude, MD; Paul J. Kim, MS, DPM; Sandy Lavery; Magnus Löndahl, MD, PhD; David J. Margolis, MD, PhD; Janice V. Mascarenhas, MBBS; Jill McNair; Lindsay Parnell; Jim A. Reekers, MD, PhD, EBIR; Nicholas A. Richmond, BS; Lee C. Rogers, DPM; Clifford P. Shearman, MS, FRCS; Wei Shen, MD, PhD; Alejandra C. Vivas, MD; Dane Wukich, MD.

The planning committee, staff, authors and editors listed below have identified financial relationships or relationships to products or devices they or their spouse/life partner have with commercial interest related to the content of this CME activity:
Robert S. Kirsner, MD, PhD is a consultant/advisor for Organogenesis Inc. and Shire, and has a research grant from Healthpoint.

Lawrence A. Lavery, MPH, DPM is on speakers bureau for Innovative Therapies Inc., Pamlab, Inc., KCL Licensing, Inc.; and Shire Regenerative Medicine; is consultant advisor for Innovative Therapies Inc., Pamlab, Inc. and KCI Licensing, Inc; has stock ownership in Diabetica Solutions Inc. and Prizm Medical Inc.; has research grants from Osiris Therapeutics Inc, Thermotek, MacroCure, GlaxoSmithKline, Innovative Therapies Inc, Pamlab, Inc. and KCI Licensing, Inc.; and has royalties/patents with Diabetica Solutions.

Benjamin A. Lipsky, MD, FACP, FIDSA, FRCP is on speakers bureau for Merck & Co., Inc. and Novartis Pharmaceuticals Corporation; is a consultant/advisor for Innocll, Cerexa, Inc. and Novartis Pharmaceuticals Corporation; and has a research grant from Innocll.

Edgar J.G. Peters, MD, PhD has a research grant from Fonds Nuts Ohra.

UNAPPROVED/OFF-LABEL USE DISCLOSURE
The EOCME requires CME faculty to disclose to the participants:
1. When products or procedures being discussed are off-label, unlabelled, experimental, and/or investigational (not US Food and Drug Administration (FDA) approved); and

2. Any limitations on the information presented, such as data that are preliminary or that represent ongoing research, interim analyses, and/or unsupported opinions. Faculty may discuss information about pharmaceutical agents that is outside of FDA-approved labelling. This information is intended solely for CME and is not intended to promote off-label use of these medications. If you have any questions, contact the medical affairs department of the manufacturer for the most recent prescribing information.

TO ENROLL
To enroll in the *Medical Clinics of North America* Continuing Medical Education program, call customer service at 1-800-654-2452 or sign up online at http://www.theclinics.com/home/cme. The CME program is available to subscribers for an additional annual fee of USD $267.

METHOD OF PARTICIPATION
In order to claim credit, participants must complete the following:
1. Complete enrolment as indicated above.
2. Read the activity.
3. Complete the CME Test and Evaluation. Participants must achieve a score of 70% on the test. All CME Tests and Evaluations must be completed online.

CME INQUIRIES/SPECIAL NEEDS
For all CME inquiries or special needs, please contact elsevierCME@elsevier.com

MEDICAL CLINICS OF NORTH AMERICA

NOW AVAILABLE FOR YOUR iPhone and iPad

Contributors

EDITOR

ANDREW J.M. BOULTON, MD, DSc (Hon), FACP, FRCP
Professor of Medicine, Centre for Endocrinology and Diabetes, Faculty of Medical and Human Sciences, Manchester Diabetes Centre, Consultant Physician, Manchester Royal Infirmary, University of Manchester, Manchester, United Kingdom; Visiting Professor, Voluntary Professor of Medicine, Diabetes Research Institute, University of Miami, Miami, Florida; President, European Association for the Study of Diabetes, Dusseldorf, Germany

AUTHORS

MOSTAFA A. ALBAYATI, MBBS, BSc
Department of Vascular Surgery, University Hospital Southampton, Southampton, Hampshire, United Kingdom

DAVID G. ARMSTRONG, DPM, MD, PhD
Professor of Surgery and Director, Southern Arizona Limb Salvage Alliance (SALSA), Department of Surgery, University of Arizona College of Medicine, Tucson, Arizona

ANDREW J.M. BOULTON, MD, DSc (Hon), FACP, FRCP
Professor of Medicine, Centre for Endocrinology and Diabetes, Faculty of Medical and Human Sciences, Manchester Diabetes Centre, Consultant Physician, Manchester Royal Infirmary, University of Manchester, Manchester, United Kingdom; Visiting Professor, Voluntary Professor of Medicine, Diabetes Research Institute, University of Miami, Miami, Florida; President, European Association for the Study of Diabetes, Dusseldorf, Germany

ROBERT G. FRYKBERG, DPM, MPH
Chief, Podiatry Section, Phoenix VA Healthcare System, Phoenix, Arizona

FRANCES L. GAME, FRCP
Consultant Diabetologist and Honorary Associate Professor, Department of Diabetes and Endocrinology, Derby Hospitals NHS Trust, Derby, United Kingdom

ADAM L. ISAAC, DPM
Southern Arizona Limb Salvage Alliance (SALSA), Department of Surgery, University of Arizona College of Medicine, Tucson, Arizona

WILLIAM JEFFCOATE, MRCP
Professor, Department of Diabetes and Endocrinology, Nottingham University Hospitals Trust, Nottingham, United Kingdom

EDWARD B. JUDE, MD
Consultant Physician and Reader in Medicine, Tameside Hospital NHS Foundation Trust, Ashton-under-Lyne, Lancashire; University of Manchester, Manchester, United Kingdom

PAUL J. KIM, MS, DPM
Associate Professor, Department of Plastic Surgery, Georgetown University School of Medicine, Georgetown University Hospital, Washington, DC

ROBERT S. KIRSNER, MD, PhD
Professor, Vice Chairman and Stiefel Laboratories Chair, Department of Dermatology and Cutaneous Surgery, University of Miami Miller School of Medicine, Miami, Florida

JAVIER LA FONTAINE, MS, DPM
Associate Professor, Department of Plastic Surgery, The University of Texas Southwestern Medical Center, Dallas, Texas

LAWRENCE A. LAVERY, MPH, DPM
Professor, Department of Plastic Surgery, The University of Texas Southwestern Medical Center, Dallas, Texas

BENJAMIN A. LIPSKY, MD, FACP, FIDSA, FRCP
Visiting Professor of Medicine, University of Geneva, Switzerland; Professor, University of Washington, Seattle, Washington

MAGNUS LÖNDAHL, MD, PhD
Department of Clinical Sciences, Lund University; Department of Endocrinology, Skane University Hospital, Lund, Sweden

DAVID J. MARGOLIS, MD, PhD
Departments of Biostatistics and Epidemiology, and Dermatology, University of Pennsylvania School of Medicine, Philadelphia, Pennsylvania

JANICE V. MASCARENHAS, MBBS
Clinical Research Fellow, Department of Endocrinology, St. John's National Academy of Health Sciences, Bangalore, Karnataka, India

EDGAR J.G. PETERS, MD, PhD
Department of Internal Medicine, VU University Medical Center, Amsterdam, The Netherlands

JIM A. REEKERS, MD, PhD, EBIR
Department of Radiology, Academic Medical Center, Teaching Hospital, University of Amsterdam, Amsterdam, The Netherlands

NICHOLAS A. RICHMOND, BS
Wound Research Fellow, Department of Dermatology and Cutaneous Surgery, University of Miami Miller School of Medicine, Miami, Florida

LEE C. ROGERS, DPM
Co-Director, Amputation Prevention Center, Valley Presbyterian Hospital, Los Angeles, California; Assistant Professor, College of Podiatric Medicine, Western University of Health Sciences, Pomona, California

CLIFFORD P. SHEARMAN, MS, FRCS
Professor, Department of Vascular Surgery, University Hospital Southampton, Southampton, Hampshire, United Kingdom

WEI SHEN, MD, PhD
University of Pittsburgh Medical Center Comprehensive Foot and Ankle Center, Pittsburgh, Pennsylvania

ALEJANDRA C. VIVAS, MD
Postdoctoral Clinical Research Associate, Department of Dermatology and Cutaneous Surgery, University of Miami Miller School of Medicine, Miami, Florida

DANE WUKICH, MD
University of Pittsburgh Medical Center Comprehensive Foot and Ankle Center, Pittsburgh, Pennsylvania

Contents

Osteomyelitis of the foot in diabetes is common and frequently undiagnosed. Diagnosis should be clinical and based on signs of infection, the size of the lesion, and the visibility of bone in the first instance but supported by the results of radiologic examination. The gold standard for diagnosis is histologic and microbiological examination of bone, which is not possible or necessary in all patients. There is no consensus as to whether management should be primarily medical or surgical; the pros and cons of each approach must be taken into account on an individual basis and after discussion with patients.

Hyperbaric oxygen therapy (HBO) is a short-term, high-dose oxygen inhalation and diffusion therapy, delivered systemically through airways and blood under high pressure using hyperbaric chambers. HBO stimulates angiogenesis, reduces edema, augments granulation tissue formation by enhancing fibroblasts, and improves leukocyte function by elevating the partial pressure of oxygen in tissue. The number of clinical trials evaluating the effect of HBO on the healing of diabetic foot ulcers is increasing, and to date two double-blind randomized controlled trials have been published, both showing improved long-term healing after HBO.

Preface

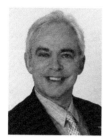

Andrew J.M. Boulton, MD, DSc (Hon), FACP, FRCP
Editor

A recent article from the United Kingdom reported that guidelines on diabetic foot care are not being adhered to, resulting in a variation in the rates of potentially preventable amputations across the country.[1] Many patients with diabetic foot lesions present late in the natural history of the condition, often because they have lost the "gift of pain" as a consequence of neuropathy. Foot ulcers and amputations result in reduced quality of life, often prolonged hospital in-patient stays, and increased morbidity and mortality. Cavanagh et al revised comparative costs of treating diabetic foot lesions in five different countries[2]; looking at the cost burden for the individual patient, they reported that whereas treatment of a simple foot ulcer in the United States would cost the equivalent of six days of average income; a below-knee amputation in India would cost the equivalent of nearly six years of income. Thus, in this issue of the *Medical Clinics of North America*, the first few articles review the pathways to ulceration, epidemiology of foot problems, and the potential for prevention. As outlined by Jeffcoate and Margolis, problems with the definition and ascertainment of diabetes as well as differences in the measurement of amputation may partially explain variations in amputation not only between centers but also between countries.

Research in diabetic foot problems is a relatively new discipline, and the whole area has been plagued by a lack of evidence-based reports and randomized controlled trials of putative new therapies. This has partly been a consequence of the rarity of certain of the sequelae of diabetic neuropathy. Thus three reviews focus on Charcot neuroarthropathy, the commonest cause of which in the 21st century is diabetes: a recent systematic review of surgical management of Charcot neuroarthropathy confirmed that the 95 articles included were generally case reports or series classed as level 4 or 5 evidence.[3] However, randomized controlled trials of potential therapies are extremely challenging to execute as the condition is relatively rare and no center would be able to enroll sufficient cases; multicenter trials are therefore required. In other areas such as offloading, systematic reviews and meta-analyses have been possible.[4]

The debate over surgical versus interventional radiologic treatments of lower extremity peripheral vascular disease rages on: two articles discuss potentially different management options.

Med Clin N Am 97 (2013) xiii–xiv
http://dx.doi.org/10.1016/j.mcna.2013.05.003
0025-7125/13/$ – see front matter © 2013 Published by Elsevier Inc.

medical.theclinics.com

The management of diabetic foot infections continues to be debated and this is covered by Peters and Lipsky, who also discuss the recent clinical practice guidelines on this topic.[5] The controversial topic of medical versus surgical management of osteomyelitis is discussed in two articles.

Finally, a number of new therapies and the ongoing controversy over the role of hyperbaric oxygen are debated in two reviews. During the preparation of this issue, an important article on the efficacy of hyperbaric oxygen was published[6] and comment on this is now included in the review by Londahl.

It is hoped that this issue of *Medical Clinics of North America* will update the readership on these common medical problems, but most important of all, despite all the guidelines that exist, it is vital to remember as very recently pointed out in an editorial on diabetes management,[7] to treat the patient as a whole, not only as the feet!

Andrew J.M. Boulton, MD, DSc (Hon), FACP, FRCP
Department of Medicine
Centre for Endocrinology and Diabetes
Faculty of Medical and Human Sciences
Manchester Diabetes Centre
193 Hathersage Road
Manchester, M13 0JE, UK

Department of Medicine
Diabetes Research Institute
Miami, FL 33101, USA

European Association for the Study of Diabetes
Dusseldorf, Germany

E-mail address:
ABoulton@med.miami.edu

REFERENCES

1. McInnes AD. Diabetic foot disease in the United Kingdom: about time to put feet first. J Foot Ankle Res 2012;11:26.
2. Cavanagh P, Attinger C, Abbas Z, et al. Cost of treating diabetic foot ulcers in five different countries. Diabetes Metab Res Rev 2012;28(Suppl 1):107–1011.
3. Lowery NJ, Woods JB, Armstrong DG, et al. Surgical management of Charcot neuroarthropathy of the foot and ankle: a systematic review. Foot Ankle Int 2012;33:113–21.
4. Morona JK, Buckley ES, Jones S, et al. Comparison of the clinical effectiveness of different off-loading devices for the treatment of neuropathic foot ulcers in patients with diabetes: a systematic review and meta-analysis. Diabetes Metab Res Rev 2013;29:183–93.
5. Lipsky BA, Berendt AR, Cornia PB, et al. 2012 Infectious Diseases Society of America clinical practice guideline for the diagnosis and treatment of diabetic foot infections. Clin Infect Dis 2012;54:132–73.
6. Margolis DJ, Gupta J, Hoffstad O, et al. Lack of effectiveness of hyperbaric oxygen therapy for the treatment of diabetic foot ulcer and the prevention of amputation: a cohort study. Diabetes Care 2013;36 [Epub ahead of print] Feb 19.
7. McLaren LA, Quinn TJ, McKay GA. Diabetes control in older people. BMJ 2013; 346:f2625.

The Pathway to Foot Ulceration in Diabetes

Andrew J.M. Boulton, MD, DSc (Hon), FRCP[a,b,c,*]

KEYWORDS

- Diabetic foot ulceration • Diabetic neuropathy • Peripheral vascular disease
- Foot pressures • Risk factors

KEY POINTS

- Risk factors for foot lesions include peripheral and autonomic neuropathy, peripheral vascular disease, history of ulceration or amputation, other microvascular complications (particularly end-stage renal disease on dialysis), foot deformity, and abnormalities of foot pressures.
- Peripheral neuropathy, foot deformity, and trauma (often from ill-fitting footwear) represent the commonest causal pathway to foot ulceration.
- All patients with diabetes require an annual foot screen, and those found to be at risk require specialist foot care and preventive foot-care education.
- Recent developments in foot screening include the Ipswich Touch Test, the Vibratip, and the Neuropad. An understanding of the implications of the loss of protective sensation is essential if we are to succeed in reducing the all too high incidence of foot problems in diabetes.

INTRODUCTION

"Coming events cast their shadow before"
— Thomas Campbell.

Foot ulcers in diabetic patients are common but eminently preventable, and occur in both main types of diabetes. From a global perspective, although diabetic foot ulcers (DFU) are seen in every race and country, the pathways resulting in foot lesions do vary according to the geographic location. It has been estimated that the lifetime risk of a patient with diabetes developing a foot ulcer may be as high as 25%,[1] and at any one time in Western countries 2% to 3% of diabetic patients are likely to have active foot ulceration.[2,3] It has also been estimated that up to 80% of all amputations in diabetes are preceded by DFU, therefore any success in reducing the incidence of DFU will also

[a] European Association for the Study of Diabetes, Düsseldorf, Germany; [b] Manchester Royal Infirmary, University of Manchester, Manchester, UK; [c] University of Miami, Downtown, FL, USA
* Manchester Diabetes Centre, 193 Hathersage Road, Manchester M13 0JE, UK.
E-mail address: ABoulton@med.miami.edu

Med Clin N Am 97 (2013) 775–790
http://dx.doi.org/10.1016/j.mcna.2013.03.007
0025-7125/13/$ – see front matter © 2013 Elsevier Inc. All rights reserved.

medical.theclinics.com

have some impact on amputation rates. A thorough understanding of the pathways leading to foot ulceration is therefore vital if any reduction in the incidence of these feared complications is to be achieved. The words of Campbell, although clearly not referring to foot ulceration or amputation, can be applied to the etiopathogenesis of foot ulceration. There are many "shadows" or signs that may be detected in patients with diabetes that would suggest they may be at increased risk of developing foot lesions. DFU rarely occur spontaneously, so it is a combination of several contributory factors that ultimately result in the development of an ulcer. Foot ulceration invariably occurs as a consequence of an interaction of specific abnormalities in the lower extremity acting in conjunction with environmental hazards. Lower extremity problems are one of the commonest precipitants of hospitalization in diabetic patients, and there are therefore potential economic benefits to be gained by preventive strategies. The cost of DFU has been reviewed,[4] and the potential economic benefits of prevention strategies have been calculated.[5]

Several contributory factors that are important in the pathogenesis of DFU are considered in this review, followed by a description of the pathways that might result in ulceration. The value of screening for patients with diabetes for risk factors for foot ulceration and potential preventive strategies are then discussed; finally, the challenges of living with sensory loss are explained.

ETIOPATHOGENESIS OF DIABETIC FOOT ULCERATION

As already noted, DFU rarely result from a single pathologic factor; the large number of potential contributory factors that might result in breakdown of the high-risk foot are discussed in this section (**Fig. 1**). The breakdown of the diabetic foot was traditionally considered to result from an interaction between peripheral vascular disease (PVD), distal symmetric polyneuropathy, and infection. However, whereas both PVD and

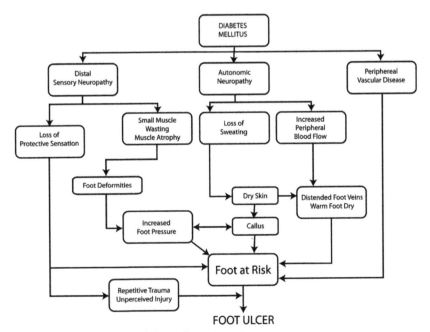

Fig. 1. Potential pathways to diabetic foot ulceration.

neuropathy are confirmed risk factors for foot ulceration, there is no evidence that infection is a contributory factor; rather, infection occurs as a result of ulceration. Thus, the question of infection in the diabetic foot, discussed in detail articles elsewhere in this issue, are not further described in this article.

Peripheral Vascular Disease

That PVD is common in patients with diabetes has been confirmed by large epidemiologic studies.[6–8] The DARTS Study from Scotland confirmed the enormous burden of macrovascular disease in type 2 diabetes, and showed that the incidence rates of peripheral vascular disease per 1000 patients in this population-based study were 5.5 for type 1 diabetes and 13.6 for type 2 diabetes.[6] The large National Health and Nutrition Examination Survey reported the prevalence of PVD in the general population of the United States to be 4.3%, and having diabetes was positively associated with prevalent PVD (odds ratio 2.8).[7] In the Fremantle Diabetes Study, a population-based study of peripheral arterial disease in type 2 diabetes in Australia, the reported prevalence for PVD in this population was 13.6%. In a 5-year follow-up, the incidence of new PVD was 3.7 per 100 patient-years.[8] Prevalent and incident PVD were both strongly and independently associated with other factors such as total serum cholesterol and smoking. In the Fremantle Study, PVD was also shown to predict cardiac death.[8] In most studies of PVD in diabetes, simple screening techniques such as foot pulse evaluation and using a handheld Doppler stethoscope to calculate the ankle brachial index (ABI) have frequently been used.[9] However, peripheral arteries in the diabetic patient frequently have medial and intimal calcification, resulting in higher ankle pressures and falsely elevated ABIs (**Fig. 2**). Therefore, measurement of toe pressures may be more reliable.[9]

In the pathogenesis of ulceration, PVD in isolation is rarely a cause of ulceration: as with neuropathy, a combination of risk factors with minor trauma more commonly leads to ulceration. A frequent scenario is a minor injury and subsequent infection, both of which go unnoticed because of coexistent neuropathy that increases the demand for blood supply beyond the circulatory capacity; neuroischemic or ischemic ulceration, and the risk of amputation, follow. In the last 2 decades there has been a change in the patterns of ulceration seen in Western countries, with the previously predominant neuropathic ulcer having been replaced by the neuroischemic ulcer as the most frequently seen in many clinics.[10] In the Eurodiale Study, more than 1000 consecutive patients presenting to specialist foot clinics in 14 European hospitals in 10 countries were investigated. PVD was present in nearly half of all subjects, with infection in more than half, and more than one-third had both PVD and infection. This finding suggests that ischemia is increasingly common in the pathogenesis of diabetic foot ulcers, often in combination with neuropathy.[10] In a follow-up of the Eurodiale Study, the presence of infection and peripheral arterial disease (PAD) emerged as a predictor of nonhealing.[11] This finding led the investigators to propose that DFU with or without concomitant PVD should be defined as 2 separate disease states. When assessing determinants of minor amputations in diabetes, PAD, as well as ulcer depth and male sex, was a significant predictor of amputation, suggesting that early referral of patients to a diabetic foot clinic is indicated in those with PVD and infection.[12]

In summary, PVD is a common contributory factor to the genesis of DFU in diabetic patients. Although the role of blood glucose in the genesis of macrovascular disease is controversial, there is no doubt that educational strategies aimed at the cessation of smoking and control of hypercholesterolemia remain extremely important in the prevention of PVD in diabetes.

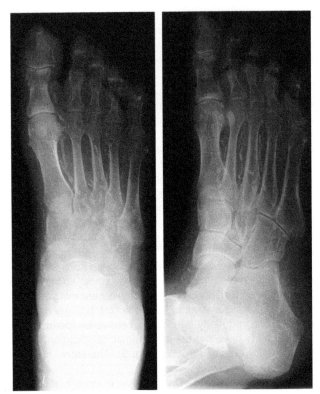

Fig. 2. Radiograph of the foot of a neuropathic diabetic patient showing extensive medial arterial calcification down to the digital vessels. Such calcification is also present in larger proximal vessels, and will lead to false elevation of the ankle brachial index.

Diabetic Peripheral Neuropathy

The diabetic neuropathies are among the commonest of all the long-term diabetic complications, and may present with diverse clinical manifestations.[13] One of the important functions of the sensory peripheral nervous system is to protect the extremities from injury: small afferent nerve fibers carry the sense of pain and temperature, whereas larger fibers conduct sensory abnormalities including vibration and sensation of joint position. Chronic sensorimotor diabetic peripheral neuropathy (DPN) is the commonest of all the neuropathies and this, together with peripheral autonomic sympathetic neuropathy, plays an important part in the development of foot ulceration. Much about the pathogenesis and management of insensitive foot lesions has been learned from the writings of Paul Brand, a surgeon working with leprosy patients in South India in the last century. It was Brand who described pain as "God's greatest gift to mankind." Although the pathologic causes of sensory loss in leprosy in diabetes are very different, the end results are the same, namely the insensitive high-risk foot. Sympathetic autonomic neuropathy affecting the lower extremities leads to reduced sweating, resulting in dry skin that is prone to crack or fissure but also to increased blood flow (in the absence of PVD) caused by the release of sympathetic controlled vasoconstriction. That both DPN and peripheral sympathetic neuropathy are important in the genesis of foot ulcers in diabetes has been recognized for many years,[14] and each is now described in further detail.

Chronic Sensorimotor Diabetic Peripheral Neuropathy

The frequency of DPN in the diabetic population is well described in both clinic-based[15] and population-based[16] studies, which report a prevalence varying from approximately 25% to 35%. It can be safely assumed that at least half of older type 2 diabetic patients have significant sensory loss.[13,17] The diagnosis must never be made without a careful clinical examination of the lower limbs, as absence of symptoms can never be equated with absence of signs.[13]

DPN is of gradual or insidious onset, and up to 50% of patients may never experience any typical neuropathic symptoms.[13] For those who do experience symptoms, the commonest include altered temperature perception (feet feel on fire, burning, or freezing), sharp stabbing electrical-type sensations, paresthesias, and hyperesthesias, all of which are prone to nocturnal exacerbation. Clinical examination typically reveals a sensory deficit in a stocking distribution with signs of motor dysfunction, including small-muscle wasting and absence of ankle reflexes. A well-recognized situation originally described by Ward is the "painful-painless leg," in which patients experience severe neuropathic symptomatology, but on examination there is loss of sensation to all modalities. Such patients are at high risk of insensitive injury. The explanation for this observation is that there is severe distal loss of nerve fibers, but that electrical ("neuroma"-like) activity proximally is interpreted by the patient as originating from where the peripheral nerve used to innervate.[18]

The threshold of sensation that protects normal feet from injury is difficult to define. As described by Brand,[19] the purpose of pain sensation is not to cause discomfort but to enable the body to use its strength to the maximum, short of damage. A person with reduced sensation therefore has not totally lost the ability to perceive pain, but simply feels the discomfort at a higher level of stimulation. It thus requires more pressure or temperature, or more prolonged ischemia, before the residual nerve fibers are activated to warn higher centers. It is therefore important to realize that neuropathic ulceration may occur in patients who still have some ability to perceive stimuli to various modalities. As it is extremely difficult to define a "significant loss of sensation," or at what level sensory loss becomes "critical," it is usual therefore to set levels of sensory loss for the purpose of screening conservatively, as it is preferable to have more false positives (ie, those who are identified as being at risk because of sensory loss but in fact have sufficient protective sensation) than false negatives.

DPN is a sensorimotor neuropathy and, although the symptoms are predominantly sensory, motor dysfunction commonly occurs in this condition and is important in the genesis of foot ulceration. A long-term follow-up study of type 1 diabetic patients confirmed that muscular atrophy in DPN occurs early in the feet and progresses steadily, potentially leading to weakness at the ankle.[20] Using quantitative tests for the assessment of muscle function, patients with both type 1 and type 2 diabetes have been detected to have weakness at the ankle and even the knee. This motor dysfunction leads to an increased risk of developing foot ulcers, owing to secondary alterations in the biomechanics of the feet caused by muscle atrophy.[21]

Peripheral Sympathetic Autonomic Neuropathy

DPN is typically accompanied by distal sympathetic autonomic neuropathy, signs of which are often found on examination. These signs include dryness of the skin with a propensity to callus formation under high-pressure areas, and a warm foot in the absence of large-vessel PVD. The warm, insensitive, and dry foot that results from a combination of somatic and autonomic dysfunction may provide the patient with a false sense of security, as most patients have a "vascular model," believing that most problems in the lower limb occur as a consequence of PVD.

Neuropathy in the Pathway to Ulceration

Although it has been stated for more than 200 years that loss of sensation results in foot ulceration, it is only in the last 2 decades that prospective studies have confirmed that this is indeed the case. The first single-center prospective study to confirm neuropathy as a risk factor for foot ulcers assessed vibration perception threshold (VPT) as measured by the biothesiometer (Biomedical Instrument Co, Newbury, OH, USA) in a population of diabetic patients with no history of ulcers. In a 4-year prospective study, those patients with a baseline threshold above 25 V were 7 times more likely to develop foot ulcers.[22] These observations were subsequently confirmed in a larger multicenter study that showed a significant increase in risk with each volt increase of VPT over 25 V.[23] A large study in northern United Kingdom (the North West Diabetes Foot Care Study) followed a cohort of 10,000 patients for 2 years and confirmed, using a simple neuropathy disability score (NDS), that those with an NDS of 6 or more had a 6% annual incidence of first ulcers, compared with 1% in those with a baseline NDS of less than 6.[23] Other prospective trials have confirmed the key role of both large-fiber (proprioceptive/vibration deficits) and small-fiber (loss of pain and temperature sensation) neurologic deficits in the pathogenesis of ulceration.[13,24]

OTHER RISK FACTORS FOR DIABETIC FOOT ULCERATION
Demographics

1. *Age.* The risk of ulcers and amputations increases with age and duration of diabetes.[1–3,17] The average age of patients presenting with new foot ulcers tends to be on average 10 years more than in those presenting with new Charcot neuroarthropathy.[25]
2. *Gender.* The male sex has been associated with a 1.6-fold increased risk of ulcers in most,[3,4,10,26] but not all[2] studies from Western countries. Amputation rates also appear to be higher in the male sex[26]: mechanisms by which the male sex is at greater risk of these lower extremity complications have yet to be explained.
3. *Ethnicity.* Within Europe, it appears that diabetic patients of European origin have higher risks of both foot ulcers and amputations than those patients with Indian subcontinent, Asian, or African-Caribbean ancestry.[27] Explanations for these differences, particularly in the Asian population, probably relate to several factors including better foot care in certain religious groups, reduced foot pressures, and the fact that diabetic neuropathy appears to be less prevalent in this population.[27,28]

Similar data exist in United States populations, with ulceration and amputation more common in Hispanic Americans and Native Americans than in non-Hispanic whites.[29] Similarly, amputation rates are higher in African Americans.

History of Foot Ulceration or Amputation

Patients with a history of foot ulcers or amputations are at the highest risk of recurrent foot ulcer. In some series, the annual recurrence rate is as high as 50%. Certainly in the North West Diabetes Foot Care Study, a history of ulcers was the strongest predictor of development of new ulceration.[3] A recent systematic review has confirmed the importance of previous ulcer or lower extremity amputation as predictors of future risk of foot problems.[30]

Other Diabetic Microvascular Complications

1. *Retinopathy*. Not surprisingly, poor vision, mainly as a consequence of diabetic retinopathy, was shown to be a significant predictor of the risk of foot ulceration in the Seattle Diabetic Foot Study (**Box 1**).[31]
2. *Nephropathy*. It has been known for many years that patients at all stages of diabetic nephropathy, even microalbuminuria, appear to have an increased risk of foot ulceration.[32] However, the very high risk of ulceration and amputation among patients with end-stage renal disease has recently been the focus of several studies. Game and colleagues[33] first showed a temporal association between the initiation of dialysis treatment in diabetic patients and the increased incidence of foot ulceration. In subsequent collaborative studies between the United Kingdom and the United States, dialysis has been shown to be an independent risk factor for foot ulceration in diabetic patients,[34] and the same group also confirmed that the ethnic protection from neuropathy and risk of foot ulcer is lost when diabetic patients of Asian origin are on long-term dialysis therapy.[35] Of note, even nondiabetic patients in dialysis units have observed the high risk of foot ulcers and amputations in the dialysis unit: Carey wrote "throughout dialysis, patients suddenly appear with amputations: very often with heavily managed feet rapidly followed by crutches and then wheelchairs."[36] Thus diabetic patients on dialysis must be regarded as being at extremely high risk of lower extremity complications, and warrant regular foot-care education and podiatry.

Peripheral edema

The presence of peripheral edema, presumably because of impairment of local blood flow, has been associated with an increased risk of ulceration.[37]

Callus

The presence of plantar callus, as already noted, a consequence of peripheral sympathetic dysfunction in the neuropathic foot, is strongly associated with risk of ulceration.

Box 1
Risk factors for foot ulceration

- Diabetic neuropathy
  - Distal sensorimotor neuropathy
  - Peripheral sympathetic neuropathy
- Peripheral vascular disease
- Foot deformity
- Callus under weight-bearing areas
- History of foot ulceration
- Previous amputation
- Other microvascular complications
  - Proliferative retinopathy/visual impairment
  - End-stage renal disease
  - Any dialysis treatment
  - Postrenal transplant
- Poor glycemic control
- Smoking

In one prospective study ulceration only occurred at sites of callus, representing an infinite increase in risk.[38]

Deformity

Deformities are frequently present in the neuropathic foot in diabetes, and may occur as a consequence of an imbalance between flexor and extensor muscles, giving rise to prominence of the metatarsal heads and clawing of the toes.[21] In the neuropathic foot, Charcot prominences are a not infrequent cause of ulceration, and the presence of other potentially nonrelated abnormalities such as hallux valgus will increase the risk of breakdown in the insensate foot. Prospective follow-up in the North West Diabetes Foot Care Study showed that foot deformities were independently related to the risk of new ulcers.[3]

THE PATHWAY TO FOOT ULCERATION

As described earlier, a single pathologic factor, such as insensitive feet secondary to diabetic neuropathy, does not itself result in ulceration. It is therefore a combination of risk factors that ultimately results in the pathway to skin breakdown. Pecoraro and colleagues[39] and then later Reiber and colleagues[37] used the Rothman model for causation, and applied this first to amputation and later to foot ulceration in diabetes. The model used is the concept that a single component cause (eg, neuropathy or foot deformity) is not sufficient on its own to result in ulceration; when several component causes act together, this combines to form a sufficient cause that inevitably will lead to ulceration. In the first study on amputation, 5 component causes were described to lead to amputation: neuropathy, minor trauma, ulceration, faulty healing, and gangrene.[39] When applied to the pathogenesis of DFU, several causal pathways were identified, with several component causes working together to result in ulceration. In this particular study, 3 component causes working together (neuropathy, deformity, and trauma) were present in nearly 2 out of every 3 incident cases of ulceration. Most of the other risk factors for foot ulceration (see **Box 1**) also featured as component causes in this observational study.[37]

Simple examples of a 2-component pathway would be the patient with an insensitive foot that ulcerates after placing his or her foot, which is perceived to be cold, against a radiator (component causes: neuropathy plus thermal injury). An example of a 3-component pathway would be a patient with insensitive feet and clawing of the toes who wears a shoe with an insufficiently deep toe-box and develops dorsal ulcers in the interphalangeal area of the toes (component causes: neuropathy plus deformity plus trauma).

Abnormalities of pressures and loads under the diabetic foot have been recognized for many years,[1,14] and these may form a component cause on the pathway to ulceration. Pressure ulcers on the plantar surface of the foot are the consequence of pressure that would not normally cause ulceration, but which, because of intrinsic abnormalities of the neuropathic foot, leads to plantar ulceration when repetitively applied. Thus, the combination of insensitivity, abnormally high foot pressures, and repetitive stress from, for example, walking, may lead to breakdown under high-pressure areas such as the metatarsal head region. Autonomic neuropathy leading to dry skin and callus build up at such sites, and can also be regarded as a component cause. A prospective study by Veves and colleagues[40] observed a 28% incidence of ulceration in neuropathic feet with high plantar pressures during a 2.5-year follow-up period. By contrast, no ulcers developed in patients with normal pressure. Therefore biomechanics, the branch of science concerned with the consequences of forces applied to living tissue, is clearly relevant to diabetic foot disease because many neuropathic foot ulcers result from repetitive stress that is not perceived by the patient.

Several methodologies that may be useful in research studies are available to assess plantar pressures.[41] Simple, semiquantitative estimation of pressure distribution under the foot can be used in clinical practice. The Pressure Stat or Podotrack is a simple, inexpensive, semiquantitative footprint mat that was validated by comparing with the then gold standard, the optical pedobarograph.[42] Such a simple, inexpensive, semiquantitative footprint mat has the potential for use as a screening tool for high pressures in clinical practice. The same group described the potential of reducing plantar pressures in patients with active foot ulcers using a pressure-relieving dressing[43]; no such dressing is yet available for therapeutic use, but the technology could be applied in the future.

Using the Rothman model for causation has provided a better understanding of factors that result in incident ulcers, and suggests the possibility of prevention of foot ulcers by identifying potential component causes and preventing them occurring together in any one patient. Thus, for example, regular podiatry with removal of callus could reduce high foot pressures and remove that single component cause.[38] Similarly, use of appropriate orthotics in appropriate footwear can reduce foot pressures.

IDENTIFICATION OF THE FOOT AT RISK OF ULCERATION

"The trouble with doctors is not that they do not know enough, but that they do not see enough"

—*Sir Dominic Corrigan.*

The words of Corrigan, best known for his description of the collapsing pulse in aortic valve disease, can be usefully applied to the identification of the foot at risk of ulceration in diabetic patients. Brand later observed that the most important step in reducing amputations in diabetes is that every time a patient with diabetes is seen by the physician, the shoes and socks should be removed and the feet examined carefully.[19] It is likely that many patients' feet are not examined because they have no specific complaints; as already noted, up to 50% of patients with diabetic neuropathy may have no symptoms of the condition whatsoever. Again, it was Brand who described that the insensitive foot is not only painless, but often feels as if it does not belong to the individual. Screening for "at-risk feet" is the job of all of those caring for people with diabetes. Every diabetic patient warrants an annual review whereby symptoms and signs suggestive of the development of the late complications of diabetes are assessed. A Taskforce of the American Diabetes Association (ADA) reported in 2008 on what the central components of the Comprehensive Diabetic Foot Examination (CDFE) should be.[44] The main attributes of the CDFE are now summarized, and recommendations for screening according to the level of care are provided in **Table 1**.

History

Although the medical history is a pivotal component of any risk assessment, a careful examination of the foot remains the key component of the foot check in the diabetic patient.

1. Any history of past or present neuropathic symptoms?
2. History of ulcer or minor/major amputation?
3. Other diabetic complications, especially visual impairment or end-stage renal failure (on dialysis or posttransplant)
4. History of any lower extremity vascular problem (intermittent claudication/rest pain/ history of bypass surgery or angioplasty)
5. Social factors (living alone? blood glucose control? cigarette smoking?)

Table 1
Screening for the high-risk foot according to level of care

	Primary Care	Secondary Care	Clinical Research
History (eg, past ulcer, neuropathy, peripheral vascular disease)	+++	+++	+++
Clinical examination	+++	+++	+++
Monofilament	+++	++	+
Vibration perception	++	++	+++
Ipswich Touch Test	+++	+	−
Vibratip	++	++	−
Quantitative sensory tests	−	+	++
Neuropad	++	++	+
Electrophysiology	−	−	++
Pressure mat (eg, Pressure Stat)	++	++	++
Quantitative foot pressure	−	+	++

Key: +++, recommended; ++, useful if available; +, occasionally required, −, not indicated.

Clinical Examination: An Essential Component of the Annual Check

1. Inspection after shoes and socks removed
   a. Skin status: color, thickness, callus, dryness, cracking?
   b. Normal sweating?
   c. Any signs of bacterial/fungal infection? Always check between toes
   d. Any breaks in skin/ulceration?
   e. Foot deformities: check for Charcot changes/clawing of the toes/prominent metatarsal heads, and so forth
   f. Foot shape
   g. Small muscle wasting?
   h. Skin temperature? Compare both feet. A unilateral warm swollen foot with intact skin should be considered to be an acute Charcot neuroarthropathy until proven otherwise
   i. Check patients' footwear for suitability
2. Neurologic assessment

The CDFE report by the ADA[44] recommends the use of 2 simple tests to identify the patient with loss of protective sensation (LOPS). One of these should be pressure perception using a 10-gauge monofilament, which has been shown in several prospective studies to be a useful predictor of foot ulceration.[44,45] The recommended sites for assessment of pressure perception are the first, third, and fifth metatarsal heads, and the plantar surface of the distal hallux. The patient should be asked if he or she perceives the sensation of pressure when the monofilament buckles. Failure to detect the perception of pressure at 1 or more sites in each foot would be considered to be an abnormal response.

The result of the monofilament pressure perception test should then be confirmed by using 1 of the following for simple tests of sensory perception:

1. *Vibrating 128-Hz tuning fork.* This vibration should be tested over the apex of the hallux bilaterally, and an abnormal response would occur when the patient fails to perceive vibration.

2. *Pin-prick sensation.* The inability of a patient to detect pin-prick sensation can be tested using a disposal pin, again over the apex of the halluces. An abnormal result would be failure to perceive pin-prick sensation on either tested site.
3. *Ankle reflexes.* Absence of ankle reflexes in either leg would be regarded as an abnormal response.
4. *Vibration perception threshold.* As many Centers in North America and Europe possess a biothesiometer or similar vibration detection instrument, it was agreed that this could be 1 of the 4 other tests required to confirm the monofilament test. Again, this is tested over the apex of the hallux: an abnormal result would be a VPT of 25 V or more as determined by previous studies.[22,23]
5. *Vascular assessment.* A vascular examination would normally comprise palpation of the posterior tibial and dorsalis pedis pulses: the pulses should be described as being either "present" or "absent"; assessing a pulse as "reduced" is notoriously inaccurate.

Bedside assessment of the circulation using a Doppler ultrasound probe can be useful, although it is recognized that because of arterial calcification as noted earlier, the ABI is less accurate; waveform analysis and toe pressures are likely to be more effective.[46]

Other Assessments

Quantitative sensory testing
Detailed quantitative sensory testing (QST) is not indicated for the annual screen of diabetic patients.[44] However, vibration perception using the biothesiometer may be helpful if available. Other detailed QST and electrophysiology are generally indicated only in clinical research studies, although they may occasionally be useful in the secondary care (hospital) setting.

Foot-pressure studies
Use of devices such as the Pressure Stat, which is a simple, inexpensive, semiquantitative footprint mat that takes a minute or two to measure plantar pressures, may be helpful in identifying specific high-risk areas under the diabetic foot, but these may also be used as an educational tool.[42]

Recently Described Screening Tests
Several potentially useful screening tests have been described since the publication of the 2008 ADA CDFE Guidelines, and these are briefly described here.

1. *Ipswich Touch Test (IpTT).* The simplest of all screening tests, the IpTT was developed to promote more foot screening of inpatients with diabetes. The IpTT simplifies sensory testing to lightly touching the tips of the first, third, and fifth toes of each foot. This simple procedure has been validated by comparing its results with well-validated tests such as the monofilament. On direct comparison, the agreement between the IpTT and the monofilament was virtually perfect ($\kappa = 0.88$: $P<.0001$).[47] This test may be particularly useful in developing countries where availability of any equipment is limited, and also has the advantage of having no cost whatsoever.
2. *Vibratip* (**Fig. 3**). The Vibratip is a pocket-sized disposal device for testing the integrity of the sensory nervous system, and has been specifically designed to overcome barriers associated with other methods such as the high cost for purchase and replacement as well as the requirement for training. A recent study validated

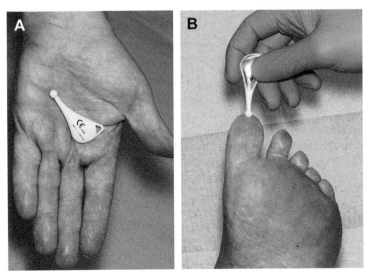

Fig. 3. The Vibratip, a new handheld disposal device for testing vibration perception. This battery-operated disposal device is shown in (A). In (B) it is shown being tested on a patient's hallux: Squeezing the top of the device leads to vibration in the tip, which is then reported by the patient. The test is reported as positive (ie, complete loss of vibration perception) or normal (normal vibration perception).

this device by comparing it with gold-standard tests including the monofilament, the NDS, and VPT using the biothesiometer. Again, almost perfect agreement was found when comparing the Vibratip and its ability to predict the risk of ulcers with the other standard tests.[48]

3. *Neuropad.* The Neuropad[49] is a simple, noninvasive indicator test that has been developed for the assessment of sweating and, hence, autonomic innovation of the diabetic foot. This plaster-like device is applied to the plantar surface of the foot; with normal sweating, callus changes from blue to pink. Absence of sweating results in no color change. The diagnostic ability of Neuropad to identify absent sweating has been shown to have excellent reproducibility, with high sensitivity and negative predictive value. In a study comparing the Neuropad assessment with quantitative sensory and autonomic function testing as well as intraepidermal nerve-fiber density in foot skin biopsies, this test was confirmed to be sensitive in detecting clinical neuropathy.[50]

In summary, there are several well validated tests that can be used in the screening of diabetic patients for evaluation of their risk of foot ulceration. Whereas the simpler tests summarized in the CDFE[44] are entirely appropriate for screening patients in the community, the more sophisticated tests described here might be used in hospital care and in clinical research settings.

SUMMARY

It should now be possible to achieve a reduction in the incidence of foot ulceration and amputations as knowledge about pathways that result in both these events increases.[51] However, despite the universal use of patient education and the hope of reducing the incidence of ulcers in high-risk patients, there are no appropriately designed large, randomized controlled trials actually confirming that education works. It has been recognized for some years that education as part of a multidisciplinary approach to care of the diabetic foot can help to reduce the incidence of amputations in certain settings.[52–54] Ultimately, however, a reduction in neuropathic foot problems will only be achieved if we remember that the patients with neuropathic feet have lost their prime warning signal—pain—that ordinarily brings patients to their doctor. Very little training is offered to health care professionals as to how to deal with such patients. Much can be learned about the management of such patients from the treatment of individuals with leprosy[19]: if we are to succeed, we must realize that with loss of pain there is also diminished motivation in the healing of and prevention of injury.

REFERENCES

1. Singh N, Armstrong DG, Lipsky BA. Preventing foot ulcers in patients with diabetes. JAMA 2005;293:217–28.
2. Müller IS, de Grauw WJ, van Gerwen WH, et al. Foot ulceration and lower limb amputation in Type 2 diabetic patients in Dutch primary health care. Diabetes Care 2002;25:570–4.
3. Abbott CA, Carrington AL, Ashe H, et al. The North-West Diabetes Foot Care Study: incidence of, and risk factors for new diabetic foot ulceration in a community-based patient cohort. Diabet Med 2002;20:377–84.
4. Boulton AJ, Vileikyte L, Ragnarson-Tennvall G, et al. The global burden of diabetic foot disease. Lancet 2005;366:1719–24.
5. Ollendorf DA, Kotsanos JG, Wishner WJ, et al. Potential economic benefits of lower-extremity amputation prevention strategies in diabetes. Diabetes Care 1998;21:1240–5.
6. McCalpine RR, Morris AD, Emslie-Smith A, et al. The annual incidence of diabetic complications in a population of patients with type 1 and type 2 diabetes. Diabet Med 2005;22:348–52.
7. Selvin E, Erlinger TP. Prevalence of and risk factors for peripheral arterial disease in the United States: results from the National Health and Nutrition Examination Survey, 1999-2000. Circulation 2004;110:738–43.
8. Norman PE, Davis WA, Bruce DG, et al. Peripheral arterial disease and risk of cardiac death in type 2 diabetes: the Fremantle Diabetes Study. Diabetes Care 2006;29:575–80.
9. Gibbons GW, Shaw PM. Diabetic vascular disease: characteristics of vascular disease unique to the diabetic patient. Semin Vasc Surg 2012;25:89–92.
10. Prompers L, Huijberts M, Apelqvist J, et al. High prevalence of ischaemia, infection and serious co-morbidity in patients with diabetic foot disease in Europe. Baseline results from the Eurodiale study. Diabetologia 2007;50:18–25.
11. Prompers L, Schaper N, Apelqvist J, et al. Prediction of outcome in individuals with diabetic foot ulcers: focus on the differences between individuals with and without peripheral arterial disease. The Eurodiale study. Diabetologia 2008;51: 747–55.
12. van Battum P, Schaper N, Prompers L, et al. Differences in minor amputation rate in diabetic foot disease throughout Europe are in part explained by differences in disease severity at presentation. Diabet Med 2011;28: 199–205.
13. Boulton AJ, Malik RA, Arezzo J, et al. Diabetic somatic neuropathies: a technical review. Diabetes Care 2004;27:1458–86.

14. Boulton AJ, Hardisty CA, Betts RP, et al. Dynamic foot pressure and other studies as diagnostic and management aids in diabetic neuropathy. Diabetes Care 1983;6:26–33.
15. Young MJ, Boulton AJ, MacLeod AF, et al. A multicentre study of the prevalence of diabetic peripheral neuropathy in the UK hospital clinic population. Diabetologia 1993;36:150–4.
16. Ziegler D, Rathmann W, Dickhaus T, et al. Prevalence of polyneuropathy in pre-diabetes and diabetes is associated with abdominal obesity and macroangiopathy: the MONICA/KORA Augsburg Surveys S2 and S3. Diabetes Care 2008;31:464–9.
17. Kumar S, Ashe H, Fernando DJ, et al. The prevalence of foot ulceration and its correlates in type 2 diabetic patients: a population-based study. Diabet Med 1994;11:480–4.
18. Ward JD. The diabetic leg. Diabetologia 1982;22:141–7.
19. Brand PW. Diabetic foot. In: Ellenberg M, Rifkin H, editors. Diabetes mellitus: theory and practice. 3rd edition. New York: Medical Examination Publishing; 1983. p. 829–49.
20. Andreassen CS, Jakobsen J, Ringgaard S, et al. Accelerated atrophy of lower leg and foot muscles—a follow-up study of long-term diabetic polyneuropathy using magnetic resonance imaging (MRI). Diabetologia 2009;52:1182–91.
21. Anderson H. Motor dysfunction in diabetes. Diabetes Metab Res Rev 2012;28:89–92.
22. Young MJ, Veves A, Breddy JL, et al. The prediction of diabetic neuropathic foot ulceration using vibration perception threshold: a prospective study. Diabetes Care 1994;17:557–60.
23. Abbott CA, Vileikyte L, Williamson S, et al. Multicenter study of the incidence of and predictive risk factors for diabetic neuropathic foot ulceration. Diabetes Care 1998;21:1071–8.
24. Boulton AJ. Diabetic neuropathy: is pain God's greatest gift to mankind? Semin Vasc Surg 2012;25:61–5.
25. Jeffcoate WJ. Charcot neuro-osteoarthropathy. Diabetes Metab Res Rev 2008;24:S62–5.
26. Mayfield JA, Reiber GE, Sanders LJ, et al. Preventative foot care in people with diabetes. Diabetes Care 1998;12:2161–78.
27. Abbott CA, Garrow AP, Carrington A, et al. Foot ulcer risk is lower in South Asian and African-Caribbean compared to European diabetic patients in the UK: the North West Diabetes Foot Care Study. Diabetes Care 2005;28:1869–75.
28. Abbott CA, Chaturvedi N, Malik RA, et al. Explanations for the lower rates of diabetic neuropathy in Indian Asians versus Europeans. Diabetes Care 2010;33:1325–30.
29. Lavery LA, Armstrong DG, Wunderlich RP, et al. Diabetic foot syndrome: evaluating the prevalence and incidence of foot pathology in Mexican-Americans and non-Hispanic whites from a diabetes management cohort. Diabetes Care 2003;26:1435–8.
30. Monteiro-Soares M, Boyko EJ, Ribeiro J, et al. Predictive factors for diabetic foot ulceration: a systematic review. Diabetes Metab Res Rev 2012;28:574–600.
31. Boyko EJ, Ahroni JH, Cohen V, et al. Prediction of diabetic foot ulcer occurrence using commonly available clinical information: the Seattle Diabetic Foot Study. Diabetes Care 2006;29:1202–7.
32. Fernando DJ, Hutchinson A, Veves A, et al. Risk factors for non-ischaemic foot ulceration in diabetic nephropathy. Diabet Med 1991;8:223–5.

33. Game FL, Chipchase SY, Hubbard R, et al. Temporal association between the incidence of foot ulceration and the start of dialysis in diabetes mellitus. Nephrol Dial Transplant 2006;21:3207–10.
34. Ndip A, Rutter MK, Vileikyte L, et al. Dialysis treatment is an independent risk factor for foot ulceration in patients with diabetes and stage 4 or 5 chronic kidney disease. Diabetes Care 2010;33:1811–6.
35. Ndip A, Lavery LA, Lafontaine J, et al. High levels of foot ulceration and amputation risk in a multiracial cohort of diabetic patients on dialysis therapy. Diabetes Care 2010;33:878–80.
36. Carey R, Harker M. Kidney dialysis—the need for humanity. Br Med J 2012;342: e4492.
37. Reiber GE, Vileikyte L, Boyko EJ, et al. Causal pathways for incident lower extremity ulcers in patients with diabetes from two settings. Diabetes Care 1999; 22:157–62.
38. Murray HJ, Young MJ, Boulton AJ. The association between callus formation, high foot pressures and neuropathy in diabetic foot ulceration. Diabet Med 1996;13:979–83.
39. Pecoraro RE, Reiber RE, Burgess EM. Pathways to diabetic limb amputation: basis for prevention. Diabetes Care 1990;13:510–21.
40. Veves A, Murrary HJ, Young MJ, et al. The risk of foot ulceration in diabetic patients with high foot pressure: a prospective study. Diabetologia 1992;35:660–3.
41. Boulton AJ, Kirsner RS, Vileikyte L. Neuropathic diabetic foot ulcers. N Engl J Med 2004;351:48–55.
42. van Schie CH, Abbott CA, Vileikyte L, et al. A comparative study of the Podotrack, a simple semi-quantitative plantar pressure measuring device, and the optical paedobarograph in the assessment of pressures under the diabetic foot. Diabet Med 1999;16:154–9.
43. van Schie CH, Rawat F, Boulton AJ. Reduction of plantar pressure using a prototype pressure-relieving dressing. Diabetes Care 2005;28:2236–7.
44. Boulton AJ, Armstrong DG, Albert SF, et al. Comprehensive foot examination and risk assessment: a report of the task force of the foot care interest group of the American Diabetes Association, with endorsement by the American Association of Clinical Endocrinologists. Diabetes Care 2008;31:1679–85.
45. Mayfield JA, Sugarman JR. The use of the Semmes-Weinstein monofilament and other threshold tests for preventing foot ulceration and amputation in persons with diabetes. J Fam Pract 2002;49(Suppl 11):S17–29.
46. Khan NA, Rahim SA, Anand SS, et al. Does the clinical examination predict lower extremity peripheral arterial disease? JAMA 2006;295:536–46.
47. Rayman G, Vas PR, Baker N, et al. The Ipswich Touch Test: a simple and novel method to identify inpatients with diabetes at risk of foot ulceration. Diabetes Care 2011;34:1517–8.
48. Bowling FL, Abbott CA, Harris WE, et al. A pocket-sized disposable device for testing the integrity of sensation in the outpatient setting. Diabet Med 2012;29: 1550–2.
49. Papanas N, Boulton AJ, Malik RA, et al. Neuropad (®): A simple new non-invasive sweat indicator test for the diagnosis of diabetic neuropathy. Diabet Med 2012. http://dx.doi.org/10.1111/dme.12000.
50. Quattrini C, Jeziorska M, Tavakoli M, et al. The Neuropad test: a visual indicator test for human diabetic neuropathy. Diabetologia 2008;51:1046–50.
51. Malik RA, Tesfaye S, Ziegler D. Medical strategies to reduce amputation in patients with type 2 diabetes. Diabet Med 2013. http://dx.doi.org/10.1111/dme.12169.

52. Dargis V, Pantelejeva O, Jonushaite A, et al. Benefits of a multi-disciplinary approach in the management of recurrent diabetic foot ulceration in Lithuania: a prospective study. Diabetes Care 1999;22:1428–31.
53. Krishnan S, Nash F, Baker N, et al. Reduction in diabetic amputations over eleven years in a defined UK population: benefits of multi-disciplinary team work and continuous prospective audit. Diabetes Care 2008;31:99–101.
54. Kuehn BM. Prompt response, multi-disciplinary care: key to reducing diabetic foot amputation. JAMA 2012;308:19–20.

Epidemiology of Foot Ulceration and Amputation

Can Global Variation be Explained?

David J. Margolis, MD, PhD[a,b,*], William Jeffcoate, MRCP[c]

KEYWORDS

- Epidemiology • Lower extremity amputation • Diabetes • Global variation
- Incidence

KEY POINTS

- Global variation in the incidence of amputation exists.
- Amputation is an imperfect measure of diabetic foot disease.
- Variation may be partially explained by differences in the measurement of amputation and the type of amputation, as well as the ascertainment of diabetes.
- Variation may also be partially explained by race/ethnicity, treatment of diabetes, the management of diabetic foot disease, societal factors, patient behavior and mood, access to care, and aspects of specialist care.

There is evidence of variation in the incidence of amputation both between countries and within them.[1–6] Such variation may derive from differences in (1) the populations cared for, (2) the culture and social conditions, (3) patient behavior, and (4) aspects of professional management. Before considering these aspects in detail, it is important to put into perspective the use of amputation as a measure of outcome of foot disease, and of diabetic foot ulcers in particular.

MEASURES OF OUTCOME OF DIABETIC FOOT DISEASE

When examining outcome measures for disease of the foot in diabetes, the principal interest lies in the outcome of foot ulcers, and other conditions (including the acute Charcot foot) need to be considered separately. Various measures can be used to

[a] Department of Biostatistics and Epidemiology, University of Pennsylvania School of Medicine, Philadelphia, PA, USA; [b] Department of Dermatology, University of Pennsylvania School of Medicine, Philadelphia, PA, USA; [c] Department of Diabetes and Endocrinology, Nottingham University Hospitals Trust, Nottingham, NG5 1PB, UK
* Corresponding author. Department of Dermatology, University of Pennsylvania School of Medicine, Philadelphia, PA.
E-mail address: margo@upenn.edu

Med Clin N Am 97 (2013) 791–805
http://dx.doi.org/10.1016/j.mcna.2013.03.008
0025-7125/13/$ – see front matter © 2013 Elsevier Inc. All rights reserved.

document the quality of management, but if the data used for systematic audit are to be reliable, it is important either that the necessary details can be recorded easily within the course of routine care or that they are already being documented as part of hospital management systems.[7] Records that require extensive documentation of new clinical details will be in danger of being incomplete and, therefore, of minimal value.

In large population studies the outcome most often recorded on a routine basis is the occurrence of amputation, rather than the more preferred outcome of wound healing; however, amputation as an outcome of interest needs to be carefully interpreted.[2] Data on the incidence of amputation should not ideally be taken in isolation, but should properly be linked to information on mortality, function, and well-being. However, apart from mortality such detail is very difficult to collect, and hence cannot be used for routine audit and study. It is also important to acknowledge that amputation is not a measure of the natural history of disease but is simply a treatment, and that the selection of treatment varies according to health care provider, medical necessity, medical need, and patient preference.

TECHNICAL ISSUES IN COUNTING AMPUTATIONS

To properly compare the rates of lower extremity amputation between populations, it is necessary to understand what is being measured. Incidence and prevalence are very basic epidemiologic terms: incidence is the number of new events that occur over a period of time among those at risk, whereas prevalence refers to the number of individuals with an event among the population under study. Prevalence is important when trying to understand the burden of a disease on a population because it estimates how many people have a disease at a given time. Incidence, however, is more germane when trying to understand the onset of a disease, its risk factors and its pathophysiology, and the influence of early diagnosis and effective treatment.

Numerator and Denominator

Both incidence and prevalence are expressed using a numerator (the number of events) and a denominator (the population being considered). Incidence is also expressed in terms of time: the period over which the new events occur, usually over one year. The choice of numerator and denominator varies widely between different publications, making it difficult to make valid comparisons.

Numerator

In the case of amputation incidence, the numerator may be the number of new major amputations (with definition of "major" also varying between different groups, but usually taken as operations undertaken above the ankle), minor amputations (which may or may not include amputations limited to digits), or all amputations (major and minor combined). The term lower extremity (or limb) amputation (LEA, LLA) usually refers to the combination of major and minor operations but may be used less specifically on occasion, as, for instance, in the title of published articles. Comparison between reports can also be made more difficult by reports being restricted, or not, to those which are "first ever," or gender specific, defined by age or diabetes type, or are adjusted in 1 of a variety of ways. Investigators usually (but not always) exclude observations in those who have an amputation as the result of either malignancy or trauma.

While it is generally believed that the hospital activity/discharge data will furnish a more or less complete account of the number of amputations undertaken, there has always been a problem with the reliability of how diabetes is documented at the time of discharge, the exception being in health care systems that ensure a differential rate of payment (whether from private practice, insurance reimbursement, the internal "virtual" market currently used in the UK National Health Service, or in the US Medicare system where incorrect billing can be prosecuted). Failure to document that an amputee also has diabetes will lead to an inevitable underrecording of diabetes-related operations.

Denominator

The denominator for amputation incidence should be expressed in terms of the total population at risk for the area, i.e., in terms of the population who have diabetes, and over a chosen time period such as 1 year. Given the rarity with which accurate data exist relating to the local population known to have diabetes, it is very much easier to report the incidence of amputation in terms of the total (with and without diabetes) population, and usually expressed per 10^5 persons per year. In the setting of incidence of first amputation among those with diabetes, the population at risk should have diabetes and no previous amputation.

Reasonably complete data on the prevalence of diabetes in an unselected community exist only in a small number of countries. Almost all other reports in which the incidence of amputation is expressed in terms of the population at risk (ie, the population with diabetes) are derived either from specific research projects in circumscribed communities or from selected groups, as, for instance, those insured by a particular private insurer or covered by a particular health care scheme (eg, Veterans Health Administration or Medicare in the United States). Such populations will be selected variously by age, disability, affluence, and social deprivation, as well as gender.

Definition of Diabetes

The definition of diabetes has changed several times over the past 20 years. Definitions have been changed by country-specific professional societies as well as by world bodies. These changes in diagnostic criteria for diabetes have usually decreased the magnitude of the fasting blood sugar, decreased the magnitude of the glycemic elevation for a glucose tolerance test, and/or accepted hemoglobin A1c as a diagnostic test, and hence have tended to increase the number of individuals diagnosed with the disease. It is also highly likely that the new, larger, population at risk from diabetes will include an increased prevalence of those with disease with lesser degrees of hyperglycemia and shorter duration of disease. Because these individuals will be at lesser risk of amputation, there will be an inevitable reduction in the incidence on amputation in this new, expanded, at-risk population.

For example, the World Health Organization and American Diabetes Association changed the criteria used to make a diagnosis of diabetes in 1997, 2003, and 2010. Among those with diabetes, the incidence of amputation in the United States was close to 10 per 1000 individuals in 1996 and dropped to 8 per 1000 individuals in 1998. It was 7 per 1000 individuals in 2002 and dropped to 5.5 per 1000 individuals in 2004 (http://www.cdc.gov/diabetes). An illustration of this potential phenomenon was presented more recently by Li and colleagues.[8]

A similar effect will also have occurred in communities that have adopted community-wide screening for, and earlier detection of, diabetes, which is often asymptomatic. The influence of screening, like that of the changes of definition, will mean that the apparent decline in incidence that has been observed in many countries over the last 10 to 15 years cannot necessarily be entirely attributed to improvements in disease management.

In some cases, the denominator is determined by a history of having been prescribed glucose-lowering therapy, albeit sometimes supplemented with a record of the diagnosis being recorded in the patient record. This figure may exclude a sizable number of those with diet-controlled disease, and therefore inflate the apparent incidence or prevalence of amputation in the at risk population.

VARIATION IN THE OBSERVED INCIDENCE OF AMPUTATION IN DIABETES
Variation in Incidence of Total Amputations

Reviews published on the prevalence and incidence of diabetic foot ulcer and amputation show marked variation worldwide in the rates of foot ulcer and amputation.[9,10] However, many of the reported studies were more than 10 years old, and the most comprehensive published epidemiologic record came from North America and Europe. Overall, the incidence of LEA was shown to vary from about 2 to 21 per 1000 person-years of individuals with diabetes.[9,10] This wide variation was confirmed in a recent systematic review by Moxey and colleagues[6] of data from 1989 to 2010, which reported that incidence rates varied from 0.46 to 96 per 1000 with diabetes. As already noted, it is very important to carefully interpret these rates given that definitions of diabetes and amputation vary widely in these studies.

Incidences of total amputations (LEA) reported in the last 10 years and expressed in terms of people with diabetes have ranged from 1.76 to 3.44 per 1000 patient-years in Europe, and was 2.2 per 1000 in the United States.[8] The incidence was 2.7 per 1000 in Alaskan Natives following the introduction of a designated foot-care pathway.[11] A figure of 3.8 per 1000 was reported from Western Australia, but this referred to amputations undertaken over a longer period from 1996 to 2005.[12]

Other surveys from the United States have been restricted to populations for which reliable data on the prevalence of diabetes exist, principally those in the Veterans Health Administration (VHA) and/or those receiving health care from Medicare or Medicaid. These populations are at greater risk, and the reported incidence of both major and total amputations (LEA) is correspondingly higher (**Table 1**).[4,5,13–18]

Variation in Incidence of Major Amputation

The only data from the last decade whereby the incidence of major amputation is expressed in terms of the "at risk" (ie, those with diabetes), but otherwise more or less unselected, populations are derived from Europe and the United States. Thus, the incidences of major (above the ankle) amputation per 1000 patient-years were recently reported to be 1.11 and 0.97 in Scotland and England, respectively, and as low as 0.76 and 0.67 in particular towns in the United Kingdom: Middlesbrough and Ipswich.[1,19–21] Incidences recently reported from Trondheim (Norway), Tayside (Scotland), Andalusia (Spain), and Ireland were: 2.4, 2.9, 3.4 and 1.76 per 1000 patient-years, respectively.[22–25]

Variation in the Relative Risk of Amputation in People with Diabetes when Compared with Those Without Diabetes

While all reports confirm that the incidence of amputation is high in diabetes, the relative risk (RR) ranged from a 7.4-fold increase for first major amputation in Finland to 22-fold for any major amputation in both England and Ireland, compared with those without diabetes.[1,22,26] Johannesson and colleagues[27] reported the RR for amputations other than of the digit in people with peripheral arterial disease (PAD) to be 8-fold higher in Sweden, whereas Jonasson and colleagues[28] found the RR for all amputations in people with type 1 diabetes alone to be 86-fold higher in the same country.

Table 1
Incidence of lower extremity amputation by country

	Authors,[Ref.] Year	Year of Data	At Risk per 10^3	Total per 10^5 Total Population	Comments
Major	Tseng et al,[15] 2004	1999	4.5		USA VHA
	Tseng et al,[15] 2004	1999	8.6		USA VHA plus Medicare plus Medicaid
	Kennon et al,[19] 2012	2008	1.11	4.43	Scotland
	Vamos et al,[62] 2010	2008	1.02		Hospital episode statistics England
	Witsø et al,[23] 2010	2004–2007	2.4		Trondheim
	Canavan et al,[20] 2008	2000	0.67		Middlesbrough, England
	Krishnan et al,[21] 2008	2005	0.76		Ipswich, England
	Schofield et al,[24] 2009	2006	2.9		Tayside, Scotland
	Tseng et al,[18] 2011	2004	1.59		USA VHA First ever amputation
Minor	Tseng et al,[15] 2004	1999	3.1		USA VHA
	Tseng et al,[15] 2004	1999	5.5		USA VHA plus Medicare plus Medicaid
	Vamos et al,[62] 2010	2008	1.49		Hospital episode statistics England
	Kennon et al,[19] 2012	2008	1.03	4.10	Scotland
LEA	Kennon et al,[19] 2012	2008	2.13	8.53	Scotland
	Almaraz et al,[25] 2012	2006	3.44		Standardized incidence, age >30 y Andalusia, Spain
	Vamos et al,[62] 2010	2008	2.5		Hospital episode statistics England
	Margolis et al,[4] 2011	2006–2008	5.0		USA Medicare Data Points # 2
	Fosse et al,[68] 2009	2003		3.78	France
	Davis et al,[12] 2006	1996–2005	3.8		Fremantle T2DM only
	Li et al,[8] 2012	2008	2.13		CDC USA
	Buckley et al,[22] 2012	2012	1.76		Ireland
	Goldberg et al,[14] 2012	2006	4.4		USA Medicare
	Schraer et al,[11] 2004	1998	2.7		Alaska Natives Following new health care program

Abbreviations: CDC, Centers for Disease Control and Prevention; LEA, lower extremity amputation; T2DM, type 2 diabetes mellitus; VHA, Veterans Health Administration.

Variation in the Incidence of Amputation in Diabetes Within Countries

Variation within a country has been reported in several carefully conducted investigations. In 1996/1997, Wrobel and colleagues[29] found an 8.6-fold variation in the incidence of amputation in the Medicare population, and opined that the variation could be associated with regional variation in care. More recently, Margolis and colleagues[5] again reported the annual incidence of lower extremity amputation to be on the order of 4 to 5 per 1000 person-years in 5 million beneficiaries with diabetes in the US Medicare population between 2006 and 2008. The investigators noted 3- to 5-fold geographic variation in the incidence of amputation, and that areas of higher and lower incidence appeared to cluster in specific geographic regions. Areas of higher incidence of amputation neighbored other areas of higher incidence, and areas of lower incidence neighbored areas of lower incidence. The clustering was maintained after adjusting for variations in race, income, education, physician access, age of the population, incidence of diabetes, and frequency of microvascular and macrovascular complications. It was concluded that variation could be due to the disease process, implementation of guidelines, health care provider training and/or therapeutic preference, or patient preference.[30] Similarly, a study in 2012 by Holman and colleagues[1] demonstrated an 8-fold variation in the rate of all amputations (LEA) and a 10-fold variation in major amputations among the Primary Care Trusts (PCTs) in England. The investigators also noted close correlations between PCTs in the incidences of major and of minor amputations in people with and without diabetes, indicating that geographic variation in the incidence of amputation was unrelated to diabetes. Because National Health Service care is freely available to all, variation was unlikely to be related to access to care, although it could be related in part to social deprivation and ethnicity. These findings conflict to some extent with those of Tseng and colleagues,[31] who demonstrated different outlier centers for high rates of incidence of major and of minor amputation in Medicare beneficiaries in the VHA system, both with and without diabetes. Variation noted in Australia has been linked to socioeconomic status by Bergin and colleagues.[32]

FACTORS CONTRIBUTING TO OBSERVED VARIATION IN INCIDENCE OF AMPUTATION IN DIABETES

Factors may contribute to the incidence of amputation by having an impact on the development of diabetes, on the development of diabetes-related complications, and on the rate of healing of foot ulcers once they arise.

Factors Related to the Incidence of Diabetes

If the incidence of amputation is expressed in terms of the total (community-wide) population, it will be heavily influenced by the prevalence of diabetes, and especially of type 2 diabetes. The current rapid increase in prevalence of known diabetes is also relevant, being partly caused by increasing ascertainment resulting from more systematic screening, but largely the result of change in diet and lifestyle leading to obesity and reduced physical fitness. There are obviously a large number of factors that may determine the varying prevalence of diabetes in different communities.

Factors Related to the Incidence of New Foot Ulcers

Foot ulcers are more likely in those whose diabetes is less well managed.[33,34] Many factors will obviously contribute to poor glycemic control: awareness of the diagnosis and its implications, education, availability of effective primary care and treatments, social deprivation with worse health care–related behavior, lack of adequate footwear, and conflicting societal pressures.[32]

Factors Related to the Adverse Outcome of Established Ulcers

Many factors affect the rate of healing of different ulcers, in addition to the obvious causative or complicating influences and PAD. All of these could contribute to any variation in healing observed between different communities.

Available evidence suggests that any newly presenting ulcer should be assessed as quickly as possible by someone with specialist knowledge to ensure prompt treatment of particular factors identified as contributing to presentation, with the main principles of care being to treat complicating infection and underlying PAD, cleansing of the wound bed, protection of the wound from unnecessary trauma by provision of effective off-loading, and arranging frequent review.[35–38]

Social and Societal Factors

A person with a new foot ulcer may not realize the need for prompt assessment, and may delay seeking help because of other pressures (eg, financial: both maintaining income and avoiding the costs of care), or advice from friends and/or elders and religious leaders. Access to primary care advice and expert assessment may be limited.

Patient Behavior

Behavior will reflect societal pressures and the individual's ability to cope with illness. Behavior may also be affected by fear in those who are aware of the potential significance of new foot ulceration. Some may also delay seeking advice because of guilt, being aware that the new ulcer appeared because they failed to exercise the protective precautions they had been told to take. Others may feel guilt because they have failed to stop smoking when they have been threatened that smoking may cause them to lose a leg. Scollan-Koliopoulos and colleagues[39] noted the effect of a previous family history of amputation on the foot-care response to fear of the impact of foot disease. It is also important to consider that health literacy, which is often associated with socioeconomic status, race/ethnicity, and glycemic control, is associated with poor glycemic control and patients' ability to manage their illness.[40–42]

Glycemic Control

Long-term hyperglycemia is associated with increased risk of amputation, presumably primarily through its importance in the development of neuropathy, but there is no convincing evidence that differences in glycemic control at presentation are independently associated with outcome,[33,34,43,44] although Christman and colleagues[45] did recently show an association between a slower healing rate and glycemic control.

Mood

Depression, as either a consequence or a potential cause of amputation, has received relatively little attention, although Williams and colleagues[46] have demonstrated a strong association between depression and subsequent major (but not minor) amputation in a VHA population.

Race and Ethnicity

The impact of race is complex because it overlaps with social and societal factors (see earlier discussion) as well as to poverty, deprivation, and restricted access to health care services, both in developing countries and among ethnic minorities in developed countries.

Asians in the United Kingdom may have a reduced incidence of foot ulceration that, at least in part, results from a decreased incidence of distal neuropathy.[47,48] However, the potentially beneficial impact of other aspects of racially mediated behavior (such as walking barefoot or the use of only slippers in the house, or the ritual washing of feet by Muslims) is not known.

Black (African-derived) races have an increased risk of diabetes when compared with Caucasians, but this is not sufficient to explain the much increased incidence of amputation among African Americans, although this contrasts with the findings from London, England, which showed that the incidence of amputation among black males was only one-third that of Caucasians.[49] This finding suggests that much of the increased incidence in African Americans may relate more to social factors and to reduced access to effective health care services. It has been shown that African Americans (both with and without diabetes) are less likely than whites to have operative debridement and revascularization before amputation.[50] On the other hand, Rucker-Whitaker and colleagues[51] reported that in a population with PAD, the increased incidence of amputation among African Americans (both with and without diabetes) was largely the result of a much increased likelihood of repeat major amputation.

Genetic Factors

Genetic variation may underlie some aspects of individual and racial variation in the healing of wounds, as reflected, for instance, in the known predisposition of certain races to keloid formation. Evidence is also available on the possible importance of polymorphisms relating to the expression of vascular endothelial growth factor and of neuronal nitric oxide synthase accessory protein, but the field is in its infancy.[52]

The Structure and Effectiveness of Health Care Services

Access to effective primary care will be reduced or absent in many developing nations or in poorer communities in others, and the incidence of amputation has been shown to drop dramatically when programs are introduced to correct this.[11,53] In some countries the only available health care service is private, and the costs of care can be relatively enormous.[54,55] In countries where health care is largely financed through insurance reimbursement, there will be inequalities that result from the extent of insurance cover and, indirectly, wealth. Regional differences in spending on diseases of the foot in diabetes have been reported in the Medicare population, although this does appear to link directly with associated differences in the incidence of amputation.[5,49,56]

ASPECTS OF PROFESSIONAL CARE

Because the contribution of aspects of professional training, belief, and practice to the outcome of diabetic foot disease has received relatively little scrutiny hitherto, this is considered separately.

Professional Belief and Practice

Health care professionals practice according to the codes of conduct they have learned, but their education will always have been subject not just to the accepted principles prevalent on the country, community, or culture but also to the beliefs of their trainers, which are themselves based on personality and experience. The result is that where firm scientific evidence to underpin the management of disease of the foot is lacking (as is the case for virtually aspect of care of diabetic foot disease[57,58]), it is very likely that variation will exist.

Study Evidence of Links Between Professional Belief and the Incidence of Amputation

The first article to suggest that professional belief contributed, at least in part, to up to a 4-fold variation in LEA observed in centers in England was a study by Connelly and colleagues[59] based on responses to questions posed to vascular surgical teams about the management of several hypothetical cases.

Variation in the Incidence of Amputation for Osteomyelitis of the Foot

Evidence is also apparent from the reported incidence of major amputation for people who present with osteomyelitis, whereby differences occur between those experts who believe that surgical excision of infected bone is an essential part of management and those who believe that surgical intervention should be reserved for the minority in whom there is a clear indication.[60,61] These differences in opinion divide along national lines to some extent, and clearly reflect the training of the clinicians.

Geographic Clustering of Areas of Low and High Amputation in the United States

Evidence to highlight the likely importance of training comes from the analysis of geographic variation in the incidence of amputation that can be observed in different areas of the United States.[5] It is possible that clustering of centers according to their overall incidence of amputation reflects, to some extent, the influence of local undergraduate and postgraduate training, although other factors may play a part.

Geographic Clustering of Major and Minor Amputation, and of Amputation in People both With and Without Diabetes in the United Kingdom

The recent study by Holman and colleagues[1] reported a 10-fold variation in the incidence of major amputation between PCTs in England, and also demonstrated a correlation between the incidence of major and of minor amputation as well as between the incidence of both types of operation in people with and without diabetes. These data suggest that there are areas where the threshold for surgical intervention is relatively low and others where it is not, and that this might relate more to professional belief than to variation in case mix.

Improvement in Care

The last strand of evidence to suggest the importance of professional belief and practice is the widespread evidence that the incidence of amputation is falling in many industrialized countries of the world. Given, however, the rapidly rising prevalence of diabetes (and of type 2 diabetes in particular), and the inevitable increase in incidence of amputation when expressed in terms of the total population, it is necessary to select only studies that report the incidence of amputation in terms of the at-risk population, and this requires information on the prevalence of diabetes in the area.[62]

Such studies indicate, however, that the incidence of both LEA and major amputation alone is decreasing (**Table 2**). Reports in the last decade of a decrease in incidence of all amputations in diabetes (LEA, expressed in terms of the at-risk population) are available from unselected populations in the United States, Scotland, Germany, Finland, Spain, and the England, even though no decrease was reported from Andalusia and Ireland.[8,19–22,25,63–65] Decreases in incidence of LEA have similarly been reported in selected patient groups in the United States.[4,8,14,31]

Data on major amputation are even more striking, with considerable decreases reported in the last 10 to 15 years in Scotland, Norway, Finland, Germany, and in patients cared for by the VHA in the United States.[19,23,24,26,31,63] Perhaps the most impressive results were those reported by 2 community hospitals in England, in which the incidence of major amputation decreased over a period of 4 to 5 years from

Table 2
Studies of change in incidence by country over time

	Authors,[Ref.] Year	Period	Change in Incidence per 1000	Location and Comments
Major	Schofield et al,[24] 2009	2000–2006	5.1 to 2.9	Tayside, Scotland. Age, sex, duration adjusted
	Tseng et al,[18] 2011	2000–2004	3.06 to 1.59	USA VHA First ever amputation
	Witso et al,[23] 2010	1994–1997 to 2004–2007	4.0 to 2.4	Trondheim, Norway
	Kennon et al,[19] 2012	2004–2008	1.87 to 1.11	Scotland
	Vamos et al,[62] 2010	2004–2008	No change	Hospital episode statistics England
	Lopez-de-Andres et al,[64] 2011	2001–2008	Decrease in T1DM but not T2DM	Spain
	Ikonen et al,[26] 2010	1997–2007	48.8%	First major
	Canavan et al,[20] 2008			Middlesbrough, England
	Krishnan et al,[21] 2008			Ipswich, England
	Tseng et al,[18] 2011	2000–2005	BKA 1.08 to 0.87 AKA 1.41 to 0.72	VHA Age and gender standardized First ever amputation
	Trautner et al,[69] 2007	1990–2004	Decrease	Small community in Germany: Leverkusen
	Canavan et al,[20] 2008	1995–2000	3.11 to 0.76	Middlesbrough, England
	Krishnan et al,[21] 2008	1995–2005	3.64 to 0.67 and 7.4 to 2.8	Ipswich, England
Minor	Tseng et al,[18] 2011	2000–2004	4.59 to 2.49	US Veterans hospital system: First ever amputation
All LEA	Li et al,[8] 2012	1996–2008	11.2 to 2.9	USA: age >40 y
	Schofield et al,[24] 2009	2000–2006	Decrease	Tayside, Scotland Age, sex, duration adjusted
	Kennon et al,[19] 2012	2004–2008	3.04 to 2.13	
	Almaraz et al,[25] 2012	1998–2006	No change	Standardized incidence. Age >30 y Andalusia, Spain
	Vamos et al,[62] 2010	2004–2008	No change	Hospital episode statistics England
	Buckley et al,[22] 2012	2005–2009	1.44 to 1.76	Ireland
	Tseng et al,[18] 2011	2000–2005	7.08 to 4.65	US VHA: first ever amputation
	Goldberg et al,[14] 2012	1999–2006	4.8 to 4.4	USA Medicare
	Trautner et al,[69] 2007	1990–2004	Reduction 37%	Leverkusen. Amputations of digit only excluded
	Eskelinen et al,[65] 2006	1990–2002	Reduction 33%	Helsinki, Finland
	Krishnan et al,[21] 2008	1995–2005	5.32 to 1.60	Ipswich, England
	Canavan et al,[20] 2008	1995–2000	5.64 to 1.76	Middlesbrough, England

Abbreviations: AKA, above-knee amputation; BKA, below-knee amputation.

3.11 to 0.76 per 1000 patient-years in Middlesbrough and 3.64 to 0.67 per 1000 patient-years in Ipswich.[20,21]

It must be noted that these, sometimes massive, decreases in incidence have taken place in the absence of any significant advance in the treatments available for the care of chronic foot ulcers. These decreases are also far greater than could be accounted for by changes in the criteria used for the diagnosis of diabetes or by the impact of screening programs. In other words, they may have resulted to a very large extent simply from a restructuring of clinical services.

Improvements have also been reported in Finland following the introduction of a National Development Program to improve the prevention and care of diabetes, and the incidence of first major amputation has decreased by 48.8% from 1997 to 2007.[26]

The impact of structuring care has also been demonstrated in a randomized controlled trial conducted in Taiwan, which showed that urgent surgical debridement was associated with a reduced incidence of amputation in people with infected diabetic foot ulcers.[66]

Association Between Reduced Incidence of Amputation and Increased Use of Revascularization

It is suggested by some (eg, Paulus and colleagues[67]) that the decreasing incidence of amputation relates to the increased use of revascularization, especially with an endovascular approach. Although the decrease in amputation incidence and the increase in revascularization procedures are undeniable, it is not yet possible to conclude that there is a causative relationship between them.

SUMMARY

Amputation is a treatment, and not simply part of the natural history of foot disease. However, assessment of amputation incidence is the measure most frequently used to document an outcome reflecting the management of diabetic foot disease, mainly because the data are already captured in most health care systems. Nevertheless, interpretation of the results requires great care. Many centers have recorded decreases in the incidence of amputation in recent years and have concluded that this reflects improvement in clinical care. Although improvement in clinical care is clearly of a priority, it is important not to underestimate the extent to which the at-risk population (those with diabetes) may have changed as a result of changing criteria for the diagnosis of diabetes, as well as the increasing implementation of systematic and opportunistic screening.

The incidence of amputation can be calculated and expressed in many ways, with different groups using different criteria for deciding both the numerator and the denominator, and studying populations that may differ in several different ways. Given that the incidence of amputation can also be influenced by a wide variety of clinical and social factors, it is not surprising that considerable variation exists between published studies from different countries. For these reasons it is currently difficult to make meaningful comparisons between data from different countries.

On the other hand, the demonstration of wide variation within a single country or between countries or communities that have very similar populations, health care systems, and procedures for documenting amputation incidence is of greater interest. When 8- to 10-fold variation exists within similar health care systems, a risk as large as any published risk factor for amputation, it is essential that the reasons are explored. While race and social deprivation both make an important contribution to variation, another is likely to relate to aspects of the structure of care, including the training and beliefs of individual clinicians, patients' access to care, preferences of patients, and the ability of a patient to understand the need for care and execute a care plan. This area of study requires further investigation.

REFERENCES

1. Holman N, Young RJ, Jeffcoate WJ. Variation in the recorded incidence of amputation of the lower limb in England. Diabetologia 2012;55:1919–25.
2. Jeffcoate WJ, van Houtum WH. Amputation as a marker of quality of care. Diabetologia 2004;47:2051–8.
3. Jeffcoate WJ, Young B, Holman N. The variation in incidence of amputation throughout England. Practical Diabetes Int 2012;29:205–7.
4. Margolis D, Malay DS, Hoffstad OJ, et al. Incidence of diabetic foot ulcer and lower extremity amputation among Medicare beneficiaries, 2006 to 2008. Rockville (MD): Agency for Healthcare Research and Quality; 2011.
5. Margolis DJ, Hoffstad O, Nafash J, et al. Location, location, location: geographic clustering of lower-extremity amputation among Medicare beneficiaries with diabetes. Diabetes Care 2011;34:2363–7.
6. Moxey PW, Gogalniceanu P, Hinchliffe RJ, et al. Lower extremity amputations—a review of global variability of incidence. Diabet Med 2011;28:1144–53.
7. Jeffcoate WJ, Chipchase SY, Ince P, et al. Assessing the outcome of management of diabetic foot ulcers using ulcer-related and person-related measures. Diabetes Care 2006;29:1784–7.
8. Li Y, Burrow NR, Gregg EW, et al. Declining rates of hospitalization for nontraumatic lower-extremity amputation in the diabetic population aged 40 years or older: US 1988-2008. Diabetes Care 2012;35:273–7.
9. Boulton AJ, Vileikyte L, Ragnarson-Tennvall G, et al. The global burden of diabetic foot disease. Lancet 2005;366:1719–24.
10. Boulton AJ. The diabetic foot: grand overview, epidemiology and pathogenesis. Diabetes Metab Res Rev 2008;24(Suppl 1):S3–6.
11. Schraer CD, Weaver D, Naylor JL, et al. Reduction of amputation rates among Alaska Natives with diabetes following the development of a high-risk foot program. Int J Circumpolar Health 2004;63:114–9.
12. Davis WA, Norman PE, Bruce DG, et al. Predictors, consequences and costs of diabetes-related lower extremity amputation complicating type 2 diabetes: the Fremantle Diabetes Study. Diabetologia 2006;49:2634–41.
13. Margolis D, Malay DS, Hoffstad OJ, et al. Prevalence of diabetes, diabetic foot ulcer, and lower extremity amputation among Medicare beneficiaries, 2006 to 2008. Rockville (MD): Agency for Healthcare Research and Quality; 2010.
14. Goldberg JB, Goodney PP, Cronewett JL, et al. The effect of risk and race on lower extremity amputations among Medicare diabetic patients. J Vasc Surg 2012;56:1663–8.
15. Tseng CL, Greenberg JD, Helmer D, et al. Dual-system utilization affects regional variation in prevention quality indicators: the case of amputations among veterans with diabetes. Am J Manag Care 2004;10:886–92.
16. Tseng CL, Rajan M, Miller D, et al. Use of administrative data to risk adjust amputation rates in the national cohort of medicare-enrolled veterans with diabetes. Med Care 2005;43(1):88–92.
17. Jones WS, Patel MR, Dai D, et al. Temporal trends and geographic variation of lower-extremity amputation in patients with peripheral artery disease: results from U.S. Medicare 2000-2008. J Am Coll Cardiol 2012;60:2230–6.

18. Tseng CL, Rajan M, Miller DR, et al. Trends in initial lower extremity amputation rates among Veterans Health Administration health care system users from 2000 to 2004. Diabetes Care 2011;34:1157–63.
19. Kennon B, Leese GP, Cochrane L, et al. Reduced incidence of lower-extremity amputations in people with diabetes in Scotland: a nationwide study. Diabetes Care 2012;35:2588–90.
20. Canavan RJ, Unwin NC, Kelly WF, et al. Diabetes and non-diabetes related lower extremity amputation incidence before and after the introduction of better organized diabetes foot care: Continous longitudinal monitoring using a standard method. Diabetes Care 2008;31:459–63.
21. Krishnan S, Nash F, Baker N, et al. Reduction in diabetic amputations over 11 years in a defined UK Population. Diabetes Care 2008;31:99–101.
22. Buckley CM, O'Farrell A, Canavan RJ, et al. Trends in the incidence of lower extremity amputations in people with and without diabetes over a five-year period in the Republic of Ireland. PLoS One 2012;7:e41492.
23. Witsø E, Lium A, Lydersen S. Lower limb amputations in Trondheim, Norway. Acta Orthop 2010;81:737–44.
24. Schofield CJ, Yu N, Jain AS, et al. Decreasing amputation rates in patients with diabetes—a population-based study. Diabet Med 2009;26:773–7.
25. Almaraz MC, Gonzalex-Romero S, Bravo M, et al. Incidence of lower limb amputations in individuals with and without diabetes mellitus in Andalusia (Spain) from 1998 to 2006. Diabetes Res Clin Pract 2012;95:399–405.
26. Ikonen TS, Sund R, Venermo M, et al. Fewer major amputations among individuals with diabetes in Finland in 1997-2007: a population study. Diabetes Care 2010;33:2598–603.
27. Johannesson A, Larsson GU, Ramstrand N, et al. Incidence of lower-limb amputation in the diabetic and nondiabetic general population: A 10-year population-based cohort study of initial unilateral and contralateral amputations and reamputations. Diabetes Care 2009;32:275–80.
28. Jonasson JM, Ye W, Sparen P, et al. Risks of nontraumatic lower-extremity amputations in patients with type 1 diabetes. Diabetes Care 2008;31:1536–40.
29. Wrobel JS, Mayfield JA, Reiber GE. Geographic variation of lower-extremity major amputation in individuals with and without diabetes in the Medicare population. Diabetes Care 2001;24:860–4.
30. Chin ML, Drum ML, Jin L, et al. Variation in treatment preferences and care goals among older patients with diabetes and their physicians. Med Care 2008;46:275–86.
31. Tseng CL, Helmer D, Rajan M, et al. Evaluation of regional variation in total, major, and minor amputation rates in a national health-care system. Int J Qual Health Care 2007;19:368–76.
32. Bergin SM, Brand CA, Colman PG, et al. Diabetes related foot disease; "Know thine enemy". J Foot Ankle Res 2011;4(Suppl 1):O8.
33. Adler AI, Erqou S, Lima TA, et al. Association between glycated haemoglobin and the risk of lower extremity amputation in patients with diabetes mellitus—review and meta-analysis. Diabetologia 2010;53:840–9.
34. Sahakyan K, Klein BE, Lee KE, et al. The 25-year cumulative incidence of lower extremity amputations in people with type 1 diabetes. Diabetes Care 2011;34:649–51.
35. Ince P, Kendrick D, Game F, et al. The association between baseline characteristics and the outcome of foot lesions in a UK population with diabetes. Diabet Med 2007;24:977–81.

36. Margolis DJ, Gelfand JM, Hofstad O, et al. Surrogate endpoints for the treatment of diabetic neuropathic foot ulcers. Diabetes Care 2003;26:1696–700.
37. Margolis DJ, Taylor LA, Hofstad O, et al. Diabetic neuropathic foot ulcers: predicting which ones will heal. Am J Med 2003;115:627–31.
38. Jeffcoate WJ. Wound healing—a practice algorithm. Diabetes Metab Res Rev 2012;28:85–8.
39. Scollan-Koliopoulos M, Walker EA, Bleich D. Perceived risk of amputation, emotions, and foot self-care among adults with type 2 diabetes. Diabetes Educ 2010;36:473–82.
40. Feinglass J, Shively VP, Martin GJ, et al. How 'preventable' are lower extremity amputations? A qualitative study of patient perceptions of precipitating factors. Disabil Rehabil 2012;34:2158–65.
41. Rothman RL, DeWalt DA, Malone R, et al. Influence of patient literacy on the effectiveness of a primary care-based diabetes disease management program. JAMA 2004;292:1711–6.
42. Marden S, Thomas PW, Sheppard ZA, et al. Poor numeracy skills are associated with glycaemic control in Type 1 diabetes. Diabet Med 2012;29:662–9.
43. Margolis DJ, Kantor J, Santanna J, et al. Risk factors for delayed healing of neuropathic diabetic foot ulcers: a pooled analysis. Arch Dermatol 2000;136:1531–5.
44. O'Connor DJ, Gargiulo NJ III, Jang J. Hemoglobin A1c as a measure of disease severity and outcome in limb threatening ischemia. J Surg Res 2012;174:29–32.
45. Christman AL, Selvin E, Margolis DJ, et al. Hemoglobin A1c predicts healing rate in diabetic wounds. J Invest Dermatol 2011;131:2121–7.
46. Williams LH, Miller DR, Fincke G, et al. Depression and incident lower limb amputations in veterans with diabetes. J Diabetes Complications 2011;25:175–82.
47. Abbott CA, Garrow AP, Carrington AL, et al. Foot ulcer risk is lower in South-Asian and African-Caribbean compared with European diabetic patients in the U.K.: the North-West Diabetes Foot Care Study. Diabetes Care 2005;28:1869–75.
48. Chaturvedi N, Abbott CA, Whalley A, et al. Risk of diabetes-related amputation in South Asians vs. Europeans in the UK. Diabet Med 2002;19:99–104.
49. Leggetter S, Chaturvedi N, Fuller JH, et al. Ethnicity and risk of diabetes-related lower extremity amputation: a population-based, case-control study of African Caribbeans and Europeans in the United Kingdom. Arch Intern Med 2002;162:73–8.
50. Holman KH, Henke PK, Dimick JB, et al. Racial disparities in the use of revascularization before leg amputation in Medicare patients. J Vasc Surg 2011;54:420–6.
51. Rucker-Whitaker C, Feinglass J, Pearce WH. Explaining racial variation in lower extremity amputation: a 5-year retrospective claims data and medical record review at an urban teaching hospital. Arch Surg 2003;138:1347–51.
52. Margolis DJ, Gupta J, Thom SR, et al. Diabetes, lower extremity amputation, loss of protective sensation, and NOS1AP in the CRIC study. Wound Repair Regen 2013;21:17–24.
53. Rith-Najarian SJ, Stolusky T, Gordes DM. Identifying diabetic patients at high risk for lower-extremity amputation in a primary care setting. Diabetes Care 1992;15:1386–9.
54. Ali SM, Fareed A, Humail SM, et al. The personal cost of diabetic foot disease in the developing world—a study from Pakistan. Diabet Med 2008;25:1231–3.
55. Cavanagh P, Attinger C, Abbas Z, et al. Cost of treating diabetic foot ulcers in five different countries. Diabetes Metab Res Rev 2012;28(Suppl 1):107–11.

56. Sargen MR, Hoffstad O, Margolis DJ. Geographic variation in Medicare spending and mortality for diabetic patients with foot ulcers and amputations. J Diabetes Complications 2012;26:301–7.
57. Dumville JC, Soares MO, O'Meara S, et al. Systematic review and mixed treatment comparison: dressings to heal diabetic foot ulcers. Diabetologia 2012;55: 1902–10.
58. Game FL, Hinchliffe RJ, Apelqvist J, et al. A systematic review of interventions to enhance the healing of chronic ulcers of the foot in diabetes. Diabetes Metab Res Rev 2012;28(Suppl 1):119–41.
59. Connelly DJ, Airey M, Chell S. Variation in clinical decision making is a partial explanation for geographical variation in lower extremity amputation rates. Br J Surg 2001;88:529–35.
60. Game FL, Jeffcoate WJ. Primarily non-surgical management of osteomyelitis of the foot in diabetes. Diabetologia 2008;51:962–7.
61. Henke PK, Blackburn SA, Wainess RW, et al. Osteomyelitis of the foot and toe in adults is a surgical disease: conservative management worsens lower extremity salvage. Ann Surg 2005;241:885–92.
62. Vamos EP, Bottle A, Edmonds ME, et al. Changes in the incidence of lower extremity amputations in individuals with and without diabetes in England between 2004 and 2008. Diabetes Care 2010;33:2592–7.
63. Trautner C, Haastert B, Giani G, et al. Amputations and diabetes: a case-control study. Diabet Med 2002;19:35–40.
64. Lopez-de-Andres A, Martinez-Huedo MA, Carrasco-Garrido P, et al. Trends in lower-extremity amputations in people with and without diabetes in Spain, 2001-2008. Diabetes Care 2011;34:1570–6.
65. Eskelinen E, Eskelinen A, Alback A, et al. Major amputation incidence decreases both in non-diabetic and in diabetic patients in Helsinki. Scand J Surg 2006;95:185–9.
66. Chiu CC, Huang CL, Weng SF, et al. A multidisciplinary diabetic foot ulcer treatment programme significantly improved the outcome in patients with infected diabetic foot ulcers. J Plast Reconstr Aesthet Surg 2011;64:867–72.
67. Paulus N, Jacobs M, Greiner A. Primary and secondary amputation in critical limb ischemia patients: different aspects. Acta Chir Belg 2012;112:251–4.
68. Fosse S, Hartemann-Heurtier A, Jacqueminet S, et al. Incidence and characteristics of lower limb amputations in people with diabetes. Diabet Med 2009;26: 391–6.
69. Trautner C, Haastert B, Mauckner P, et al. Reduced incidence of lower-limb amputations in the diabetic population of a German city, 1990-2005: results of the Leverkusen Amputation Reduction Study (LARS). Diabetes Care 2007;30: 2633–7.

Preventing the First or Recurrent Ulcers

Lawrence A. Lavery, MPH, DPM[a],*, Javier La Fontaine, MS, DPM[a],
Paul J. Kim, MS, DPM[b]

KEYWORDS

• Diabetes • Ulcer • Infection • Prevention

KEY POINTS

- Prevention is best achieved within a multispecialty group of providers that have a common objective.
- The basic elements of prevention involve education, foot examination, risk classification, therapeutic shoes and insoles, and regular foot care.
- High-risk patients need additional assessment for vascular disease and intensive disease management, and corrective vascular and foot surgery when necessary.
- Basic interventions can reduce the incidence of foot ulcers by more than 50%.

INTRODUCTION

Prevention in the diabetic foot is often neglected, even in very high-risk patients. The simple elements of the "standard of care" for prevention are not well understood by most clinicians, educators, or patients. The benefit of a team approach to prevent foot ulceration and reduce amputations has been described multiple times in the United States and Europe.[1–4] The standard approach to prevent ulceration requires little advanced technology or expensive testing procedures. The basic elements of prevention include screening, risk classification, regular foot care, protective shoes and insoles, and diabetic foot education. Most of the published work on prevention targets patients with diabetes that have had a previous ulcer. This is because their risk of experiencing another event is very high. Only about 3% to 4% of patients that have sensory neuropathy without a previous ulceration or peripheral arterial disease develop a foot ulcer in a year, so a large number of patients have to be evaluated

Disclosures: None.

[a] Department of Plastic Surgery, The University of Texas Southwestern Medical Center, 1801 Inwood Road, Dallas, TX 75390–9132, USA; [b] Department of Plastic Surgery, Georgetown University School of Medicine, Georgetown University Hospital, 3800 Reservoir Rd, Washington, DC 20007, USA
* Corresponding author.
E-mail address: Larry.Lavery@utsouthwestern.edu

Med Clin N Am 97 (2013) 807–820
http://dx.doi.org/10.1016/j.mcna.2013.05.001
0025-7125/13/$ – see front matter © 2013 Elsevier Inc. All rights reserved.

medical.theclinics.com

to be able to measure the effects of treatment. Therefore, there is very little evidence about the ability to prevent the first foot ulcer in people with diabetes.

The cause of ulcerations in diabetes is associated with the presence of peripheral sensory neuropathy and repetitive trauma caused by normal walking activities to areas on the foot that are subject to moderate or high pressures and shear.[5] Pressure sites on the sole of the foot are often associated with limited joint mobility of the foot or ankle or structure deformities, such as hammer toes and hallux valgus deformity. The goal of prevention is to interrupt this pathway as often as possible.

RISK CLASSIFICATION

The first challenge in prevention is to identify who to target first, or where to target resources. Classifying patients into groups based on risk status is a pivotal process to help identify the highest-risk patients and direct dwindling medical resources appropriately. Unfortunately, in most centers even basic foot risk assessment is not performed even though the criteria and procedures are inexpensive, practical, and easy to execute. A trained technician can perform the screening history and testing and place patients into the correct risk stratification.

There are several risk stratification tools that have been used to identify and treat high-risk patients. Some systems use a simple low- and high-risk scheme,[4,6,7] whereas others provide four to five specified risk categories and suggested prevention strategies for each. The International Working Group on the Diabetic Foot's (IWGDF) risk classification was designed from a consensus panel, and it has been adopted as an international tool. The most important factors for risk classification include assessment of sensory neuropathy; peripheral arterial disease; severe foot deformity; and history of foot pathology, such as ulceration, amputation, or Charcot neuroarthropathy.

Mayfield, Lavery, and Peters used risk classifications similar to the IWGDF risk classification to demonstrate that the frequency of foot complications increases as risk criteria increases.[8-10] The highest-risk groups to develop ulceration are patients with a previous ulcer or amputation. These patients have a 36-fold increased risk of developing a foot ulcer in the next year compared with patients without neuropathy or peripheral arterial disease.[8,9,11] Lavery and coworkers[10] evaluated a cohort of 1666 patients with diabetes that participated in a diabetes disease management program. In the program, patients received foot-specific education, therapeutic shoes and insoles, and regular foot care over a 2-year period. The IWGDF classification was expanded within current risk tiers to evaluate the contribution of various factors (**Table 1**). Lavery and coworkers[10] reported no difference in ulceration in patients with neuropathy, and neuropathy and foot deformity (risk group 1 and 2). There was a significant increase in the yearly incidence foot ulceration, reulceration, infection, amputation, and hospitalization in patients with peripheral arterial disease, compared with patients with neuropathy, and neuropathy and foot deformity. In addition, there were more ulcers in patients with a history of ulcers and amputations (risk group 3).[10] Overall, there were increasing trends in foot ulcers, infections, and amputations as risk tiers increased based on the criteria described in the IWGDF risk classification (see **Table 1**).

Targeting the correct risk group is important to provide cost-effective preventative care. In a prevention program with limited resources, the highest-risk groups should be the main focus for prevention services. Patients in risk group 3 can be easily identified from administrative data. This small minority (15%) accounts for a disproportionate number of wounds, infections, and hospitalizations (see **Table 1**). The

Table 1		
The incidence of ulcers and amputation based on the International Working Group for the Diabetic Foot risk classification		
N = 1666	**Ulcer**	**Amputation**
0 No sensory neuropathy No peripheral arterial disease No complication history	2%	0.04%
1 Sensory neuropathy No peripheral arterial disease No complication history	4.5%	0
2 Sensory neuropathy and foot deformity or limited joint mobility No complication history	3%	0.7%
peripheral arterial disease No complication history	13.8%	3.7%
3 Ulcer history	31.7%	2.2%
Amputation history	32.2%	20.7%

Data from Peters EJ, Lavery LA. Effectiveness of the diabetic foot risk classification system of the International Working Group on the Diabetic Foot. Diabetes Care 2001;24(8):1442–7.

benefit of intensive prevention services to patients in lower-risk groups has not been specifically addressed in the medical literature.

EDUCATION

The diabetic foot is wrapped in mythology and misinformation for patients, their families, and clinicians. Education is a key component to get the patient and their family to participate in the prevention process. By itself, education is unlikely to be effective. The high-risk patient needs to have education as one of the primary layers of prevention, but other elements, such as therapeutic shoes and insoles, professional foot care, and systemic disease modification, must be included. It is difficult to evaluate education as a single intervention in a randomized clinical trial unless the other aspects of care are standardized. Several studies to evaluate diabetic foot education incorporate standard prevention strategies; however, many do not specify if these services are available or how they were provided.[12,13]

There are three randomized clinical studies that evaluated clinical outcomes with an education intervention.[12,14,15] Most studies evaluate a change in patient knowledge as the primary outcomes. It is unclear if better knowledge translates into sustained changes in behavior and a reduction in ulcers, infections, or amputations. Understanding the disease process is not enough. The diabetic foot is a mechanical problem more than a medical problem. If the abnormal biomechanics of the foot are not addressed, the high-risk patient's understanding of the disease process alone will be insufficient to prevent repetitive ulcers, infections, and amputations. Usually, the education message to patients is to inspect their feet, avoid going barefoot, avoid hot surfaces, avoid hot water, and seek professional foot care on a regular basis. These instructions are not practical or effective for most high-risk patients. Many patients are obese with poor vision and limited mobility of their back, hip, knee, and ankle. Most patients are unable to provide any meaningful self-inspection.[9] Because of obesity or limited joint range of motion, they cannot physically position themselves to see the bottom of their feet. As a consequence of poor vision, they cannot see the bottom of their feet or recognize subtle changes that identify tissue damage. For instance, in a study by Lavery and colleagues[9] 48% of study patients had impaired vision and 41% lacked the flexibility to adequately position the foot so it could be examined. Locking-Cusolito and colleagues[16] evaluated similar criteria in a dialysis population and found that 25% of study patients had impaired vision and 45% lacked flexibility to correctly position the lower extremity so it could be visualized.[9] Perhaps a more rational approach is to assess the skills of the patient, and if they are unable to see the top and bottom of the foot, someone else in the family could help with this type of assessment.

If patients have good vision and they can position themselves to see their feet, they still may not be able to identify any changes that are meaningful. The early changes to the skin before an ulcer develops are too subtle for a patient or their caregiver to recognize. However, they may be able to identify an ulcer as soon as it develops. Lavery and colleagues[17] reported the results of a randomized clinical study where the control group received therapeutic shoes and insoles, education, and regular foot care. Patients were instructed to contact the study nurse if they identified any abnormalities during visual inspection. A list of local signs they should look for was provided, such as changes in color, or temperature, or swelling. An ulcer had already developed in most cases (97%) by the time the patient saw something that was "abnormal." Visual changes and self-inspection may not be effective for most patients to prevent foot ulcers if warning signs are too subtle to see.[18]

Malone and colleagues,[14] Lincoln and colleagues,[15] and Litzelman and colleagues[12] used education in randomized clinical trials of high-risk patients to prevent ulcers and amputations.[19] Malone and colleagues[14] randomized patients into an education group (N = 103) and a group with no education (N = 100). The educational intervention was based on a single education session. Provision of therapeutic shoes and insoles was not reported. However, during the follow-up period there were significantly few ulceration (education 8, no education 26; $P<.005$) and amputation (education 7, no education 21; $P = .025$).

Lincoln and colleagues[15] used a similar approach to that described by Malone and colleagues.[14] Lincoln randomized 172 patients with newly healed DFUs (diabetic foot ulcers) to receive usual care or one-to-one education. Patients that received the "education intervention" participated in a single session. Lincoln reported that subjects in the education group demonstrated improved knowledge compared with the control group. However, clinical outcomes were no different. There was no difference in foot ulcers or amputations among the treatment groups. The incidence of foot ulcers at 6 and 12 months was 30% and 41% in the education group and 21% and 41% in the control group.

Litzelman and colleagues[12] randomized 395 patients with diabetes to be assigned to either an education and prevention program or the standard care they would normally receive. The education intervention group received foot education, telephone follow-up calls, and reminders to their primary care providers to do diabetic foot examinations. Patients that received "community standard care" were more likely to develop a foot ulcer, not perform recommended self-care practices, or have their feet examined by their primary care physician (education group 68%; standard of care group 28%).

THERAPEUTIC SHOES AND INSOLES

Special shoes and insoles are a mainstay of ulcer prevention in high-risk patients with diabetes. In the United States, the Therapeutic Shoe Bill has provided shoes and insoles for high-risk Medicare beneficiaries with diabetes since 1993. Unfortunately, these services are dramatically underused. Only 7% to 16% of high-risk patients are prescribed therapeutic shoes and insoles. After they are prescribed, only about a third of patients wear the shoes for more than 12 hours a day.[20,21] Some reports suggest that 30% of high-risk patients prefer to go barefoot or wear slippers or stockings while at home.[22]

Several[23,24] studies have shown a significant reduction in foot ulcers in patients that receive therapeutic shoes compared with shoes patients would normal select themselves. There is little clinical evidence to help in understanding the effectiveness of the types of therapeutic shoes and insoles that are commonly used to prevent foot complications. There are a variety of insole materials and material combinations and different accommodations that can be built into the insole. Likewise, the type of shoe and outer sole accommodations are numerous. Most of the decisions for protective shoes and insoles are left to technicians that have little working knowledge of the medical literature. When patients reulcerate they do not return to the pedorthist or shoe maker for care, so these providers have no follow-up to determine if their approach is effective.

There are four randomized clinical trials and two prospective cohort studies that describe the benefit of various types of shoes and insoles for high-risk patients with diabetes (**Table 2**).[25] Most studies include patients with a previous foot ulcer and use a control group of patients with self-selected footwear. In some studies this is because they cannot afford therapeutic shoes,[26] they refuse recommended shoes,[27] or their insurance does not pay for shoes and insoles.[28] Reulceration is much higher

Table 2 Studies of therapeutic shoes and insoles				
Reiber et al,[32] 2002	RCT 24 mo	121 119 160	Custom cork and neoprene Prefabricated polyurethane insole Self-selected shoes, no insole	15% 14% 17%
Uccioli et al,[33] 1995	RCT 12 mo	33 36	Custom-made shoe and insoles Self-selected shoes, no insole	28% 58%
Lavery et al,[25] 2012	RCT 18 mo	150 149	Standard design ethyl vinyl acetate insoles, therapeutic shoes Shear design ethyl vinyl acetate insoles, therapeutic shoes	7% 2%
Rizzo et al,[30] 2012	RCT 60 mo	150 148	Standard of care Custom made orthosis with shoes	23.5% 72%
Busch and Chantelau,[28] 2003	Prospective cohort 12 mo	60 32	Rocker sole shoe and standard insole Self-selected shoes, no insole	15% 60%
Dargis et al,[29] 1999	Prospective cohort 24 mo	56 89	Therapeutic shoes and insole Self-selected shoes, no insole	30% 58%

Abbreviation: RCT, randomized controlled trial.

among patients that do not use therapeutic shoes and insoles. About 60% of patients reulcerate with self-selected shoes. Among patients that receive therapeutic shoes and insoles, there is a twofold to fourfold reduction in reulceration compared with patients that use shoes they have selected. Even with standard preventative care, such as therapeutic shoes and insoles, education, and regular foot care, about 24% to 50% of patients develop another foot ulcer within the next year.[18,29–31]

The four randomized clinical studies that evaluate therapeutic shoes and insoles provide a glimpse into the complexity of evaluating this intervention to prevent ulcers. Reiber and colleagues[32] compared two insole constructs with off-the-shelf footwear with patient-selected shoes. Uccioli and colleagues[33] compared custom-made shoes and insoles with patient-selected shoes (Table 3). Lavery and colleagues[34] randomized patients to receive a shear-reducing insole compared with a standard insole and off-the-shelf shoe, and education and regular foot care. Rizzo and colleagues[30] assessed the impact of a structured follow-up program on the incidence of diabetic foot ulceration in high-risk patients with diabetes.

Reiber and colleagues[32] compared custom bilaminar cork and neoprene insoles (N = 121), prefabricated polyurethane insoles (N = 119), and a control group (N = 160) in which patients selected their own shoes. Reiber's study was the only negative study of therapeutic shoes and insole for high-risk patients with diabetes. The study population had a high proportion of subjects without sensory neuropathy measured with a 10-g Semmes-Weinstein monofilament.[32] Many patients would not be considered "high risk" by most risk classification criteria. It was also the study with the lowest ulceration rate in the control arm treated with self-selected shoes (17%). During the 2-year evaluation, 15% of patients developed ulcers in the custom insole group, 14% developed ulcers in the prefabricated insole group, and 17% developed ulcers in the self-selected shoe group. The rate of ulceration was lower in the control arm of Reiber's study than many of the therapeutic shoe treatment groups in other studies (see Table 2).

Uccioli and coworkers[33] conducted a multicenter randomized controlled trial of patients with previous foot ulceration for 1 year. Patients were randomized to custom made shoes and insoles (N = 33) or self-selected shoes (N = 36). Reulceration was

Table 3
Foot surgery to prevent ulcer recurrence

Author	Study Population	Treatment Groups	Recurrent Foot Ulcers
Mueller et al,[31] 2003	Randomized controlled trial 7 mo follow-up	1. Achilles tendon lengthening, N = 30	15%
		2. Total contact cast, N = 33	59%
Lin et al,[45] 1996	Retrospective cohort study 17 mo follow-up	1. Achilles tendon lengthening, N = 15	0%
		2. Total contact cast, N = 21	19%
Armstrong et al,[41] 2003	Retrospective cohort study 6 mo follow-up	1. Arthroplasty of the great toe, N = 21	5%
		2. Standard care, N = 20	35%
Lin et al,[53] 2000	Retrospective cohort study 4.2 mo follow-up	1. Arthroplasty of the great toe, N = 14	0%
		2. Total contact cast, N = 21	0%

significantly lower in the custom shoe treatment group (27.7%) compared with patients that selected their own footwear (58.2%; $P = .009$). Most patients that require therapeutic shoes and insoles do not require a custom-made shoe. Usually custom shoes are only necessary when the foot is so deformed that the foot does not fit in a ready-made shoe.

Lavery and colleagues[25,34] reported the results of a randomized clinical study that compared a standard insole and therapeutic shoe with a shear-reducing insole and shoe. In the study 299 patients with diabetic neuropathy, foot deformity, or history of foot ulceration were randomized into a standard therapy group that received therapeutic shoes and insoles, education, and regular foot care (N = 150) or a shear-reducing insole instead of a standard accommodative insole (N = 149). A multilaminar insole was constructed of a 35-durometer ethyl vinyl acetate upper pad 3 mm thick, a 45-durometer ethyl vinyl acetate lower pad 3 mm thick, and a 20-durometer Plastozote top cover 1.5 mm thick. The only difference between the groups was that the shear-reducing insole used elastic binders and two thin Teflon sheets, so the top layers could slide on the bottom layers, thereby reducing pressure and shear. The standard insole materials were glued together with adhesive. Insoles were changed every 4 months. During 18 months of evaluation there were fewer ulcers in the shear-reducing insole group (N = 3; 2%) compared with the standard insole group (N = 10; 6.7%), Standard therapy patients were 3.5 times more likely to develop an ulcer compared with the shear-reducing insole group (hazard ratio, 3.47; 95% confidence interval, 0.96–12.67).[25] The rate of ulceration was low in this study because only a small proportion of the study population had a history of foot ulceration (27.5% and 23.5%).

Rizzo and colleagues[30] reported the longest study in this area. A total of 1874 patients with diabetes referred to the Diabetic Foot Unit of the University of Pisa were ranked based on the ulcerative risk score proposed by the International Consensus on Diabetic Foot. A total of 334 patients (17.8%) were randomized into two groups: one group received standard treatment, and the second group received custom-made orthosis and shoes as a part of a structured prevention program. During the first 12-month follow-up, 11.5% of patients that received shoes and insoles developed a DFU compared with 38.6% in the standard therapy group ($P<.0001$). In the extended follow-up, the cumulative incidence of ulceration in the standard therapy group was 61% and 17.6% in the group that received shoes as part of their intervention ($P<.0001$) at 3 years and at 5 years 72% of subjects in the standard therapy group ulcerated compared with 23.5% in the treatment group ($P<.0001$).

TEMPERATURE SELF-ASSESSMENT

Temperature assessment has been used in clinical practice to diagnose neuropathy and soft tissue injury in patients with neuropathy, and it has been used as a tool for self-assessment and monitoring. Clinicians have used temperature assessment to evaluate foot ulcers and Charcot neuroarthropathy. The rationale to use temperature as part of a daily foot assessment is that temperatures could provide an objective measurement of tissue injury. A change in skin temperature could be used to identify tissue that is inflamed. It is a similar thought process as described in the National Pressure Ulcer Advisory Panel ulcer classification. A stage 1 pressure ulcer is recognized as having signs of tissue injury before there is a break in the epithelium. It can be characterized by changes in temperature, in color, or in texture of the skin.

There are three randomized clinical studies that compare standard prevention therapies consisting of therapeutic shoes and insoles; regular foot care by a podiatrist; and a standard, foot-specific education to temperature home monitoring intervention in addition to standard care. All three studies demonstrated a 3- to 10-fold reduction in reulceration when patients used home temperature evaluation compared with standard prevention practices. All three studies used a similar approach. Patients used an infrared thermometer to record the temperatures from 10 sites on the foot and then compare temperatures at corresponding anatomic sites on the right and left feet to see if there was greater than 4°F difference. This temperature difference was used to define a high temperature that was believed to be associated with soft tissue injury that could lead to ulceration. Patients were to reduce their activity by 50% until temperatures normalized. If they did not return to a normal range in a set time frame, they called the study coordinator to be seen by the study physician.

FAT PAD AUGMENTATION

Several researches have explored the idea of reducing foot pressure with an "internal orthotic device" by injecting the subcutaneous tissue with material that increases the fat pad on the ball of the foot.[35–37] Balkin[38,39] reported the use of injectable silicon for the treatment of metatarsalgia, callus, scars, and diabetic foot ulcer since 1964. He reported data on a cohort of 1585 patients that were treated for metatarsalgia and diabetic foot ulcers. Balkin reported no long-term adverse events related to these injections based on close clinical monitoring and postmortem specimens.

Boulton's group prospectively evaluated a cohort of patients with diabetes over a 2-year period. Twenty-eight patients with diabetes were randomized to active treatment with six injections of 0.2 mL liquid silicone in the plantar surface of the foot or sham treatment with saline. Patients treated with silicone oil had a significant increase in plantar tissue thickness compared with the placebo group (1.8 vs 0.1 mm) and a greater plantar pressures reduction (232 vs 25 kPa) at 3, 6, and 12 months.[36,37] There are several different materials that might be used instead of silicone; however, currently there are no randomized clinical studies to support the clinical effectiveness of this approach to reduce foot ulceration in high-risk patients.

SURGERY TO HEAL ULCERS AND PREVENT RECURRENCE

Another option to prevent ulcer recurrence is to surgically correct the underlying biomechanical defect, such as hallux rigidus, hammer toe deformities, and equinus (**Fig. 1**). The goal of surgery is to reduce the long-term risk for reulceration by increasing joint motion where it is limited, reducing abnormal pressure points, and

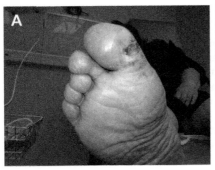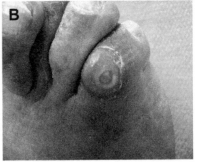

Fig. 1. (*A, B*) Limitation of hallux dorsiflexion and contracture of lesser digits increases pressure and leads to ulceration.

repairing structural foot deformities when they are an underlying cause of ulceration. The literature has several reports of retrospective case series, but there is only one randomized clinical trial that reports clinical outcomes with this type of approach. In general, surgery seems to be safe and effective at healing recalcitrant ulcers and reducing the risk of reulceration.

The question for physicians and patients is whether the risks of surgery are better than the risk of having a chronic foot ulcer. The risks of infection and amputation from a nonhealing foot ulcer are high. Approximately 10% to 20% of diabetic foot ulcers end in amputation[12,13]; 56% are treated for infection; and 20% develop osteomyelitis.[9-11] Ulcer recurrence is about 30% per year when standard preventative therapies are provided. The incidence of ulceration is 50% to 80% when no additional prevention is provided. However, several authors have reported the results of planned surgical procedures to heal foot ulcers. These studies suggest a high rate of wound healing (91%–100%) and a low rate of ulcer recurrence after 2 years (0%–39%).[40-42] If surgery is simply viewed as a prevention tool, in the correct subpopulation, surgery has the lowest reulceration rate.

Achilles Tendon Pathology

Several papers have reported results of percutaneous Achilles tendon lengthening to heal recalcitrant forefoot ulcers. Equinus deformity has been associated with high pressures on the sole of the foot and increased risk of foot ulceration in persons with diabetes.[31,43,44] Lengthening of the Achilles tendon reduces pressures on the forefoot and thereby decreases the risk of recurrent foot ulcers. Mueller and colleagues[31] and Lavery and coworkers[43] reported a 27% reduction in peak pressures on the ball of the foot in patients with diabetes after the Achilles tendon was lengthened. The procedure is very effective to heal recalcitrant forefoot ulcers, and there is a very low rate of ulcer recurrence.

Mueller and colleagues[31] conducted a randomized clinical study that compared Achilles tendon lengthening with immobilization in a total contact cast. Equinus was defined as ankle dorsiflexion less than five degrees. A higher proportion of patients healed in the surgery group (surgery 100% vs cast group 88%). Perhaps the greatest benefit to the surgery was the low rate of ulcer recurrence. The rate of reulceration was significantly lower in the surgery group at 7 months (surgery 15% vs cast group 59%) and at 24 months (surgery 38% vs cast group 83%). Lin reported similar results. After Achilles lengthening there were no cases of reulceration after 17 months.[45]

Achilles tendon surgery is not without complications. Deciding on an operational definition of equinus is difficult. A variety of different measurements and criteria have been reported.[46-48] There is no evidence-based criteria to help clinicians determine how much ankle joint motion is pathologic and how much correction is needed to make the procedure safe and effective. Over-lengthening the Achilles tendon is associated with ulcers on the heel. Holstein and coworkers[49] reported that 18% of patients with more than 10 degrees of ankle dorsiflexion after surgery developed a heel ulcer. Mueller and colleagues[31] reported similar findings; 16% of patients developed heel ulcers after undergoing an Achilles tendon lengthening procedure.[50] The average increase in ankle joint dorsiflexion was 15 degrees in Mueller and colleagues'[31] randomized clinical study.

Great Toe Ulcers Associated with Hallux Rigidus

Another example of selective foot surgery to reduce the risk of ulcer recurrence involves ulcers of the great toe. Foot ulcers of the great toe are commonly associated with hallux rigidus, or a reduced range of motion of the first metatarsophalangeal joint.[51,52] One of the most common surgical approaches to address hallux rigidus in persons with diabetes is a resectional arthroplasty of the first metatarsophalangeal joint, or more specifically resection of a portion of the base of the proximal phalanx of the great toe. This is also referred to as a Keller bunionectomy. The Keller resectional arthroplasty removes the arthritic joint and allows a pseudoarthrosis to develop in its place. Like the surgery described to increase ankle joint range of motion by lengthening the Achilles tendon (**Fig. 2**), arthroplasty of the great toe has been reported to increase healing of ulcers that have failed other therapies with a much lower rate of ulcer recurrence.

Armstrong and coworkers[41] reported the results of a cohort study of 41 patients with diabetes with great toe ulcers. Patients received either resectional arthroplasty of the great toe or standard wound care. The surgery group had faster healing (24 vs 67 days) and few recurrent ulcers after the surgery (5% vs 35%). Lin and coworkers reported similar results.[53] He treated 14 patients with great toe ulcers that failed to heal with aggressive off-loading in a total contact cast. All of the ulcers healed after the resectional arthroplasty was performed, and none of the patients had an ulcer recurrence after 26 weeks.

Lesser Toe Ulcers Associated with Hammer toe Deformity

Ulcers on the tip of the toe or on the top of the toe are often associated with hammer toe or mallet toe deformity (**Fig. 3**). Ulcers on the distal portion of the toe are especially prone to recurrence because the deformity causes the patient to bear weight on the tip of the toe.[29,41] Several authors have described a percutaneous flexor tenotomy of the long flexor tendon to heal recalcitrant ulcers and reduce ulcer recurrence.[52,54,55] Kearney and coworkers[55] described the results of 58 tenotomies for distal toe ulcers. Ninety-eight percent of ulcers healed and only 12% recurred after surgery after an

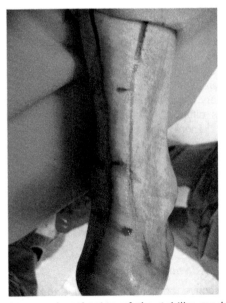

Fig. 2. A simple, percutaneous, lengthening of the Achilles tendon increases range of motion at the ankle joint and decreases forefoot pressure.

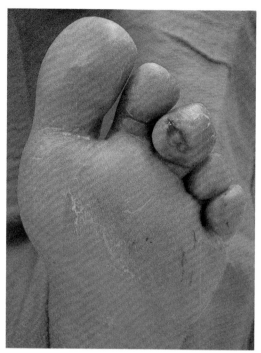

Fig. 3. Clawtoe deformity with neuropathy commonly leads to ulceration at the tip of the toe.

average of 28 months evaluation period. Two patients (3.4%) eventually had amputation of a portion of the toe.

Ulcers on the dorsum of the toe are usually associated with a hammer toe deformity. A joint resection of the proximal interphalangeal joint to correct the hammer toe deformity has been described to heal the ulcer and reduce the risk of reulceration. Armstrong and coworkers[42] compared the results of 31 patients with diabetes with hammer toe surgery. Ninety-six percent of ulcers healed; 14% of patients developed postoperative infections. However, after surgery none of the patients with an ulcer developed a recurrent foot ulcer in the next year.

These studies indicate that surgery to heal ulcers and prevent ulcer recurrence is safe in comparison with the natural course of the disease process. By increasing joint range of motion or correcting structural deformity, the pathway to ulcerations is more dramatically interrupted than with other interventions, such as therapeutic shoes and insoles or education. Many high-risk patients are not good candidates for surgery because of poor healing potential, poor glucose control, and inability to comply with the requirements of self-care after surgery. Patient selection is one of the most important aspects of successful surgery.

SUMMARY

Prevention is overlooked and underused, even in very high-risk patients. Prevention is best achieved within a multispecialty group of providers that have a common objective. Ideally, the team approach should include educators; physical therapists; nurses; internist; pedorthists; and vascular, orthopedic, and podiatric surgeons. The basic elements involve education, foot examination, risk classification, therapeutic shoes and insoles, and regular foot care. High-risk patients need additional assessment for vascular disease and intensive disease management, and corrective vascular and foot surgery when necessary. Basic interventions can reduce the incidence of foot ulcers by more than 50%.

REFERENCES

1. Ronnemaa T, Hamalainen H, Toikka T, et al. Evaluation of the impact of podiatrist care in the primary prevention of foot problems in diabetic subjects. Diabetes Care 1997;20(12):1833–7.
2. Plank J, Haas W, Rakovac I, et al. Evaluation of the impact of chiropodist care in the secondary prevention of foot ulcerations in diabetic subjects. Diabetes Care 2003;26(6):1691–5.
3. Armstrong DG, Harkless LB. Outcomes of preventative care in a diabetic foot specialty clinic. J Foot Ankle Surg 1998;37(6):460–6.
4. Leese GP, Stang D, Pearson DW. A national approach to diabetes foot risk stratification and foot care. Scott Med J 2011;56(3):151–5.
5. Brand P. The diabetic foot. In: Ellenberg M, Rifkin H, editors. Diabetes mellitus, theory and practice. New York: Medical Examination Publishing; 1983. p. 803–28.
6. Leese G, Schofield C, McMurray B, et al. Scottish foot ulcer risk score predicts foot ulcer healing in a regional specialist foot clinic. Diabetes Care 2007;30(8): 2064–9.
7. Monteiro-Soares M, Boyko EJ, Ribeiro J, et al. Risk stratification systems for diabetic foot ulcers: a systematic review. Diabetologia 2011;54(5):1190–9.
8. Mayfield JA, Reiber GE, Nelson RG, et al. A foot risk classification system to predict diabetic amputation in Pima Indians. Diabetes Care 1996;19(7):704–9.
9. Lavery LA, Armstrong DG, Vela SA, et al. Practical criteria for screening patients at high risk for diabetic foot ulceration. Arch Intern Med 1998;158(2):157–62.
10. Lavery LA, Peters EJ, Williams JR, et al. Reevaluating the way we classify the diabetic foot: restructuring the diabetic foot risk classification system of the International Working Group on the Diabetic Foot. Diabetes Care 2008;31(1): 154–6.
11. Peters EJ, Lavery LA. Effectiveness of the diabetic foot risk classification system of the International Working Group on the Diabetic Foot. Diabetes Care 2001; 24(8):1442–7.
12. Litzelman DK, Slemenda CW, Langefeld CD, et al. Reduction of lower extremity clinical abnormalities in patients with non-insulin-dependent diabetes mellitus. A randomized, controlled trial. Ann Intern Med 1993;119(1):36–41.
13. Donohoe ME, Fletton JA, Hook A, et al. Improving foot care for people with diabetes mellitus–a randomized controlled trial of an integrated care approach. Diabet Med 2000;17(8):581–7.
14. Malone JM, Snyder M, Anderson G, et al. Prevention of amputation by diabetic education. Am J Surg 1989;158(6):520–3 [discussion: 523–4].
15. Lincoln NB, Radford KA, Game FL, et al. Education for secondary prevention of foot ulcers in people with diabetes: a randomised controlled trial. Diabetologia 2008;51(11):1954–61.
16. Locking-Cusolito H, Harwood L, Wilson B, et al. Prevalence of risk factors predisposing to foot problems in patients on hemodialysis. Nephrol Nurs J 2005; 32(4):373–84.

17. Lavery LA, Higgins KR, Lanctot DR, et al. Home monitoring of foot skin temperatures to prevent ulceration. Diabetes Care 2004;27(11):2642–7.
18. Lavery LA, Higgins KR, Lanctot DR, et al. Preventing diabetic foot ulcer recurrence in high-risk patients: use of temperature monitoring as a self-assessment tool. Diabetes Care 2007;30(1):14–20.
19. Dorresteijn JA, Kriegsman DM, Assendelft WJ, et al. Patient education for preventing diabetic foot ulceration. Cochrane Database Syst Rev 2010;(5):CD001488.
20. Lavery LA, Armstrong DG. Temperature monitoring to assess, predict, and prevent diabetic foot complications. Curr Diab Rep 2007;7(6):416–9.
21. Armstrong DG, Holtz-Neiderer K, Wendel C, et al. Skin temperature monitoring reduces the risk for diabetic foot ulceration in high-risk patients. Am J Med 2007; 120(12):1042–6.
22. Reiber GE, Smith DG, Wallace CM, et al. Footwear used by individuals with diabetes and a history of foot ulcer. J Rehabil Res Dev 2002;39(5):615–22.
23. Ndip A, Rutter MK, Vileikyte L, et al. Dialysis treatment is an independent risk factor for foot ulceration in patients with diabetes and stage 4 or 5 chronic kidney disease. Diabetes Care 2010;33(8):1811–6.
24. Lavery LA, Hunt NA, Lafontaine J, et al. Diabetic foot prevention: a neglected opportunity in high-risk patients. Diabetes Care 2010;33(7):1460–2.
25. Lavery LA, LaFontaine J, Higgins KR, et al. Shear-reducing insoles to prevent foot ulceration in high-risk diabetic patients. Adv Skin Wound Care 2012; 25(11):519–24 [quiz: 525–6].
26. Viswanathan V, Madhavan S, Gnanasundaram S, et al. Effectiveness of different types of footwear insoles for the diabetic neuropathic foot: a follow-up study. Diabetes Care 2004;27(2):474–7.
27. Edmonds ME, Blundell MP, Morris ME, et al. Improved survival of the diabetic foot: the role of a specialized foot clinic. Q J Med 1986;60(232):763–71.
28. Busch K, Chantelau E. Effectiveness of a new brand of stock 'diabetic' shoes to protect against diabetic foot ulcer relapse. A prospective cohort study. Diabet Med 2003;20(8):665–9.
29. Dargis V, Pantelejeva O, Jonushaite A, et al. Benefits of a multidisciplinary approach in the management of recurrent diabetic foot ulceration in Lithuania: a prospective study. Diabetes Care 1999;22(9):1428–31.
30. Rizzo L, Tedeschi A, Fallani E, et al. Custom-made orthesis and shoes in a structured follow-up program reduces the incidence of neuropathic ulcers in high-risk diabetic foot patients. Int J Low Extrem Wounds 2012;11(1): 59–64.
31. Mueller MJ, Sinacore DR, Hastings MK, et al. Effect of Achilles tendon lengthening on neuropathic plantar ulcers. A randomized clinical trial. J Bone Joint Surg Am 2003;85-A(8):1436–45.
32. Reiber GE, Smith DG, Wallace C, et al. Effect of therapeutic footwear on foot reulceration in patients with diabetes: a randomized controlled trial. JAMA 2002;287(19):2552–8.
33. Uccioli L, Faglia E, Monticone G, et al. Manufactured shoes in the prevention of diabetic foot ulcers. Diabetes Care 1995;18(10):1376–8.
34. Lavery LA, Lanctot DR, Constantinides G, et al. Wear and biomechanical characteristics of a novel shear-reducing insole with implications for high-risk persons with diabetes. Diabetes Technol Ther 2005;7(4):638–46.
35. Bowling FL, Metcalfe SA, Wu S, et al. Liquid silicone to mitigate plantar pedal pressure: a literature review. J Diabetes Sci Technol 2010;4(4): 846–52.

36. van Schie CH, Whalley A, Armstrong DG, et al. The effect of silicone injections in the diabetic foot on peak plantar pressure and plantar tissue thickness: a 2-year follow-up. Arch Phys Med Rehabil 2002;83(7):919–23.

37. van Schie CH, Whalley A, Vileikyte L, et al. Efficacy of injected liquid silicone in the diabetic foot to reduce risk factors for ulceration: a randomized double-blind placebo-controlled trial. Diabetes Care 2000;23(5):634–8.

38. Balkin SW. Silicone injection for plantar keratoses. Preliminary report. J Am Podiatry Assoc 1966;56(1):1–11.

39. Balkin SW. Treatment of painful scars on soles and digits with injections of fluid silicone. J Dermatol Surg Oncol 1977;3(6):612–4.

40. Rosenblum BI, Giurini JM, Chrzan JS, et al. Preventing loss of the great toe with the hallux interphalangeal joint arthroplasty. J Foot Ankle Surg 1994;33(6):557–60.

41. Armstrong DG, Lavery LA, Vazquez JR, et al. Clinical efficacy of the first metatarsophalangeal joint arthroplasty as a curative procedure for hallux interphalangeal joint wounds in patients with diabetes. Diabetes Care 2003;26(12):3284–7.

42. Armstrong DG, Lavery LA, Stern S, et al. Is prophylactic diabetic foot surgery dangerous? J Foot Ankle Surg 1996;35(6):585–9.

43. Lavery LA, Armstrong DG, Boulton AJ. Ankle equinus deformity and its relationship to high plantar pressure in a large population with diabetes mellitus. J Am Podiatr Med Assoc 2002;92(9):479–82.

44. Armstrong DG, Stacpoole-Shea S, Nguyen H, et al. Lengthening of the Achilles tendon in diabetic patients who are at high risk for ulceration of the foot. J Bone Joint Surg Am 1999;81(4):535–8.

45. Lin SS, Lee TH, Wapner KL. Plantar forefoot ulceration with equinus deformity of the ankle in diabetic patients: the effect of tendo-Achilles lengthening and total contact casting. Orthopedics 1996;19(5):465–75.

46. DiGiovanni CW, Kuo R, Tejwani N, et al. Isolated gastrocnemius tightness. J Bone Joint Surg Am 2002;84-A(6):962–70.

47. Morton DJ. The human foot. New York: Columbia University Press; 1935.

48. Michael SD. Ankle equinus. In: Banks AS, Downey MS, Martin DE, et al, editors. McGlamry's comprehensive textbook of foot and ankle surgery. 3rd edition. Philadelphia: Lippincott Williams & Wilkins; 2001. p. 715–60.

49. Holstein P, Lohmann M, Bitsch M, et al. Achilles tendon lengthening, the panacea for plantar forefoot ulceration? Diabetes Metab Res Rev 2004; 20(Suppl 1):S37–40.

50. Barry DC, Sabacinski KA, Habershaw GM, et al. Tendo Achillis procedures for chronic ulcerations in diabetic patients with transmetatarsal amputations. J Am Podiatr Med Assoc 1993;83(2):96–100.

51. Boffeli TJ, Bean JK, Natwick JR. Biomechanical abnormalities and ulcers of the great toe in patients with diabetes. J Foot Ankle Surg 2002;41(6):359–64.

52. Laborde JM. Neuropathic toe ulcers treated with toe flexor tenotomies. Foot Ankle Int 2007;28(11):1160–4.

53. Lin SS, Bono CM, Lee TH. Total contact casting and Keller arthoplasty for diabetic great toe ulceration under the interphalangeal joint. Foot Ankle Int 2000; 21(7):588–93.

54. Tamir E, McLaren AM, Gadgil A, et al. Outpatient percutaneous flexor tenotomies for management of diabetic claw toe deformities with ulcers: a preliminary report. Can J Surg 2008;51(1):41–4.

55. Kearney TP, Hunt NA, Lavery LA. Safety and effectiveness of flexor tenotomies to heal toe ulcers in persons with diabetes. Diabetes Res Clin Pract 2010;89(3): 224–6.

Peripheral Arterial Disease and Bypass Surgery in the Diabetic Lower Limb

Mostafa A. Albayati, MBBS, BSc, Clifford P. Shearman, MS, FRCS*

KEYWORDS

- Diabetes • Peripheral arterial disease • Lower limb amputation
- Surgical revascularization

KEY POINTS

- Diabetes is a major risk factor for the development of atherosclerotic peripheral arterial disease (PAD) and patients with diabetes are 4 times more likely to develop PAD.
- One of the commonest and most costly causes of admission to hospital for a person with diabetes is foot and lower limb complications, which often lead to amputation.
- One of the most difficult decisions is deciding when to revascularise a limb and this should be made by a multidisciplinary team.
- Revascularisation can be achieved by open surgical techniques (bypass or endarterectomy) or by endovascular procedures such as angioplasty with or without a stent.
- Surgical revascularisation can achieve good results but careful patient selection, operative planning and the use of autologous vein are necessary. Revascularisation if needed should be carried out early.

BACKGROUND

By 2030 it is estimated that there will be 439 million people in the world living with diabetes.[1] In England alone, this number is now in excess of 3 million and 5.5% of the adult population have been diagnosed with diabetes with a further 2% remaining undiagnosed.[2] As the control of diabetes and management of infective complications have improved, the commonest cause of death has become cardiovascular disease.[3] Diabetes is a major risk factor for the development of atherosclerotic peripheral arterial disease (PAD) and patients with diabetes are 4 times more likely to develop PAD.[4] It is estimated that, even at the time of diagnosis, 8% of people with type 2 diabetes already have PAD and one-third of patients with diabetes over the age of 40 years will have PAD.[5] The presence of PAD in a patient with diabetes is associated with a

Department of Vascular Surgery, University Hospital Southampton, Tremona Road, Southampton, Hampshire SO16 6YD, UK
* Corresponding author.
E-mail address: cps@soton.ac.uk

Med Clin N Am 97 (2013) 821–834
http://dx.doi.org/10.1016/j.mcna.2013.03.009
0025-7125/13/$ – see front matter © 2013 Elsevier Inc. All rights reserved.

70% to 80% increased risk of dying from cardiovascular disease compared with a person with diabetes and no PAD. In addition, the risk of lower limb amputation is 10 to 16 times greater in people with diabetes and those with PAD have the greatest risk of limb loss.[6] One of the commonest and most costly causes of admission to the hospital for a person with diabetes is foot and lower limb complications, which often lead to amputation. The outlook for patients after amputation is generally poor and only around 30% will ambulate with a prosthetic limb; 50% will be dead within 2 years.[7,8]

Worldwide the commonest cause of amputation is complications associated with diabetes. In England, over the 3 years between 2007 and 2010, 34,109 major and minor amputations were performed in patients, 48.9% of whom had diabetes. In people with diabetes the incidence of amputation was 2.51 per 1000 person-years compared with patients without diabetes in whom the incidence was 0.11 per 1000 person-years (relative risk 23.3 for diabetes).[9] Perhaps more worrying was the 8-fold variation in the incidence of amputation depending on the where the individual lived, suggesting a wide variation in the quality of service provided. This local variation in amputation rates is also reflected internationally.[10]

Eighty percent of amputations in people with diabetes are preceded by foot ulceration. The foot in a person with diabetes is at risk of ulceration and damage due to neuropathy, ischemia, and infection. In the Eurodiale Study of 1008 patients with foot ulcers, PAD was identified in 47.5% of individuals and PAD was the strongest prognostic indicator not only of failure of the ulcer to heal (odds ratio = 2.82; confidence interval 1.88–4.22) but also of the risk of amputation and death.[11] The combination of infection and PAD had a particularly bad outlook.

Equally, patients diagnosed with PAD have a high prevalence of diabetes. In the Bypass versus Angioplasty in Severe Ischemia of the Leg (BASIL) Trial, which recruited patients more than 12 years ago, 42% of patients at that time with critical or severe limb ischemia had diabetes.[12] Even in mild PAD, 44.2% of patients had already been diagnosed with diabetes.[13]

Therefore most people treated for PAD in the next decade will inevitably have diabetes. The number of people with diabetes who develop foot complications and have PAD will increase and they are at significant risk of poor ulcer healing and limb loss. This article examines the role of surgical revascularization in these patients.

DIABETIC PERIPHERAL ARTERIAL DISEASE

In people with diabetes, atherosclerosis has several specific biologic and clinical differences to the disease in patients who are not diabetic. Before planning intervention in a patient with diabetes, it is important to understand this difference if a successful outcome is to be achieved. Most vascular services and interventions have been developed for patients without diabetes with PAD and therefore may not be appropriate to those with diabetes.

The very high prevalence of diabetic PAD may be partly explained by the specific effects that impaired glucose homeostasis has on the vasculature. Nuclear factor-κB regulates pro-inflammatory and pro-atherosclerotic genes in endothelial cells, vascular smooth muscle cells, and macrophages and is upregulated by elevated levels of glucose.[14] Elevated levels of glucose are associated with increased monocyte-vascular endothelial interaction, an early step in the development of atherosclerosis. Hyperglycemia also causes changes in proteins, producing advanced glycation end products , which are associated with oxidative stress, smooth muscle cell proliferation and migration, and increased inflammatory proteins, again important factors in the atherosclerotic process.[15] Impaired glucose homeostasis has a marked effect on lipid metabolism, resulting in an "atherogenic dyslipidemia," which is strongly associated with the development of atherosclerosis and can occur without significantly raised total serum cholesterol.[16]

Diabetes is also associated with a pro-thrombotic state with increases in fibrinogen, factor VII activity, plasminogen activator inhibitor-1, and platelet aggregation. This powerful combination of hyperglycemic vascular endothelial dysfunction, abnormal lipid profiles, and a prothrombotic state may explain the particularly aggressive nature of diabetic PAD.[17] Examination of atherosclerotic plaque in people with diabetes shows markedly different composition to nondiabetic disease. Macrophage infiltration and thrombus formation are increased and there is evidence of increased inflammation and neovascularization, which makes the plaque unstable and prone to rupture.[18] Calcification is particularly common and, although occurring in the plaque, it is also common in the media of the blood vessel.[19] Not only is calcification a marker of increased cardiovascular risk, but it also has significant implications for treatment, making the artery more fragile and prone to cracking and disruption.

One of the most characteristic features of diabetic PAD is the distribution of the disease. There is a preponderance of small-vessel disease below the knee with relative sparing of the proximal aorto-iliac segments.[20] Despite the tibial vessels being occluded, the pedal vessels usually remain patent, which again has significant implications for intervention to revascularize the limb. Blood flow needs to be established beyond the diseased crural vessels and often small-vessel angioplasty or short bypass grafts into the foot are required.

INDICATIONS FOR REVASCULARIZATION

One of the most difficult decisions is deciding when to revascularize a limb; this should be made by a multidisciplinary team, including diabetologists, surgeons, podiatrists, and wound care specialists experienced in the management of diabetic foot complications. It may be relatively easy to determine that a patient has no PAD on clinical assessment and noninvasive imaging, such as duplex ultrasound. In contrast, sometimes the ischemia is so advanced with worsening gangrene and tissue loss that the need for urgent revascularization is evident (cf **Fig. 1**). However, in many patients with PAD the degree of ischemia and need for revascularization is less clear. The interaction of large-vessel disease, microcirculatory abnormalities, and infection makes the decision to offer revascularization challenging even for an expert. However, the current problem in most cases lies not with the difficulty of assessment but in failing or delaying referral for assessment. In patients with foot ulcers, 30% to 50% of patients are referred only after the development of gangrene and up to 40% are not investigated for the presence of PAD at all. Disappointingly, 50% of patients have no vascular assessment before amputation.[21] Any patient with diabetes and a foot ulcer in whom there is any doubt about the circulation should be referred urgently to a vascular multidisciplinary team for assessment. Delay in revascularization results in worse outcomes and higher amputation rates.[22]

Vascular assessment is based, first, on detecting PAD and, second, on assessing its significance. All patients with diabetes and a foot ulcer should have an initial assessment to detect PAD. This initial assessment is based on history, clinical examination, and measurement of ankle systolic blood pressure. Symptoms such as claudication and rest pain do occur and their severity gives some indication of the disease severity, but many people with diabetes will have asymptomatic PAD, which only comes to light when they develop a foot ulcer. Clinical examination is an important first-line

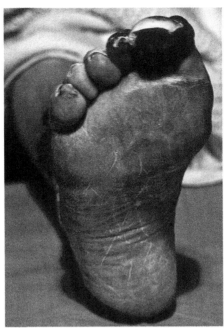

Fig. 1. Gangrene of the great and second toes caused by long-standing atherosclerotic obstruction of the femoral arteries in a patient with diabetes.

assessment and the absence of pedal pulses is related to an approximately 50% risk of the ulcer not healing. Pulse palpation can be challenging and noninvasive assessment should be undertaken in all patients with a foot ulcer, even if it is thought that the foot pulse is present. Ankle systolic blood pressure can be useful and an abnormal ankle brachial pressure index (ABPI; ratio of ankle systolic blood pressure to arm systolic blood pressure, normal range, 0.9–1.3) is strongly suggestive of PAD. In up to 40% of patients, calcification or incompressibility of the calf vessels will result in artificially raised ankle blood pressures. If there is any doubt, then simply elevating the limb while insonating the ankle vessels will detect those patients with very low perfusion pressure in the foot, as the signal will disappear and reappear on lowering the leg.[23] However, unless there is no history of cardiovascular disease, palpable foot pulses and a normal ABPI in a patient should prompt urgent referral to a specialist foot care team.

More objective tests may be used by specialist teams to determine the significance of the PAD. An ankle pressure less than 80 mm Hg, or a toe pressure less than 50 mm Hg, indicates a patient is at significant risk of amputation. Low oxygen tension in the skin of the foot (less than 50 mm Hg) using transcutaneous oxygen tension measurement ($TcPO_2$) is also associated with a poor prospect for healing.[24] However none of these assessments are strongly predictive and can only act as a guide. The extent of damage caused to the tissue by infection and the size and extent of the wound are also important factors. The speed of wound healing is also an important consideration. Impaired circulation may ultimately be sufficient to achieve wound closure but takes much longer than well-perfused tissue. During the time it takes to heal, the patient is at an increased risk of further infection and has the inconvenience of the need for regular wound care and rescued mobility. Finally, microcirculatory abnormalities may amplify the effects of

PAD, causing a lesion to be critical in a patient with diabetes, which in the patient without diabetes may have less significance.

In any patient in whom PAD is suspected or the diagnosis is still unclear, duplex ultrasound will confirm the pattern of disease and the hemodynamic significance of any lesion (cf **Fig. 2**).[25] The duplex ultrasound may also provide an indication of the optimum method of treatment, depending on the extent and pattern of disease, which can be useful in initially avoiding a major operation, for instance, in a frail patient with extensive disease who may require major surgical attempts at optimizing wound care.

In summary, any patient with a diabetic foot ulcer and in whom PAD has been detected should be considered for revascularization. Objective tests may identify patients at high risk of not healing and large wounds will need better blood supply to heal than smaller superficial wounds. However, the decision to offer revascularization can be difficult and needs expert assessment. This assessment should be obtained as soon as possible because delayed revascularization results in worse outcomes.

EVIDENCE FOR REVASCULARIZATION

The early results from Akbari and LoGerfo's unit in Boston, MA suggested that in an uncontrolled population of people with diabetes a more aggressive policy toward revascularization reduced amputation.[26] A detailed audit in Finland during a time of improving services for people with diabetes showed a 32% reduction in amputations over a 14-year period despite an increase in the number of people with diabetes being

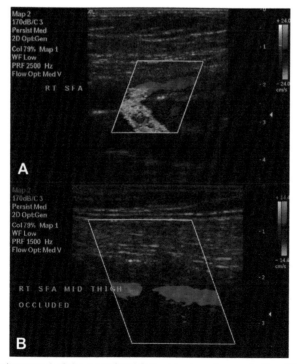

Fig. 2. Duplex ultrasound of the superficial femoral artery demonstrating (*A*) moderate stenosis with flow diversion into a large collateral vessel, and (*B*) vessel occlusion below this.

diagnosed. This reduction was inversely proportional to the number of revascularization procedures, in particular, those below the knee.[27] The systematic review performed by the International Working Group on the Diabetic Foot found that 60% of foot ulcers healed after revascularization and that this was better than patients treated medically.[28] Although the improvement in wound healing and reduction in amputation was multifactorial, it seems that revascularization is an important factor in current patient groups, who tend to present late with tissue loss and gangrene. Of course, the goal is to identify people at risk of PAD very early and manage complications before they need revascularizing but this is not achievable in the short term.

INVESTIGATIONS BEFORE REVASCULARIZATION

In most patients in whom intervention is considered to be likely, more detailed images are obtained. Most commonly this is performed with magnetic resonance angiography using gadolinium, which in patients with renal impairment can cause nephrogenic systemic fibrosis, a rare but potentially fatal complication. Computerized tomography angiography (cf **Fig. 3**) may also be used but calcification may make the images more difficult to interpret and, again, uses nephrotoxic contrast agents. The visualization of the distal circulation, particularly in the foot, which is essential for planning distal bypass surgery, is often not well shown on magnetic resonance imaging or computerized tomography angiography. In these patients, intra-arterial digital subtraction angiography still has a role.[29]

For distal bypass surgery it is essential to choose the correct vessel to use as runoff. This runoff vessel should communicate directly with the pedal vessels and supply the area (angiosome) of the foot where the wound is located. Anatomic-based imaging techniques may not always be able to identify this. Crural vessel

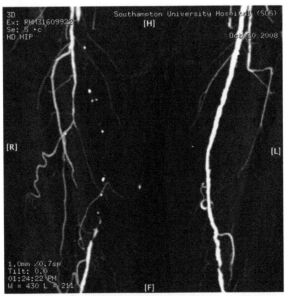

Fig. 3. Computerized tomographic angiography of a 67-year-old man demonstrating significant stenosis of the superficial femoral artery, with the vessel occluding shortly after its origin, illustrating how the branches of the profunda femoris artery have enlarged to act as collaterals to supply the lower leg.

communication with the pedal arch can be determined using a simple ultrasound technique of insonating the pedal arch with the leg in dependency and occluding the ankle vessels in turn to determine which supplies the arch.[30] There is increasing evidence to support the importance of angiosomes and ensuring that the correct one is revascularized.[31]

Finally, before undertaking distal bypass surgery, it is essential to identify a good-quality autologous vein. Preoperative duplex ultrasound vein mapping reduces operation time and allows other sources of vein to be identified if the ipsilateral long saphenous vein is not suitable or absent.

HOW TO REVASCULARIZE

Revascularization can be achieved by open surgical techniques (bypass or endarterectomy) or by endovascular procedures, such as angioplasty with or without a stent. Currently, the best option for patients with diabetic vascular disease is unclear. Excellent results from distal angioplasty have been produced from single centers with 5-year patencies of 88%.[32] However in 2 large meta-analyses of endovascular and surgical revascularization, the results were similar. At 3 years, surgery achieved a primary patency of 72.4%, a secondary patency of 62.9%, and a limb salvage rate of 82.3% compared with angioplasty rates of 48.6%, 62.9%, and 82.4%, respectively.[33,34] What does seem apparent is the higher reintervention rate in patients with diabetes due to restenosis. Although single-center studies tend to claim that results for intervention in patients with diabetes are the same as patients without diabetes, possibly due to selection, this does not seem to hold up in general. Worse outcomes for limb salvage after angioplasty[35] and surgery[36] have been reported in patients with diabetes.

This worse outcome is supported by the only randomized controlled trail to have been undertaken, the BASIL Trial. Seven hundred thirty-eight patients, 43% of whom had diabetes, were randomized to initial endovascular therapy or surgical bypass. There was no difference found between the therapies in terms of early amputation-free survival; some groups have taken this as support for an endovascular first approach. However, in longer-term follow-up, an advantage for patients who survived more than 2 years, which was 70% of the total, was confirmed in those who had a surgical bypass as the initial treatment.[37]

The BASIL Trial was conducted more than a decade ago and endovascular techniques have developed considerably. In addition, less than half of the patients involved were diabetic, which makes it difficult to extrapolate evidence from the BASIL Trial to patients with diabetes who will have predominately infrapopliteal disease. Amputation-free survival at the end of follow-up was 55% for both treatments, which is disappointing and suggests further work needs to be performed to improve these outcomes.

In reality, endovascular and open surgical techniques have different properties and one technique may be suitable for one patient but not for another. The recent guidelines from the National Institute for Health and Clinical Excellence suggest that the revascularization technique should be decided by the vascular multidisciplinary team on a case-by-case basis.[38]

SURGICAL REVASCULARIZATION

Revascularization of the lower limb is most commonly achieved by bypassing blocked arteries or removing atheroma from them, or endarterectomy. Endarterectomy was initially applied enthusiastically but restenosis of the operative site was common. However, the technique remains useful in the common femoral artery, where endovascular procedures are limited due to mobility and the close origins of the profunda and superficial femoral vessels.

Preoperative planning is essential and each step of the procedure should be considered. Surgical revascularization of a limb is best planned around the femoral artery and procedures to increase blood flow into the femoral artery are termed inflow procedures. If the arteries proximal to the common femoral artery are not affected and the femoral pulse is strong in an ischemic leg, then outflow (or infra-inguinal or distal) procedures are required. In most patients with distal disease, bypass from or below the femoral artery will be required. If the proximal superficial femoral artery is patent, this allows a shorter graft to be taken from around the level of the knee.

If the inflow is deemed to be poor, this can often be improved by angioplasty either before or at the same time as a distal bypass, which has the advantage of being less invasive and avoids implanting prosthetic material in patients with open wounds. If the inflow disease is extensive and not suitable for angioplasty, then inflow can be improved by anatomic bypass (aorto-bifemoral or ileofemoral bypass) or extra-anatomic bypass (cross-femoral or axillofemoral). Aorto-bifemoral bypass is a major operation and many patients with severe limb ischemia are not healthy enough for this operation. In most cases all of these inflow procedures use prosthetic graft material.

INFRA-INGUINAL BYPASS

Many patients requiring infra-inguinal bypass are frail with multiple comorbidities. Careful planning with the anesthetic team to optimize their condition preoperatively and plan the procedure is essential. Regional anesthesia, especially epidural, should be considered, although in some frail patients infiltrating anesthetic techniques may be all that is required.[39]

Although the focus of the surgical team will be on the possibilities of revascularization, in some patients it should be recognized that the prospects for revascularization are poor and the risks to the patient are high. In these situations it is unlikely that attempted surgical revascularization is going to be of long-term benefit to the patient and should be avoided.

Several factors have been identified that predict poor outcome, including previous myocardial infarction, stroke, tissue loss, poor radiologic runoff below the knee, low ABPI, a raised serum creatinine, and obesity.[40] Absence of a good quality vein as a bypass conduit and previous failed ipsilateral bypass are powerful predictors graft failure.[41]

The level of graft take off and target vessel for runoff must be planned preoperatively. As the outcome depends on the quality of the vein used, it is important to keep the graft as short as possible but to ensure it is taken from a good inflow and delivers in-line blood flow to the foot wound. Occasionally it may have been determined to use the profunda or proximal superficial femoral vessels if patent but usually the preferred take off for the graft will be the common femoral artery overlying the profunda origin. It is essential to make the skin incisions in the groin with great care to avoid traction on the skin and any undermining. Wound infection in this area is common and may cause graft failure as well as delayed recovery.

Below the groin, an autologous vein gives superior results in terms of patency and should always be used if possible. The quality of the vein is very important and, if it is small or diseased, it should not be used.[41] If the long saphenous vein (LSV) is not available or is small and diseased, a vein harvested from the arms gives excellent results.[42] Deep veins can be harvested to construct aortic and iliac conduits and LSV may be used for cross-femoral or obturator bypasses. The role of prosthetic grafts is limited. Not only are the patency results poor but the risk of infection in patients with tissue loss is high. Although attempts to improve patency have been made by using vein interposition cuffs or by tapering the graft, these have had limited success. One situation when prosthetic grafts may be of help is in patients with limited autologous veins and extensive distal disease but with a blind popliteal segment. A prosthetic graft is taken from the femoral vessels and anastomosed side by side with a vein graft over the popliteal vessels. The vein graft is then taken to the distal runoff vessel.[43]

If the LSV is used, it should be harvested through a series of discontinuous incisions, which reduces wound complications. The LSV may either be left in its bed (in situ) and the branches ligated and the valves cut or be taken out and reversed. There is no evidence to suggest superiority of one technique and the choice is usually determined by the operating surgeon.[44] The in situ technique places the larger vein end on the larger artery and vice versa, allowing the smaller vein end to be anastomosed to the smaller runoff artery. If the graft needs to be tunneled subcutaneously, it means that it can be performed with the graft pulsing and so avoids twists; if it occludes perioperatively, it can be easily unblocked.

The previously selected runoff vessel is then exposed and the LSV is mobilized at this level. The posterior tibial and peroneal arteries are best approached from the medial side of the leg at all levels and the anterior tibial artery is identified at the base of the anterior compartment. The dorsalis pedis and plantar arteries are approached by small incisions directly over the vessels, which are aided by preoperative marking using ultrasound. Once the graft preparation is complete, the distal anastomosis is fashioned.

On completion of the bypass, some form of quality control should be undertaken to ensure the graft is satisfactory. Most commonly this is ultrasound scanning but angiography may be used.[45] Wound closure must be accurate to promote rapid wound healing and avoid breakdown.

Finally, it must be determined whether to remove dead tissue at the same time as the bypass or to undertake this at a later date. If the tissue is infected or gangrenous, it is usually better to remove it at the time of bypass to avoid spreading infection or sepsis or the need to return a patient who has just regained mobility back to the theater, which will delay their discharge. The exception is when it is especially unclear if the tissue is viable and will recover. Delay in this situation is best.

Common Femoral Endarterectomy and Profundoplasty

Localized calcified plaque is often seen in the common femoral artery, particularly in patients with diabetes, and often extends into the profunda femoris artery as well as the superficial femoral artery. Previous studies have suggested that in patients with severe occlusive disease involving both the superficial and the profunda vessels, correcting the stenosis in the profunda femoris artery by profundoplasty significantly increases distal tissue perfusion.[46] The importance of perfusing the profunda branches is seen in **Fig. 3**.

In this approach, the femoral vessels are exposed and it is often necessary to go above the inguinal ligament to gain access to a soft segment of external iliac artery. The profunda femoris artery should be carefully assessed. If the origin is narrowed or occluded, the artery should be traced down past the first branches until a soft vessel is found. On opening the femoral vessels, it is usually possible to create a dissection plane and remove the atheromatous plaque. The endarterectomy should be extended proximally until a good size lumen is reached. Distally it should be extended into the origin of the superficial femoral artery. If the profunda is diseased, the vessel is opened and an endarterectomy is performed. Any edges are tacked down with 6-0 Prolene sutures. It is best to close the arteriotomy with a vein patch because this reduces the risk of subsequent stenosis.

Profundoplasty in the treatment of claudication can be effective and durable.[47] However, when performed to achieve limb salvage, the results are variable. Some authors have reported high limb salvage rates of 86%[48] after profundoplasty, whereas others avoided amputation in only 36% to 57%[49,50] at 12 month follow-up. With the current evidence it is therefore difficult to predict which patients would benefit from the procedure.

There has been recent interest in opening up the profunda using endovascular techniques. Donas and colleagues[51] have reported primary patency and limb salvage rates of 80% and 93.3%, respectively, in their cohort of 15 patients treated endovascularly. This approach may become an alternative option in patients with technically challenging profundoplasty in the future.

COMPLICATIONS OF SURGERY

General complications, particularly cardiovascular, are not infrequent due to the frailty and comorbidities of patients with lower limb arterial disease. It is essential to ensure that after surgery the cardiovascular risk factors of these patients are corrected. Although there is no evidence for the benefit of antiplatelet agents in vein grafts, these patients should receive these drugs in view of their cardiovascular risk.

Specific complications include wound breakdown and infection (**Fig. 4**A), graft failure, or failure to reperfuse the wound. Wound complications are common but can be reduced with prophylactic antibiotics and careful surgical technique. Graft infections

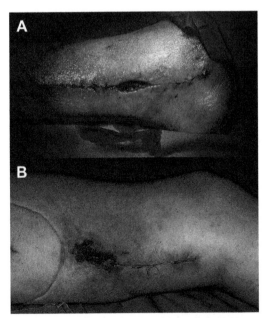

Fig. 4. (A) Postoperative wound breakdown putting the graft just below this wound at risk following femorodistal bypass surgery, and (B) persistent vein graft fistula (causing increased local venous hypertension with subsequent skin necrosis) following in situ femoropopliteal bypass surgery.

can be reduced by avoiding the use of prosthetic material when possible but particularly if infected wounds are present. Failure of wound healing despite a patent graft is due to selection of the wrong runoff vessel. Bypass grafts may also fail because of the development of aneurysms or the persistence of patent vein branches or fistulae (**Fig.** 4B).

Early graft failure is most commonly due to poor surgical technique or incorrect selection of procedure (eg, wrong runoff vessel). Failure after the first few weeks, but within 2 years, is associated with graft stenosis or thrombosis. After this time the commonest cause of graft failure is progression of vascular disease in the native vessels above or below the graft.[52]

Between 30% and 50% of patients will develop vein graft stenosis, mostly in the first 18 months after surgery, and some of these will lead to graft failure. Most units run a surveillance program using duplex ultrasound scanning to detect stenosis before they become symptomatic and intervening with angioplasty or surgery if identified.[53] Although this seems sensible, there is no evidence to show that this approach is cost-effective or of benefit to patients.

SUMMARY

PAD is very common in people with diabetes and is one of the strongest predictors of developing nonhealing foot ulcers and suffering amputation. There is strong evidence to show that early detection of PAD and revascularization will reduce amputations. Despite this, many patients have no vascular assessment even when they present with a foot ulcer or before amputation. Even when identified, patients are referred late, which worsens their outcome.

Currently there is no evidence to support surgical revascularization over endovascular treatments, but in reality the techniques are complementary and the choice of revascularization procedure should be determined by an experienced multidisciplinary vascular team. Surgical revascularization can achieve good results but careful patient selection, operative planning, and the use of autologous vein are necessary. What is clearly apparent is that at present not enough patients are being offered revascularization to prevent amputation.

REFERENCES

1. Shaw JE, Sicree RA, Zimmet PZ. Global estimates of the prevalence of diabetes for 2010 and 2030. Diabetes Res Clin Pract 2010;87(1):4–14.
2. NHS Diabetes. Inpatient care for people with diabetes: the economic case for change. Available at: www.diabetes.nhs.uk/document.php?o=3034. Accessed March 5, 2013.
3. Gu K, Cowie CC, Harris MI. Mortality in adults with and without diabetes in a national cohort study of the US population. 1971-1993. Diabetes Care 1998;21:1138–45.
4. Newman AB, Siscovick DS, Manolio TA, et al. Ankle-arm index as a marker of atherosclerosis in the Cardiovascular Health Study. Cardiovascular Heart Study (CHS) Collaborative Research Group. Circulation 1993;88:837–45.
5. Gregg EW, Sorlie P, Paulrose-Ram R, et al. Prevalence of lower extremity disease in the US adult population ≥40 years of age with and without diabetes:1999-2000 national health and nutrition examination survey. Diabetes Care 2004;27:1591–7.
6. Al-Delaimy WK, Merchant AT, Rimm EB, et al. Effect of type 2 diabetes and its duration on the risk of peripheral arterial disease among men. Am J Med 2004;116:236–40.

7. Nehler MR, Coll JR, Hiatt WR, et al. Functional outcome in a contemporary series of major lower extremity amputations. J Vasc Surg 2003;38:7–14.

8. Moulik PK, Mtonga R, Gill GV. Amputation and mortality in the new onset diabetic foot ulcers stratified by etiology. Diabetes Care 2003;26:491–4.

9. Holman N, Young RJ, Jeffcoate WJ. Variation in the recorded incidence of amputation of the lower limb in England. Diabetologia 2012;55:1919–25.

10. Moxey PW, Hofman D, Hinchliffe RJ, et al. Lower extremity amputations – a review of global variability in incidence. Diabet Med 2011;28:1144–53.

11. Prompers L, Schaper N, Apelqvist J, et al. Prediction of outcome in individuals with diabetic foot ulcers: focus on the differences between individuals with and without peripheral arterial disease. The EURODIALE Study. Diabetologia 2008; 51:747–55.

12. Basil Trial Participants. Bypass versus angioplasty in severe ischaemia of the leg (BASIL): multicentre, randomised controlled trial. Lancet 2005;366:1925–34.

13. Bhatt DL, Steg PG, Ohman E, et al. International prevalence, recognition, and treatment of cardiovascular risk factors in outpatients with atherothrombosis. JAMA 2005;295:180–9.

14. Orasanu G, Plutzky J. The pathologic continuum of diabetic vascular disease. J Am Coll Cardiol 2009;53:S35–42.

15. Eckel RH, Wassef M, Chait A, et al. Prevention conference VI: diabetes and cardiovascular disease: writing group II: pathogenesis of atherosclerosis in diabetes. Circulation 2002;105(18):e138–43.

16. Isley WL, Harris WS. Lipoprotein abnormalities. In: Marso SP, Stern DM, editors. Diabetes and cardiovascular disease. Philadelphia: Lippincott Williams and Wilkins; 2004. p. 337–52.

17. Beckman JA, Creager MA, Libby P. Diabetes and atherosclerosis: epidemiology, pathophysiology and management. JAMA 2002;287:2570–81.

18. Moreno PR, Fuster V. New aspects in the pathogenesis of diabetic atherothrombosis. J Am Coll Cardiol 2004;44(12):2293–300.

19. Everhart JE, Pettitt DJ, Knowler WC, et al. Medial arterial calcification and its association with mortality and complications of diabetes. Diabetologia 1988;31:16–23.

20. Jude EB, Chalmers N, Oyibo SO, et al. Peripheral arterial disease in diabetic and nondiabetic patients. Diabetes Care 2001;24:1433–7.

21. Moxey PW, Hofman D, Hinchliffe RJ, et al. Epidemiological study of lower limb amputation in England between 2003 and 2008. Br J Surg 2010;97:1348–53.

22. Krishnan S, Fowler D, Nash F, et al. Reduction in diabetic amputations over 11 years in a defined UK population. Diabetes Care 2008;31:99–101.

23. Smith FC, Shearman CP, Simms MH, et al. Falsely elevated ankle pressures in severe leg ischaemia: the pole test an alternative approach. Eur J Vasc Surg 1994;8:408–12.

24. Apelqvist JA, Lepantalo MJ. The ulcerated leg when to revascularize. Diabetes Metab Res Rev 2012;28(Suppl 1):30–5.

25. Andersen CA. Noninvasive assessment of lower extremity hemodynamics in individuals with diabetes mellitus. J Vasc Surg 2010;52:76S–80S.

26. Akbari CM, LoGerfo FW. Diabetes and peripheral vascular disease. J Vasc Surg 1999;30:373–84.

27. Winell K, Niemi M, Lepantalo M. The national hospital discharge register data on lower limb amputations. Eur J Vasc Endovasc Surg 2006;32:66–70.

28. Hinchliffe RJ, Andros G, Appelqvist J, et al. A systematic review of the effectiveness of revascularisation of the ulcerated foot in patients with diabetes and peripheral arterial disease. Diabetes Metab Res Rev 2012;28:179–217.

29. Pomposelli F. Arterial imaging in patients with lower extremity ischemia and diabetes mellitus. J Vasc Surg 2010;52:81S–91S.
30. Roedersheimer LR, Feins R, Green RM. Doppler evaluation of the pedal arch. Am J Surg 1981;142:601–4.
31. Neville RF, Attinger CE, Bulan EJ, et al. Revascularsiation of a specific angiosome for limb salvage: does the target artery matter? Ann Vasc Surg 2009;23: 367–73.
32. Faglia E, Dalla Paola L, Clerici G, et al. Peripheral angioplasty as the first choice revascularisation procedure in diabetic patients with critical limb ischaemia: prospective study of 993 consecutive patients hospitalised and followed between 1999-2003. Eur J Vasc Endovasc Surg 2005;29:620–7.
33. Romiti M, Albers M, Brochado-Neto FC, et al. Meta-analysis of infrapopliteal angioplasty for chronic critical limb ischaemia. J Vasc Surg 2008;47:975–81.
34. Albers M, Romitis M, Brochado-Neto FC, et al. Meta-analysis of popliteal to distal vein bypass grafts for critical ischaemia. J Vasc Surg 2006;43:498–503.
35. Bakken AM, Plachik E, Hart JP, et al. Impact of diabetes mellitus on outcomes of superficial femoral artery endoluminal interventions. J Vasc Surg 2007;46: 946–58.
36. Moxey PW, Hofman D, Hinchliffe RJ, et al. Trends and outcomes after surgical lower limb revascularisation in England. Br J Surg 2011;98:1373–82.
37. Bradbury AW, Adam DJ, Bell J, et al. Bypass versus angioplasty in severe ischaemia of the leg (BASIL) trial; analysis of amputation free and overall survival by treatment received. J Vasc Surg 2010;51(Suppl 5):18S–31S.
38. National Institute for Health and Clinical Excellence. Lower limb peripheral arterial disease: diagnosis and management. Available at: www.nice.org.uk/nicemedia/live/13856/60428/60428.pdf. Accessed March 5, 2013.
39. McKay C, Razik WA, Simms MH. Local anaesthetic for lower limb revascularisation in high risk patients. Br J Surg 1997;84:1096–8.
40. Bradbury AW, Adam DJ, Bell J, et al. Bypass versus angioplasty in severe ischaemia of the leg (BASIL) trail: a survival prediction model to facilitate clinical decision making. J Vasc Surg 2010;51:52S–68S.
41. Schanzer A, Hevelone N, Owens CD, et al. Technical factors affecting vein graft failure: observations form a large mulicenter trail. J Vasc Surg 2007;46:1180–90.
42. Vauclair F, Haller C, Marques-Vidal P, et al. Infrainguinal bypass for peripheral arterial occlusive disease: when arms save legs. Eur J Vasc Endovasc Surg 2012;43:48–53.
43. Mahmood A, Garnham A, Sintler M, et al. Composite sequential grafts for femorocrural bypass reconstruction; experience with a modified technique. J Vasc Surg 2002;36:772–8.
44. Wengerter KR, Veith FJ, Gupta SK, et al. Prospective randomised multi centre comparison of in situ and reversed vein bypasses. J Vasc Surg 1991;13:189–97.
45. Conte MS. Challenges of distal bypass surgery in patients with diabetes: patient selection, techniques and outcomes. J Vasc Surg 2010;52:96S–103S.
46. Strandness DE Jr. Functional results after revascularisation of the profunda femoris artery. Am J Surg 1970;119:240–5.
47. Towne JB, Bernhard VM, Rollins DL, et al. Profundaplasty in perspective: limitations in the long-term management of limb ischaemia. Surgery 1981;90:1037–46.
48. David TE, Drezner DA. Extended profundoplasty for limb salvage. Surgery 1978;84:758–63.
49. Morris-Jones W, Jones CD. Profundoplasty in the treatment of femoropopliteal occlusion. Am J Surg 1974;127:680–6.

50. Rollins DL, Towne JB, Bernard VM, et al. Isolated profundoplasty for limb salvage. J Vasc Surg 1985;2(4):585–90.
51. Donas KP, Pitoulias GA, Schwindt A, et al. Endovascular treatment of profunda femoris artery obstructive disease: nonsense or useful tool in selected cases? Eur J Vasc Endovasc Surg 2010;39:308–13.
52. Srithan K, Davies AH. The aetiology and management of the failed vascular bypass. In: Earnshaw JJ, Wyatt MG, editors. Complications in vascular and endovascular surgery: how to avoid them and how to get out of trouble. Castle Hill Barns (United Kingdom): TFM Publishing; 2012. p. 131–40.
53. Tinder CN, Bandyk DF. Detection of imminent vein graft occlusion: what is the optimal surveillance programme? Semin Vasc Surg 2009;22:252–60.

Interventional Radiology in the Diabetic Lower Extremity

Jim A. Reekers, MD, PhD, EBIR

KEYWORDS

- Diabetes • Diabetic foot • Ischemia • Diabetic ulcer • Arterial • Endovascular
- Interventional radiology

KEY POINTS

- Nonhealing ulcers with or without infection and gangrene are the indication for percutaneous revascularization.
- Endovascular treatment of arterial diabetic foot lesions is mainly concentrated in the below-the-knee arteries.
- Establishment of peripheral arterial disease (PAD) is the first step before revascularization can be considered in a diabetic patient with an ulcer. Positive palpation of peripheral pulses is often enough to exclude PAD.
- Endovascular treatment options below the knee in patients with critical limb ischemia have extended in the past decade and revascularization in the foot and even the plantar arch has become practice. It has been recognized that for planning of a revascularization it is important to have optimal information about outflow.

INTRODUCTION

Diabetic foot (DF) disease and interventional radiology have gained fast-growing interest over the past 10 years, because of improvements in technology and devices. In many institutions, treatment of a nonhealing ischemic diabetic ulcer is now started with an endovascular technique as first option. Despite or maybe because of this new and fast technology development, interventional radiology for diabetic vascular disease has never been very well investigated in randomized trials. The advantages of nonsurgical treatment are obvious, being a minimally invasive low-risk procedure, but the true clinical benefits have only recently become clearer. In a recent meta-analysis, it was clear that the results in terms of limb salvage in diabetic patients with an arterial ulcer are, broadly speaking, equal between surgical and nonsurgical treatments.[1] Moreover, morbidity and mortality favor interventional radiology.

Department of Radiology, Academic Medical Center, Teaching Hospital, University of Amsterdam, Amsterdam, 1105 AZ, The Netherlands
E-mail address: J.A.Reekers@amc.uva.nl

Med Clin N Am 97 (2013) 835–845
http://dx.doi.org/10.1016/j.mcna.2013.04.002
0025-7125/13/$ – see front matter © 2013 Elsevier Inc. All rights reserved.

medical.theclinics.com

DF disease has in the past always been classified in studies dealing with revascularization, either surgical or interventional, under "critical limb ischemia" (CLI). In publications on critical ischemia of the lower limb in patient demography, the number of patients with diabetes is usually mentioned, being less than 30% in most studies. DF problems have never been properly described in these studies. Nonsurgical revascularization studies including only patients with DF disease exist but are case-series without a control group.[2] There are, however, great problems with this reporting on treatment of DF when this is part of a larger, less defined patient group, such as CLI. First, peripheral arterial disease (PAD) in DF disease is fundamentally different in many ways compared with atherosclerotic PAD, which is discussed later in this article. Also, because a patient has diabetes does not directly imply that the patient's peripheral vascular disease would be diabetes related. In a general population, the total number of patients with diabetes can be very high, sometimes reaching percentages up to 20%, and these diabetic patients are also not protected against the most common vascular occlusive disease: atherosclerosis. Therefore, PAD in a patient with diabetes is not always the same as DF disease. For these reasons, the data on interventional radiology and treatment of DF are still minimal. The best data we have are based on a meta-analysis by Hinchliffe and colleagues,[1] but lacking randomized controlled trials, good or meaningful prospective data on interventional treatment of DF disease is something that remains a challenge for the future. The most used document for dissection in occlusive vascular disease is the TASC II document (Transatlantic Inter-Society Consensus for the Management of Peripheral Arterial Disease)[3]; however, in the TASC II document, the new below-the-knee (BTK) interventional techniques are not discussed.

Etiology of Ischemic Diabetic Foot Lesions

An ischemic ulcer on the DF is very often not caused by an acute or semi-acute arterial occlusion, but by a distortion of the, often long-existing, equilibrium between poor blood inflow caused by vessel disease and low blood demand. The vascular disease in diabetic patients is mostly localized in the lower leg arteries. Iliac arteries and superficial femoral arteries can also be diseased, but this is rare (<1%) and is always seen in combination with extensive BTK disease.[4] The pattern of arterial involvement in the lower limb arteries in diabetic disease is also typical and different from atherosclerotic disease. Diabetic arterial disease often shows long segmental occlusions, whereas atherosclerosis often shows short focal lesions.[4] The calcifications in diabetic disease are typical media scleroses, whereas in atherosclerosis the calcifications are diffuse intimal calcifications (**Fig. 1**). Also, there is often less disease in the foot arteries in diabetes, whereas in atherosclerosis the disease is often more pronounced in the foot with subsequent fewer endovascular options because of very poor outflow.

Diabetic foot lesions are often pain free because of the accompanying neuropathy, whereas rest pain and painful ulcers are almost always seen in atherosclerotic disease. The combination of rest pain and an ulcer can also be seen in diabetes but this is less common.

When one accepts the concept that disease in the DF is long-standing and that a misbalance of the equilibrium between inflow of blood and the oxygen demand in the DF needs to be restored, the concept of how to treat these patients is different from treatment of atherosclerotic disease, in which a more permanent patency is needed to prevent reoccurrence of complaints. It is the small skin lesion in a DF that will increase the demand for oxygen, and thereby disturbs the existing equilibrium, leading to a relative shortage of blood and oxygen needed for normal skin

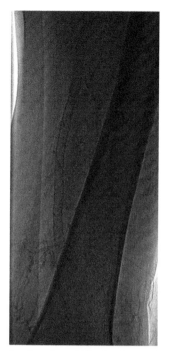

Fig. 1. Typical example of mediasclerosis or Mönckenberg sclerosis as is seen with diabetes.

healing. Infection worsens this condition by further increase of blood demand because of the increased metabolism in the wound.

To reverse this cycle, an increase in inflow of blood to the lesion area is needed to support skin healing. Of course all other supportive measurement for optimal wound care should also be taken. Revascularization is by no means a stand-alone procedure, but crucial is the temporary increase in blood flow to the lesion area to support ulcer healing. That is why some have started to call this treatment for DF lesions a "temporary percutaneous bypass."[5] When the lesion is cured, and the skin closed, the extra blood supply is no longer needed to keep the skin intact. That is why limb salvage is always reported as being much higher than the patency of the actual revascularization.

Interventional treatment in relation to DF
As previously mentioned, diabetic lower limb vascular disease is very typical and different from atherosclerotic disease. There are no data to prove that the angiographic morphology of diabetic vascular disease is also pathognomonic for diabetes, but one could not deny that the angiographic features of the disease are typical.[4]

The angiographic features of DF disease are described in the following sections.

Distribution Distribution of the disease is predominantly and more often exclusively seen in the lower leg arteries, starting from the distal popliteal artery to the foot. Often the iliac and femoral arteries show no to minimal disease on angiography. Also in DF disease, the foot arteries often seem relatively spared compared with atherosclerotic disease, in which the disease is often prominent in the foot also (**Fig. 2**).

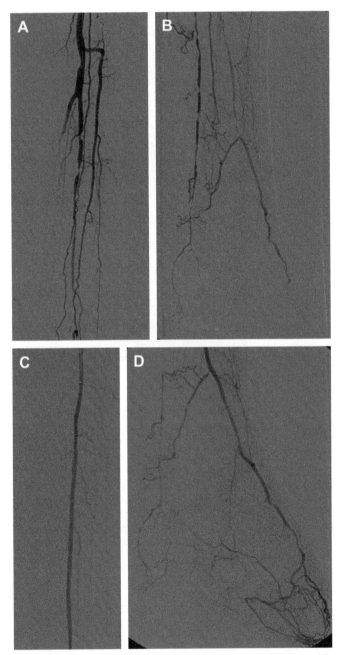

Fig. 2. Long arterial occlusive lesions in crural vessels, as is typically seen with arterial diabetic disease. (*A*) Proximal occlusion of the posterior and anterior tibial artery. Multiple stenoses in the peroneal artery. (*B*) Good filling of the dorsal pedal artery by collaterals. (*C*) Anterior tibial artery after subintimal recanalization. (*D*) Strong improvement of the outflow in the foot after recanalization of the anterior tibial artery.

Morphology Morphologic, occlusive vascular disease expressed in lower leg arteries, show long (>10 cm) segmental occlusions, often of minimal 2 lower leg arteries.

In atherosclerotic disease, the lesions tend to be much shorter (<3 cm), and there are more skip lesions (several lesions in one segment) with also more stenosis compared with occlusions. Also the collateral circulation is less developed in diabetic vascular disease.[4]

Calcification Media calcifications (Mönckenberg) (see **Fig. 1**) are typically seen in diabetic vascular disease. They show a more uniform, stockinglike, distribution. In atherosclerotic disease, the calcifications are intimal calcifications, with a nonuniform distribution. Intimal calcifications are more irregular and coarse (see **Fig. 2**). Also stenotic and occlusive lesions in atherosclerotic disease often have a direct relation in calcium deposits, which is not the case in diabetic disease.

In a patient having CLI together with diabetes, in whom these angiographic features are not present, one must consider whether the diabetes is actually the main cause of the CLI. As mentioned previously, atherosclerotic disease can also be seen in patients with diabetes.

Treatment Options

Interventional techniques are minimally invasive and can be performed under local anesthesia. This makes these techniques very applicable for these often elderly and frail patients. To make a choice for any interventional tool to overcome the vascular lesions, one has to keep in mind the aim of treatment, which is limb salvage through ulcer healing.

In general, there are 4 treatment options: conservative treatment, primary amputation, surgical bypass, and endovascular revascularization. The choice for any of these treatment options has to be made with a multidisciplinary team setting.[6] The choice between surgical or endovascular treatment is often made on the local anatomy, patient condition, and local expertise.

Indications for Treatment

Nonhealing ulcers with or without infection and gangrene are the indication for percutaneous revascularization. It is, however, essential that the limb is still viable and that the treatment will contribute to the quality of life. A bedridden patient with dementia is therefore not a primary candidate for percutaneous revascularization[7]; however, if the patient already had an amputation of the other leg, the limb now at risk can be essential for transfer and to facilitate nursing. This again underlines the importance of the multidisciplinary team, including nurses, and podiatrists, in decision making.

Also the choice between endovascular and open surgery is often the outcome of a team discussion. Local expertise plays an important role in these discussions. Arguments including high risk for surgery, nonavailability of good venous material for a conduit, no segments for surgical anastomoses, or poor outflow are often additional reasons to choose for an endovascular solution. But in many institutions, the endovascular approach is currently the first-choice treatment option.[2,8–11] The understanding that in diabetic patients "time is tissue" has the consequence that treatment of an infected ulcer in diabetic patients should be handled as an emergency procedure, to be dealt with preferably within 24 hours.

Endovascular Treatment

Endovascular treatment of arterial DF lesions is mainly concentrated in the BTK arteries.[4] Iliac and femoro-popliteal lesions are also sometimes seen in diabetic patients, but are a minority. It is even doubtful whether these lesions are not mainly associated atherosclerotic lesions. To discuss endovascular treatment, we should focus on treating BTK lesions. Diabetic lesions are often long, segmental lesions, whereas atherosclerotic lesions are more often short.[4]

Treating long, segmental diabetic lesions requires a dedicated center with ample experience, as this kind of treatment needs a personalized approach. Each procedure is tailored to the patient's needs, possibilities, and clinical situation. The end point of the treatment is ulcer healing and limb salvage.

Length and number of occlusions or calcifications are not of major importance in experienced endovascular hands. However, outflow arteries preferably should be available, although revascularization to a collateral artery can be done. For the patency of the procedure, the outflow is important, and therefore extension of a revascularization to the pedal arch and beyond, passing this pedal arch, can be important to create such outflow.[8] The latter is to be performed only in very experienced hands. Straight-line pulsatile flow to the foot is the optimal outcome, but if this is not possible, other solutions should be looked for. There are no specific morphologic guidelines to propose for an endovascular approach; basically, most lesions can be treated endovascularly. This is different from surgery in which a suitable anatomy is mandatory. The armamentarium to treat these often complex lesions has changed considerably over the past decade, and dedicated and sophisticated materials have been brought to the market. Without access to this new armamentarium, these interventions are not possible anymore. Those performing BTK treatment in patients with critical ischemia and diabetes should try to build a set of tools that works specifically for him or her, and not go with the fashion of the day.

Preferably the artery supplying the ulcer region should be revascularized; however, opening up collateral pathways can sometimes be enough to obtain good clinical success. The theory of so-called "angiosomes," specific arteries that supply areas in the foot, has gained a lot of attention recently.[12] One has to realize that angiosomes are a representation of normal anatomy in nondiseased vessels; how far this also will be true in the DF is not clear.

DIAGNOSTICS IN RELATION TO INTERVENTIONAL TREATMENT

Establishment of PAD is the first step before revascularization can be considered in a diabetic patient with an ulcer. Positive palpation of peripheral pulses is often enough to exclude PAD. Absence of palpations warrants further investigation. An ankle brachial index of less than 0.9 in the absence of marked medial arterial calcification is proof of PAD. Ankle systolic blood pressure of 50 mm Hg or lower and/or toe systolic pressure of 30 mm Hg or lower, which are the traditional criteria for critical ischemia, can be helpful but should not be decisive to plan revascularization. The combination of a nonhealing ulcer and PAD should be enough to start planning revascularization. There is still an ongoing discussion of whether imaging of the vascular tree should be done before the actual revascularization. Magnetic resonance angiography (MRA) is usually the imaging modality of choice, although computed tomography angiography (CTA) and Duplex (in experienced hands) have shown equal sensitivity and specificity. We recently performed a systematic review and meta-analysis of CTA and MRA for patients with critical ischemia (in press). From 42 eligible articles, 2 observers extracted data. Discrepancies were resolved by discussion. Data extracted were characteristics of study design, participants and imaging, and outcome measures. Methodological quality of studies was assessed using the QUADAS tool. Twelve CTA and 30 MRA studies were included, respectively evaluating 673 and 1404 participants. Summary estimates of sensitivity and specificity were respectively 96% (95% confidence interval [CI] 93%–98%) and 95% (95% CI 92%–97%) for CTA, and 93% (95% CI 91%–95%) and 94% (95% CI 93%–96%) for contrast-enhanced MRA. Median κ-value for interobserver agreement was 0.80 for CTA and 0.82 for contrast-enhanced MRA. Regression analysis showed that prevalence of CLI in individual studies was not an independent predictor for sensitivity and specificity for both modalities. The methodological quality of studies was moderate to good and publication bias was not demonstrated for both modalities. In conclusion, CTA and contrast-enhanced MRA are accurate modalities for evaluating disease severity of aortotibial arteries in patients with CLI or intermittent claudication. Significant differences in the diagnostic performance of both modalities between patients with CLI and patients with intermittent claudication were not found.

Anatomic imaging is also still done with regard to the TASC II document, which is directive to either surgical or nonsurgical revascularization. However, 90% of the vascular disease in diabetic patients is in the vessels BTK, which are not part of the TASC II document recommendations. Also the decision between surgical or open treatment very much depends on local expertise. Standard practice is to start in the lower limb with nonsurgical revascularization; direct angiography with subsequent revascularization is often the best and most direct approach.

TECHNIQUE OF DIAGNOSTIC AND THERAPEUTIC ANGIOGRAPHY

Angiography starts with puncturing the arterial system in the common femoral artery. The best way to approach the artery for diagnostic angiography and subsequent intervention is by antegrade puncture. This is the shortest and most direct way to go to the target area, which, in patients with diabetic vascular disease, is below the popliteal artery. However, for reasons unknown to me, antegrade puncture is still seen in some continents as dangerous, and not to be considered. The alternative approach is from the contralateral site with a retrograde puncture and bringing the catheter over the aortic bifurcation. For diagnostic angiography, this could produce good diagnostic images, but it needs more contrast to be used. The latter is not favorable in diabetic patients, who often also have declined renal function. Percutaneous revascularization over the bifurcation is troublesome and often impossible, as will be explained later in this article.

Angiography of the superficial femoral artery (SFA) and popliteal artery can be done from the common femoral artery in one directional plane with 10-mL low osmolar contrast in 5 seconds and an image frame rate of 2 per second. Below the popliteal artery, the best images are obtained with the catheter tip at the knee joint and 10-mL contrast in 5 seconds with a frame rate of 2 per second. Lower leg arteries need to be imaged in 2 perpendicular planes (anteroposterior and lateral). Lateral images of the foot are always needed to have a good impression of the outflow and to see if plantar revascularization is needed. Pain and cramps in the calf can be a problem with some contrast agents but are very low with iodixanol 320.

THREE-DIMENSIONAL ROTATIONAL ANGIOGRAPHY

Two-dimensional imaging may not be sufficient in severely affected and complex pedal arterial anatomy with many collaterals. Three-dimensional rotational angiography (3DRA) will give additional and detailed information of the pedal arterial anatomy. By viewing the 3D images from every desired angle, crural and pedal arterial architecture can confidently be derived.[13] Furthermore, the 3DRA acquisition can be used to find the best beam projection that visualizes the target vessel. The 3DRA of the foot contains valuable additional real-time information to better guide peripheral vascular interventions in patients with CLI and nonhealing tissue lesions. This way, optimal target artery selection can be done and patient outcome may be improved.

Interventional Treatment and the Angiosome Theory

Endovascular treatment options BTK in patients with CLI have extended in the past decade and revascularization in the foot and even the plantar arch has become practice. It has been recognized that for planning of a revascularization, it is important to have optimal information about outflow. Besides outflow, targeted revascularization of the region of interest, the location of a nonhealing tissue lesion, has become a focus of interest. Especially the angiosome theory has increased interest for more detailed information of the vascularization of the foot.[12]

INTERVENTIONAL TOOLS

There has been a revolution in revascularization tools for lower leg artery occlusions during the past decade. There are tools to overcome a chronic total occlusion (CTO), tools to get better initial results, and tools to increase patency after revascularization. However, most of these tools have never been properly tested in a controlled trial or have any long-term follow-up. Still, they are widely used and promoted. Another discussion is whether revascularization should be done through the original lumen or subintimally. A meta-analysis that studied the outcome of subintimal angioplasty showed an 80% success rate for lower limb arteries.[14] Patency of the recanalized vessel, either through transluminal or subintimal technique, seems to make a difference in favour of subintimal angioplasty in the SFA.[15] For BTK vessels there are no data available to compare the techniques. In heavily calcified vessels and longer occlusions, some or most of any recanalization will be subintimal, unintentionally.

Recanalization Tools for CTO

In many instances, a simple 0.035 guidewire, like a glidewire (Terumo, Tokyo, Japan), will be able to perform the recanalization in CTO. Subintimal is very often the only way to go. It often needs a lot of push and a subintimal J-shaped wire to get a good result. A technique often used is a combination of a wire and a percutaneous transluminal angioplasty (PTA) balloon, in which the balloon catheter is used to support the wire and to dilate the subintimal route during the revascularization. For this, a special subintimal wire, Terumo 0.035 J-shape (Terumo) half-stiff, is very helpful. Recently dedicated wires, with different tip load weight, based on cardiology techniques for CTO, have been introduced in lower limb arteries. One aim is to stay intraluminally with these wires. There are 0.014 and 0.018 wires with a variety of floppy tip lengths and also with different weights of the wire tip. Although these wires undoubtedly have less push and a higher tendency for perforation, they currently are for many interventionalists the wires of choice. There are some dedicated recanalization tools developed for the SFA that are also sometimes used BTK. Frontrunner (Cordis, Bridgewater, USA) is one of them, but BTK clinical experience is minimal with recanalization tools. Special devices include atherectomy devices, like the Fox-hollow catheter (Covidien, Mansfield, USA), which are able to take out the atheroma core of the occluded vessel. In CTO, BTK clinical experience is again limited.

Balloon angioplasty

Balloon angioplasty is still the most used technique for revascularization of lower limb arteries. New balloon technology, especially low-profile and longer balloons, have improved the technical outcome of BTK revascularization. Technical success is approximately 89%. Although the 1-year patency is between 58% and 68%, the limb salvage is much higher, at approximately 86%.[16] This is for a mixed group of patients with CLI with approximately 30% to 50% diabetic patients. Bypass surgery and PTA have a comparable 5-year limb salvage rate, which is in both groups is approximately 75%.[16–19] The number of patent runoff vessels after PTA is important for the long-term outcome.[19,20] The length of the lesions seems not to be an important determinant for outcome.[20]

Drug-eluting balloons

One of the problems after PTA is the high incidence of intima hyperplasia, resulting in early restenosis and occlusion. Antiproliferative drugs have show to be able to reduce the problem of intima hyperplasia in coronary stents. To avoid the problem of stents, paclitaxel-coated balloons have been developed to release the drug during balloon inflation on the vessel wall. Although there have been positive trials in the superficial femoral region, limited data are available for drug-eluting stents in lower limb arteries. The first studies show a better short-term result in terms of binary restenosis.[21]

Clinical follow-up exceeding 3 months is available only from one study, showing a 95% limb salvage rate.[21]

Stents A meta-analysis for stenting in infrapopliteal lesions showed on overall improvement of Rutherford class.[22] However, in the analyzed studies, most of the available data for stenting BTK come from bailout stenting.[22,23] There was no difference in outcome in this meta-analysis between balloon-expandable stents and self-expandable stents.[22,23]

In direct comparison with PTA, a significant benefit for stenting has not been demonstrated. A prospective, randomized trial by Randon and colleagues[23] found no differences at 12 months in 35 patients treating occlusions or stenoses between 2 and 15 cm in BTK arteries for limb salvage. Also other single-center and single-arm studies showed good limb salvage rates at a follow-up of 24 months.[23] However, in direct comparison with PTA, a significant benefit for stenting has not been demonstrated. Stenting has its place in infrapopliteal angioplasty if the procedure is jeopardized by a dissection or recoil.

Drug-eluting stents

Drug-eluting stents seem to have better outcome compared with bare stents regarding patency.[24] To make a comparison between paclitaxel and sirolimus is very difficult based on the current data, mostly based on bailout data. More recent studies continue to demonstrate meaningful outcomes with drug-eluting stents, with a reported 3-year amputation-free survival rate of 68% ± 5%.

SUMMARY

Most of what we know today for interventional techniques for revascularization in patients with DF disease is derived from our knowledge on CLI in patients with PAD. There are today no dedicated randomized controlled trials on interventional treatment of DF. It is, however, clear that huge progress in interventional techniques has been obtained during the past decade. In most institutions, the nonsurgical option is the current first choice. As the aim of treatment is ulcer healing through temporary increase in blood flow, it is still unclear what the contribution of new stent and drug-eluting technologies will have on the clinical outcome of DF treatment. Long-term follow-up studies, dedicated to patients with an arterial DF problem, have to be performed before we can evaluate all these new technologies.

REFERENCES

1. Hinchliffe RJ, Andros G, Apelqvist J, et al. A systematic review of the effectiveness of revascularization of the ulcerated foot in patients with diabetes and peripheral arterial disease. Diabetes Metab Res Rev 2012;28(Suppl 1): 179–217.
2. Faglia E, Mantero M, Caminiti M, et al. Extensive use of peripheral angioplasty, particularly infrapopliteal, in the treatment of ischaemic diabetic foot ulcers: clinical results of a multicentric study of 221 consecutive diabetic subjects. J Intern Med 2002;252:225–32.
3. Norgren L, Hiatt WL, Dormandy JA, et al. Inter-Society Consensus for the Management of Peripheral Arterial Disease (TASC II). Eur J Vasc Endovasc Surg 2007;33(Suppl 1):S1–75.
4. Graziani L, Silvestro A, Bertone V, et al. Vascular involvement in diabetic subjects with ischemic foot ulcer: a new morphologic categorization of disease severity. Eur J Vasc Endovasc Surg 2007;33(4):453–60.
5. Reekers JA. Percutaneous intentional extraluminal (subintimal) revascularization (PIER) for critical lower limb ischemia: too good to be true? J Endovasc Ther 2002;9(4):419–21.
6. Bakker K, Apelqvist J, Schaper NC. International Working Group on Diabetic Foot Editorial Board. Practical guidelines on the management and prevention of the diabetic foot 2011. Diabetes Metab Res Rev 2012;28(Suppl 1):225–31.
7. Taylor SH, Kalbaugh CA, Blackhurst DW, et al. Postoperative outcomes according to preoperative medical and functional status after infrainguinal revascularization for critical limb ischemia in patients 80 years and older. Am Surg 2005;71(8): 640–5.
8. Faglia E, Dalla Paola L, Clerici G, et al. Peripheral angioplasty as the first-choice revascularization procedure in diabetic patients with critical limb ischemia: prospective study of 993 consecutive patients hospitalized and followed between 1999 and 2003. Eur J Vasc Endovasc Surg 2005;29(6):620–7.
9. Jämsén T, Manninen H, Tulla H, et al. The final outcome of primary infrainguinal percutaneous transluminal angioplasty in 100 consecutive patients with chronic critical limb ischemia. J Vasc Interv Radiol 2002;13(5):455–63.
10. Uccioli L, Gandini R, Giurato L, et al. Long-term outcomes of diabetic patients with critical limb ischaemia followed in a tertiary referral diabetic foot clinic. Diabetes Care 2010;33(5):977–82.
11. Söderström MI, Arvela EM, Korhonen M, et al. Infrapopliteal percutaneous transluminal angioplasty versus bypass surgery as first-line strategies in critical leg ischemia: a propensity score analysis. Ann Surg 2010;252(5):765–73.
12. Alexandrescu V, Hubermont G. The challenging topic of diabetic foot revascularization: does the angiosome-guided angioplasty may improve outcome. J Cardiovasc Surg (Torino) 2012;53(1):3–12.
13. Jens S, Lucatelli P, Koelemay MJ, et al. Three-dimensional rotational angiography of the foot in critical limb ischemia: a new dimension in revascularization strategy. Cardiovasc Intervent Radiol 2012;36:797–802.
14. Met R, Van Lienden KP, Koelemay MJ, et al. Bipat subintimal angioplasty for peripheral arterial occlusive disease: a systematic review. Cardiovasc Intervent Radiol 2008;31(4):687–97.
15. Antusevas A, Aleksynas N, Kaupas RS, et al. Comparison of results of subintimal angioplasty and percutaneous transluminal angioplasty in superficial femoral artery occlusions. Eur J Vasc Endovasc Surg 2008;36(1):101–6.

16. Charalambous N, Schäfer PJ, Trentmann J, et al. Percutaneous intraluminal recanalization of long, chronic superficial femoral and popliteal occlusions using the Frontrunner XP CTO device: a single-center experience. Cardiovasc Intervent Radiol 2010;33(1):25–33.

17. Romiti M, Albers M, Brochado-Neto FC, et al. Meta-analysis of infrapopliteal angioplasty for chronic critical limb ischemia. J Vasc Surg 2008;47(5):975–81.

18. Blackstone E. Comparing apples and oranges. J Thorac Cardiovasc Surg 2002; 123:8–15.

19. Peregrin JH, Koznar B, Kovác J, et al. PTA of infrapopliteal arteries: long-term clinical follow-up and analysis of factors influencing clinical outcome. Cardiovasc Intervent Radiol 2010;33:720–5.

20. Schmidt A, Ulrich M, Winkler B, et al. Angiographic patency and clinical outcome after balloon-angioplasty for extensive infrapopliteal arterial disease. Catheter Cardiovasc Interv 2010;76:1047–54.

21. Schmidt A, Piorkowski M, Werner M, et al. First experience with drug-eluting balloons in infrapopliteal arteries: restenosis rate and clinical outcome. J Am Coll Cardiol 2011;58:1105–9.

22. Donas KP, Torsello G, Schwindt A, et al. Below knee bare nitinol stent placement in high risk patients with critical limb ischemia is still durable after 24 months of follow up. J Vasc Surg 2010;52:356–61.

23. Randon C, Jacobs B, De Ryck F, et al. Angioplasty or primary stenting for infrapopliteal lesions: results of a prospective randomized trial. Cardiovasc Intervent Radiol 2010;33(2):260–9.

24. Feiring AJ, Krahn RN, Nelson L, et al. Preventing leg amputations in critical limb ischaemia with below-the-knee drug-eluting stents. J Am Coll Cardiol 2010;55: 1580–9.

The Charcot Foot

Lee C. Rogers, DPM[a,b,]*, Robert G. Frykberg, DPM, MPH[c]

KEYWORDS

- Charcot foot • Neuroarthropathy • Joints • Soft tissues

KEY POINTS

- Charcot foot is primarily a clinical diagnosis at its earliest stage. Advanced imaging may aid in that diagnosis.
- Offloading and immobilization are the most important initial treatments. Success can be achieve with a total contact cast, removable cast walker, wheel chair, crutches, or bed rest.
- Surgical correction should be reserved for severely unstable cases, or in cases where non-operative treatment failed to prevent or heal and ulcer.

INTRODUCTION

In the developed world, the Charcot foot or Charcot neuroarthropathy (CN) most commonly arises in those with diabetes and peripheral neuropathy. It is a syndrome affecting the bones, joints, and soft tissues of the foot and ankle leading to dislocations, fractures, and deformity.[1] The hallmark of the deformity is the midfoot joint collapse called a rocker bottom foot, but the condition can arise in other foot and ankle joints.

There is no single cause for the development of CN and the evidence that exists is largely circumstantial. However, most experts agree that it is a combination of baseline neuropathy with an inciting trauma that sparks the syndrome.[2] Peripheral neuropathy in diabetes is a polyneuropathy, involving sensory, motor, and autonomic divisions. Sensory deficits prevent the patient from feeling the trauma and allow the patient to continue ambulating on an injured foot, increasing the trauma. Motor neuropathy causes tendon contractures, especially equinus, which increases the deforming forces on the midfoot. Autonomic neuropathy prevents autoregulation of peripheral circulation, increasing blood flow and activating bone resorption. This process has been proposed to wash out minerals from bone, leading to focal osteo-penia of the foot, as shown by reduced bone mineral density.

About 50% of patients recall a trauma that starts a period of inflammation.[3] Other triggering events could be surgery, ulceration, or infection. In some cases, Charcot foot has occurred after renal or pancreatic transplantation.[4] The inflammatory process

---

[a] Amputation Prevention Center, Valley Presbyterian Hospital, Los Angeles, CA, USA; [b] College of Podiatric Medicine, Western University of Health Sciences, Pomona, CA, USA; [c] Podiatry Section, Phoenix VA Healthcare System, Phoenix, AZ, USA
* Corresponding author. Amputation Prevention Center, Valley Presbyterian Hospital, Los Angeles, CA.
E-mail address: lee.c.rogers@gmail.com

Med Clin N Am 97 (2013) 847–856
http://dx.doi.org/10.1016/j.mcna.2013.04.003
0025-7125/13/$ – see front matter © 2013 Elsevier Inc. All rights reserved.

medical.theclinics.com

is usually unchecked, because of reduced pain from neuropathy.[5] After an injury, inflammation from a fracture or other trauma normally causes pain, and natural splinting and limping occurs. In those with loss of protective sensation, continued ambulation increases the inflammation, which sparks several chemical mediators, aggravating the process.[6]

Inflammation triggers the release of cytokines including tumor necrosis factor-alpha and interleukin-1-beta, which leads to increased expression of the polypeptide receptor activator of nuclear factor kappa-beta (RANKL). RANKL triggers the synthesis of nuclear factor kappa-beta, which stimulates the maturation of osteoclasts and reduces the function of osteoblasts by producing a decoy receptor.[7] Newer reports suggest that a genetic polymorphism may predispose individuals to developing CN.[8]

DIAGNOSIS

The diagnosis of Charcot foot begins with a heightened sense of suspicion. Diagnostic delays are common because of patient and physician unfamiliarity with the syndrome.[9] Inflammation of the foot is the earliest sign. The foot is usually red, hot, and swollen. It can be misdiagnosed as cellulitis, deep vein thrombosis, or acute gout.[10] Trauma may not be recalled, but can be minor, such as twisting or slipping. Patients often present with the complaint that the foot no longer fits in a shoe.

Foot temperature is generally hotter on the affect side, sometimes measuring a difference of 10°F or more.[11] Simple skin thermometers can be used to track temperatures, or a thermogram can give an image indicating the area of greatest difference (**Fig. 1**).

Although peripheral artery disease is common in those with diabetes, the Charcot foot usually presents with exaggerated blood flow manifested by bounding pulses.[12] Musculoskeletal deformity may or may not be present, depending on the timing of presentation. A rocker bottom deformity is usually a late sign of Charcot foot.

Imaging supplements the clinical diagnosis. Plain radiographs are usually indicated and may have to be compared with the contralateral foot to see subtle differences. Early radiographs may show no disorder, but, as the condition progresses, dislocations, fragmentation, and fractures are commonly seen. The calcaneal inclination angle is usually reduced, and can even be negative, and the talometatarsal–first metatarsal line can be broken (**Fig. 2**).[13]

If radiographs are negative and clinical suspicion is still high, consider a 3-phase bone scan or magnetic resonance imaging (MRI), which have higher sensitivity. The bone scan is generally diffusely hot across the foot in cases of acute Charcot

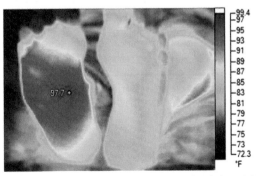

Fig. 1. A thermogram of the feet showing an active CN on the right, which is more than 10°F hotter than the left.

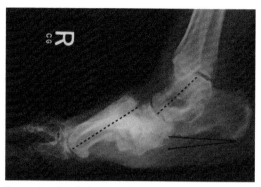

Fig. 2. A lateral radiograph of a deformed foot with CN. The calcaneal inclination angle (*solid line*) is reduced and the talometatarsal–first metatarsal line (*dashed line*) is broken.

(**Fig. 3**). MRI shows bone marrow edema and can be highly specific for Charcot foot in cases in which osteomyelitis is not suspected. When there is an ulcer, or questionable osteomyelitis, both MRI and bone scans have difficulty differentiating between the two diseases. In that case, the addition of a white blood cell–labeled bone scan or a bone biopsy might be indicated. Secondary signs can be viewed on MRI and help distinguish Charcot foot from osteomyelitis.[14] Osteomyelitis generally affects a single foot bone, is more common in the forefoot or rearfoot, and does not usually result in deformity. In addition, in cases of contiguous osteomyelitis, a tract should be found between the ulcer and the bone. In contrast, Charcot foot is more commonly diffuse, affecting many bones and joints, occurs more commonly in the midfoot, and is usually associated with deformity.

Computed tomography (CT) scans are generally useless. Further study is needed to determine the usefulness of positron emission tomography imaging and sulfur colloid marrow scan in those with Charcot foot.[15–17]

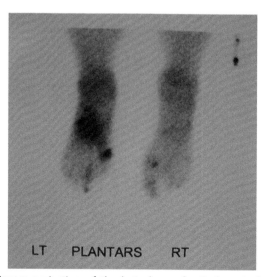

Fig. 3. A dorsal-plantar projection of the last phase of a 3-phase technetium bone scan showing diffuse uptake across the left midfoot, a common pattern in CN.

CLASSIFICATION

There are several classifications for the CN that are anatomic, radiographic, or clinical. The purpose of a disease classification should be to simplify the description, facilitate communication, direct treatment, or provide a prognosis.[18] The International Task Force on the Charcot Foot proposed a simple clinical stratification of active CN or inactive CN based on inflammation being present or absent, respectively.[19]

A frequently used classification by Sanders and Frykberg[27] describes 5 anatomic patterns (**Fig. 4**).[20] Pattern I involves the forefoot including the distal metatarsals, metatarsal-phalangeal joints, and digits. This presentation is often is found in association with other areas of involvement, rather than being isolated. Pattern II affects the tarsometatarsal (Lisfranc) joints and is the most common site for CN.[21] Pattern III is characterized by degeneration of the naviculocuneiform, talonavicular, or calcaneocuboid joints. Multiple joints are often involved within this pattern as well as in concert with radiographic changes noted in the tarsometatarsal joints. Pattern IV refers to CN of the ankle or subtalar joints and can manifest as dislocation in these sites. Pattern V, the only extra-articular presentation, involves the posterior calcaneus being fractured and superiorly located. Although not necessarily predictive of outcomes or of activity, this classification scheme subdivides the foot into distinct radiographic and anatomic regions, which facilitates ease of communication.

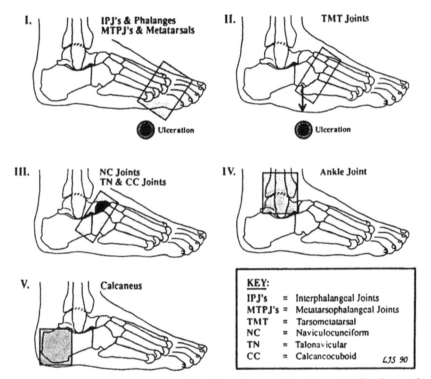

Fig. 4. The Sanders Frykberg patterns of CN. (*From* Sanders L, Frykberg RG. The Charcot foot (pied de Charcot). In: Bowker JH, Pfeiffer M, editors. Levin and O'Neal's the diabetic foot. Philadelphia: Mosby Elsevier; 2007. p. 257–83.)

The earliest known classification was introduced by Sydney Eichenholtz[22] in 1966 and is a pathology based. His writings were not specific to the foot and concentrated on the radiographic and histologic appearance of the Charcot joint. Stage I (development) is characterized by osseous fragmentation and debris formation at the articular margins. There is histologic evidence of debris embedded in the thickened synovium. Continued stress on the affected joints during this acute process leads to subluxation or dislocation. Stage II (coalescence) begins the reparative phase in which the finer debris is resorbed and edema reduces. Larger fragments may coalesce and the bone ends become sclerotic. Stage III (reconstruction) is characterized by evidence of bone healing. In 1990, Shibata and colleagues[23] added an earlier stage (stage 0) to the Eichenholtz classification to reflect the prodromal period after bone injury in which radiographic findings are normal.

Rogers and Bevilacqua[24] described a clinical classification for Charcot foot that is a 2-axis system thought to assist in predicting the outcome (**Fig. 5**). The X axis corresponds with the location of the Charcot joint (1, forefoot; 2, midfoot; 3, rearfoot/ankle) and the Y axis stages the complexity of the CN (A, acute osteoarthropathy without deformity; B, Charcot arthropathy with deformity; C, Charcot foot with deformity and ulceration; D, Charcot foot with osteomyelitis). This classification was later validated as predicting amputation.[25]

TREATMENT

Management of the Charcot foot can be divided into 2 categories: medical and surgical. The International Task Force recommended attempting medical therapy early in the course of the disease, and doing surgery in those cases in which medical therapy is unsuccessful, with a few exceptions.[26] An algorithm for treating Charcot foot that takes into account the current evidence base and practice standards was presented by the Task Force (**Fig. 6**).

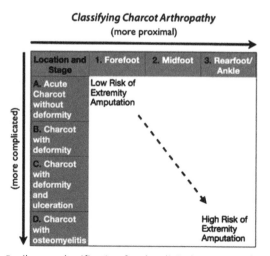

Fig. 5. The Rogers Bevilacqua classification for the clinical outcome of CN. (*Reprinted from* Rogers LC, Bevilacqua NJ. The diagnosis of Charcot foot. Clin Podiatr Med Surg 2008;25(1):43–51, vi; with permission.)

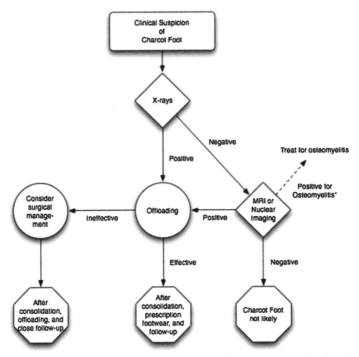

Fig. 6. The combined diagnostic and treatment algorithm recommended by the International Task Force on the Charcot Foot. (*Reprinted from* Rogers LC, Frykberg RG, Armstrong DG, et al. The Charcot foot in diabetes. Diabetes Care 2011;34:2123–9; with permission.)

The primary treatment of active CN is rest, immobilization, and offloading, thus removing the aggravating factors. Complete non–weight bearing is ideal, but unrealistic. Most investigators advocate the use of total-contact casts (TCCs) to immobilize and reduce plantar pressure (**Fig. 7**).[27] TCCs also tend to reduce the number of walking steps per day because they are cumbersome. Caution is needed with the contralateral foot because there is a 30% bilateral incidence of CN and protecting

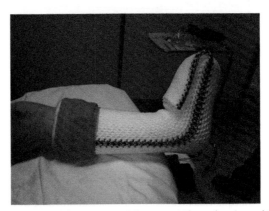

Fig. 7. A TCC (TCC-EZ, Derma Sciences, Inc., Princeton, NJ) used to immobilize and offload a Charcot foot.

the affected extremity can increase trauma to the unaffected foot.[28] The foot should be treated with offloading and immobilization until the CN becomes inactive. The duration of offloading required can be up to 6 months.[5] Monitoring foot temperatures with a dermal thermometer or thermography until the difference between feet is 4°F or less can help a clinician determine that transition,[11,29] or a prefabricated removable cast walker can be used, but patient adherence to wearing the device can be an issue.[30]

Pharmacologic therapies have been suggest to speed healing of CN in small studies. Bisphosphonate in parenteral[31–34] and oral[35] forms have been studied, but a recent large study seems to dispute their effectiveness.[36] A single small study of intranasal calcitonin suggests some benefit.[34] These therapies should be added to the standard treatment of offloading, not substitute for it. The International Task Force report was not enthusiastic about the use of existing pharmacologic therapies.[26]

Exogenous bone stimulation using pulsed electromagnetic fields has shown mediocre results without surgery.[37,38]

The role of surgery in the Charcot foot is developing. Most reports in the literature are low-quality retrospective reviews or case series.[39] In severe deformity or in the case of failure of medical therapy, surgery may be required to stabilize the foot.[40] The goals of surgery are to create a stable, plantigrade foot that reduces prominent pressure points and heals or prevents ulcers.[41,42] Surgery can be simplistic, like an Achilles tendon lengthening to reduce plantar pressure with or without an exostectomy to flatten out a bony prominence. More complex surgery involves a complete reconstruction with arthrodesis of several joints. Fixation often proves to be problematic and some surgeons prefer external ring fixators to reduce the likelihood of failure (**Fig. 8**).[40]

After the CN converts to the inactive stage, protected weight bearing can commence. The type of footwear or orthosis required generally depends on the severity of the deformity. With little or no resultant deformity, a prescription extradepth shoe with custom insert can suffice. In more severe cases, a Charcot-restraint orthotic walker, patellar-tendon bearing brace,[43] or ankle-foot orthosis may be needed.[44] Recurrence is common and the patient should be monitored occasionally for surveillance. These devices are often required for life.

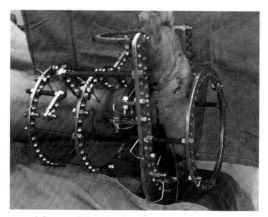

Fig. 8. A circular external fixator (RingFix, Small Bone Innovations, New York, NY) used to stabilize a Charcot foot after surgical arthrodesis.

SUMMARY

The diabetic Charcot foot is rare, but a life-changing event affecting quality of life, and it risks amputation of the limb. There is no high quality evidence base governing treatment, causing clinicians to rely on low-quality, underpowered studies and expert opinion. However, CN is a treatable condition and, with lifestyle modifications and proper footwear, it does not shorten the life span of those afflicted.

REFERENCES

1. Frykberg RG. Charcot arthropathy: pathogenesis and management. Wounds 2000;12(6 Suppl B):35B–42B.
2. Frykberg RG, Mendeszoon E. Management of the diabetic Charcot foot. Diabetes Metab Res Rev 2000;16(Suppl 1):S59–65.
3. Foltz KD, Fallat LM, Schwartz S. Usefulness of a brief assessment battery for early detection of Charcot foot deformity in patients with diabetes. J Foot Ankle Surg 2004;43(2):87–92.
4. Valabhji J. Foot problems in patients with diabetes and chronic kidney disease. J Ren Care 2012;38(Suppl 1):99–108.
5. Armstrong DG, Todd WF, Lavery LA, et al. The natural history of acute Charcot's arthropathy in a diabetic foot specialty clinic. Diabet Med 1997;14:357–63.
6. Jeffcoate WJ. Theories concerning the pathogenesis of the acute Charcot foot suggest future therapy. Curr Diab Rep 2005;5(6):430–5.
7. Boyce BF, Xing L. Functions of RANKL/RANK/OPG in bone modeling and remodeling. Arch Biochem Biophys 2008;473(2):139–46.
8. Korzon-Burakowska A, Jakobkiewicz-Banecka J, Fiedosiuk A, et al. Osteoprotegerin gene polymorphism in diabetic Charcot neuroarthropathy. Diabet Med 2012;29(6):771–5.
9. Chantelau E. The perils of procrastination: effects of early vs. delayed detection and treatment of incipient Charcot fracture. Diabet Med 2005;22(12):1707–12.
10. Armstrong DG, Peters EJ. Charcot's arthropathy of the foot. J Am Podiatr Med Assoc 2002;92(7):390–4.
11. Armstrong DG, Lavery LA. Monitoring healing of acute Charcot's arthropathy with infrared dermal thermometry. J Rehabil Res Dev 1997;34:317–21.
12. Frykberg RG. Osteoarthropathy. Clin Podiatr Med Surg 1987;4:351–6.
13. Rogers LC, Bevilacqua NJ. Imaging of the Charcot foot. Clin Podiatr Med Surg 2008;25(2):263–74, vii.
14. Ledermann HP, Morrison WB. Differential diagnosis of pedal osteomyelitis and diabetic neuroarthropathy: MR Imaging. Semin Musculoskelet Radiol 2005;9(3):272–83.
15. Sella EJ, Grosser DM. Imaging modalities of the diabetic foot. Clin Podiatr Med Surg 2003;20(4):729–40.
16. Hopfner S, Krolak C, Kessler S, et al. Preoperative imaging of Charcot neuroarthropathy in diabetic patients: comparison of ring PET, hybrid PET, and magnetic resonance imaging. Foot Ankle Int 2004;25(12):890–5.
17. Pickwell KM, van Kroonenburgh MJ, Weijers RE, et al. F-18 FDG PET/CT scanning in Charcot disease: a brief report. Clin Nucl Med 2011;36(1):8–10.
18. Frykberg RG, Rogers LC. Classification of the Charcot foot. In: Frykberg RG, editor. The diabetic Charcot foot: principles and management. Brooklandville (MD): Data Trace Publishing Company; 2010. p. 55–64.
19. Rogers LC, Frykberg RG, Armstrong DG, et al. The Charcot foot in diabetes. J Am Podiatr Med Assoc 2011;101(5):437–46.

20. Sanders LJ, Mrdjencovich D. Anatomical patterns of bone and joint destruction in neuropathic diabetics. Diabetes 1991;40(Suppl 1):529A.
21. Larsen K, Fabrin J, Holstein PE. Incidence and management of ulcers in diabetic Charcot feet. J Wound Care 2001;10(8):323–8.
22. Eichenholtz SN. Charcot Joints. Springfield (IL): Charles C. Thomas; 1966.
23. Shibata T, Tada K, Hashizume C. The results of arthrodesis of the ankle for leprotic neuroarthropathy. J Bone Joint Surg Am 1990;72:749–56.
24. Rogers LC, Bevilacqua NJ. The diagnosis of Charcot foot. Clin Podiatr Med Surg 2008;25(1):43–51, vi.
25. Viswanathan V, Kesavan R, Kavitha KV, et al. Evaluation of Rogers Charcot foot classification system in South Indian diabetic subjects with Charcot foot. J Diabetic Foot Complications 2012;4:67–70.
26. Rogers LC, Frykberg RG, Armstrong DG, et al. The Charcot foot in diabetes. Diabetes Care 2011;34:2123–9.
27. Sanders L, Frykberg RG. The Charcot foot (pied de Charcot). In: Bowker JH, Pfeiffer M, editors. Levin and O'Neal's the diabetic foot. Philadelphia: Mosby Elsevier; 2007. p. 257–83.
28. Hartsell HD, Brand RA, Saltzman CL. Total contact casting: its effect on contralateral plantar foot pressure. Foot Ankle Int 2002;23(4):330–4.
29. Lavery LA, Higgins KR, Lanctot DR, et al. Home monitoring of foot skin temperatures to prevent ulceration. Diabetes Care 2004;27(11):2642–7.
30. Hartsell HD, Fellner C, Saltzman CL. Pneumatic bracing and total contact casting have equivocal effects on plantar pressure relief. Foot Ankle Int 2001;22(6):502–6.
31. Jude EB, Selby PL, Burgess J, et al. Bisphosphonates in the treatment of Charcot neuroarthropathy: A double-blind randomised controlled trial. Diabetologia 2001;44:2032–7.
32. Jude EB, Selby PL, Burgess J, et al. Bisphosphonates in the treatment of Charcot neuroarthropathy: a double-blind randomised controlled trial. Diabetologia 2001;44(11):2032–7.
33. Selby PL, Young MJ, Boulton AJ. Bisphosphonates: a new treatment for diabetic Charcot neuroarthropathy? Diabet Med 1994;11(1):28–31.
34. Bem R, Jirkovska A, Fejfarova V, et al. Intranasal calcitonin in the treatment of acute Charcot neuroosteoarthropathy: a randomized controlled trial. Diabetes Care 2006;29(6):1392–4.
35. Pitocco D, Ruotolo V, Caputo S, et al. Six-Month Treatment With Alendronate in Acute Charcot Neuroarthropathy: a randomized controlled trial. Diabetes Care 2005;28(5):1214–5.
36. Game FL, Catlow R, Jones GR, et al. Audit of acute Charcot's disease in the UK: the CDUK study. Diabetologia 2012;55:32–5.
37. Petrisor B, Lau JT. Electrical bone stimulation: an overview and its use in high risk and Charcot foot and ankle reconstructions. Foot Ankle Clin 2005;10(4):609–20, vii–viii.
38. Wang JC, Le AW, Tsukuda RK. A new technique for Charcot's foot reconstruction. J Am Podiatr Med Assoc 2002;92(8):429–36.
39. Baravarian B, Van Gils CC. Arthrodesis of the Charcot foot and ankle. Clin Podiatr Med Surg 2004;21(2):271–89.
40. Bevilacqua NJ, Rogers LC. Surgical management of Charcot midfoot deformities. Clin Podiatr Med Surg 2008;25(1):81–94, vii.
41. Pinzur MS, Sage R, Stuck R, et al. A treatment algorithm for neuropathic (Charcot) midfoot deformity. Foot Ankle 1993;14(4):189–97.

42. Pinzur MS, Sostak J. Surgical stabilization of nonplantigrade Charcot arthropathy of the midfoot. Am J Orthop 2007;36(7):361–5.
43. Saltzman CL, Johnson KA, Goldstein RH, et al. The patellar tendon-bearing brace as treatment for neurotrophic arthropathy: a dynamic force monitoring study. Foot Ankle 1992;13:14–21.
44. Saltzman CL, Hagy ML, Zimmerman B, et al. How effective is intensive nonoperative initial treatment of patients with diabetes and Charcot arthropathy of the feet? Clin Orthop Relat Res 2005;(435):185–90.

Pathogenesis and Medical Management of Diabetic Charcot Neuroarthropathy

Janice V. Mascarenhas, MBBS[a], Edward B. Jude, MD[b],*

KEYWORDS

- Charcot neuroarthropathy • Diabetic neuropathy • Total contact cast
- Bisphosphonates (BPPs) • Calcitonin • RANKL pathway

KEY POINTS

- The Charcot foot is an acute clinical emergency that warrants immediate management in order to prevent irreversible joint destruction.
- Offloading remains the mainstay of treatment of Charcot foot; however, adjunctive therapy with antiresorptive agents may facilitate retardation and early recovery from the inflammatory destructive process.

Almost every system in the body bears the brunt from longstanding diabetes mellitus (DM). One of its profound, devastating effects is on the musculoskeletal system. This article discusses the medical management of the ever-challenging complication affecting the diabetic foot, namely the Charcot foot. Charcot foot, also known as Charcot neuroarthropathy (CN), Charcot joint disease, and diabetic neuropathic osteoarthropathy, is defined as a condition affecting the bones, joints, and soft tissues of the foot and ankle, characterized by inflammation in the earliest phase.[1] This problematic condition is also encountered as a complication in other neuropathic diseases, like tabes dorsalis, leprosy, syringomyelia, multiple sclerosis, myelomeningocele, spinal cord compression, and congenital indifference to pain. Diabetic neuropathy seems, however, to be the leading cause in majority of the cases, with 0.2% of diabetic patients affected.[2]

CN usually occurs in diabetic individuals during their sixth and seventh decades, the average age of onset being 57 years. Approximately 80% of this population has had diabetes for more than 10 years. Bilateral involvement has been reported to occur in 5.9% to 39.3% of the heterogeneous cases.[3]

[a] Department of Endocrinology, St. John's National Academy of Health Sciences, Bangalore 560034, Karnataka, India; [b] Tameside Hospital NHS Foundation Trust, Fountain Street, Ashton-Under-Lyne, Lancashire OL6 9RW, UK
* Corresponding author.
E-mail address: Edward.Jude@tgh.nhs.uk

Med Clin N Am 97 (2013) 857–872
http://dx.doi.org/10.1016/j.mcna.2013.05.002
0025-7125/13/$ – see front matter © 2013 Elsevier Inc. All rights reserved.

Several therapeutic options are available for the management of CN. Nevertheless, immobilization and reduction of weight-bearing stress (offloading) are primary key objectives when considering adjunctive medical therapy.

PATHOPHYSIOLOGY OF BONE RESORPTION

There are many predisposing conditions that are responsible for the development of CN, but because DM is accountable for majority of the cases, the evolution of CN as a complication of diabetes is elucidated. An overview of the process of osteoclastogenesis (bone resorption) is essential in order to have a better understanding of the pathophysiology of CN.

To start with, the osteoblast expresses 2 surface proteins, macrophage colony-stimulating factor and receptor activator for nuclear factor (NF)-κB (RANK) ligand (RANKL), both of which are required for stimulation of osteoclastogenesis. RANKL belongs to the tumor necrosis factor (TNF) superfamily and is responsible for the activation of mature osteoclasts. RANKL binds to its receptor, RANK, which is expressed on both osteoclast precursors and mature osteoclasts.[4] RANK belongs to the TNF receptor superfamily.

Osteoprotegerin (OPG), an inhibitor of osteoclastogenesis, however, acts as a decoy receptor for RANKL, thereby preventing the interaction of RANKL with RANK. OPG is secreted by osteoblasts and activated T cells.

Osteoclastogenesis is influenced by a balance between RANKL and OPG. If stromal or osteoblastic cells produce more RANKL than OPG, osteoclasts are formed and activated, which increases bone resorption. If stromal or osteoblastic cells produce more OPG than RANKL, OPG binds the available RANKL, and new osteoclast formation is prevented. During inflammation, T cells are activated and produce RANKL, which can stimulate osteoclast-mediated bone resorption. Cytokines, such as interleukin (IL)-1 and TNF-α can augment the effects of RANKL and macrophage colony-stimulating factor on osteoclast formation and bone resorption by directly stimulating osteoclast precursor cells and mature osteoclasts.[5]

TNF-α and IL-1β prevent apoptosis of monocytes and, hence, are protective in nature.[6,7] If inactivated, monocytes undergo apoptosis. Activated monocytes release both proinflammatory cytokines (TNF-α, IL-1β, and IL-6) and anti-inflammatory cytokines (IL-4 and IL-10). In acute Charcot, due to an accumulation of activated monocytes at the site of inflammation, there is a predominance of proinflammatory cytokines versus anti-inflammatory cytokines, resulting in a sustained inflammatory process.[8]

The RANKL/RANK pathway has also been identified in vascular diseases. It has been suggested that this cytokine system could have a possible role in mediating calcification of the arterial smooth muscle cells, which occurs in diabetic neuropathy.[9,10] A former study has also shown evidence of vascular calcification (Mönckeberg sclerosis) in 90% of patients with CN.[11] Calcification of peripheral vasculature occurs secondary to the hemodynamic changes induced by a reduction in peripheral vascular resistance, which is commonly seen in diabetic neuropathy.

Certain neuropeptides, like calcitonin gene-related peptide (CGRP) and substance P, also play a considerable role in regulating skeletal homeostasis. Both neuropeptides are found in unmyelinated C and A-δ fibers of the peripheral nervous system and are known for maintaining trabecular integrity.[12] Therefore, as expected in diabetic neuropathy, due to nerve damage, these neuropeptides are depleted and eventually osteopenia ensues. CGRP also regulates the activity of endothelial nitric oxide synthase. Endothelial nitric oxide synthase yields nitric oxide, which suppresses osteoclastic activity. The role of these mediators in preserving bone integrity has been well justified in several studies.[13,14] These studies have demonstrated a reduction of CGRP and endothelial nitric oxide synthase in bone biopsies of patients with CN. In addition, CGRP promotes monocyte apoptosis by augmenting the release of IL-10 from monocytes.[15] This suppressive effect on monocytes is lost with CGRP depletion in neuronal damage. The resultant effect is an uncontrolled release of TNF-α and IL-1β from an accumulation of activated monocytes, further perpetuating osteoclastogenesis mediated through RANKL.

A susceptible foot, like the insensate foot of diabetic neuropathy, is frequently exposed to unfavorable mechanical stress. This results in either ulceration over peak pressure point areas or fractures. An inflammatory response is initiated, which is further exacerbated with the increased blood flow that occurs with associated autonomic dysfunction. The release of proinflammatory cytokines, including TNF-α and IL-1β, leads to increased expression of RANKL. RANKL triggers the synthesis of the nuclear transcription factor, NF-κB, and this in turn stimulates the maturation of osteoclasts from osteoclast precursor cells. This localized osteolysis may inevitably become persistent if misdiagnosed during the early phase of CN, in the presence of unrecognized recurrent trauma.

As with any high bone turnover state, elevated biochemical markers of bone resorption, derived from collagen breakdown, are detectable in CN, which is evident by the presence of increased serum levels of pyridinoline cross-linked carboxy-terminal telopeptide domain of type 1 collagen (1 carboxy-terminal telopeptide) and urinary levels of cross-linked N-telopeptides of type 1 collagen. This is not accompanied, however, by a compensatory increase in bone formation markers because the serum levels of carboxy-terminal propeptide of type 1 collagen remain unchanged.[16]

Hitherto, 2 theories have been proposed that serve as a possible explanation for the development of CN.[17–19] According to the neurotraumatic theory, abnormal plantar pressures develop as a result of underlying sensorimotor neuropathy. Repetitive trauma promotes microfractures and joint and ligament instability, leading to an unstable foot. In contrast, the neurovascular theory states that an increased blood flow as a consequence of autonomic neuropathy causes bone resorption and osteopenia.

RISK FACTORS PERPETUATING THE DEVELOPMENT OF CHARCOT FOOT

The Charcot foot has been known to result from an interplay of myriad morbid risk factors, the most common being diabetic neuropathy.

Peripheral Sensorimotor Neuropathy

Peripheral sensorimotor neuropathy is characterized by loss of protective sensation, absent deep tendon reflexes, diminished vibratory perception, and muscle weakness. The insensate foot is, therefore, highly vulnerable to trauma, which may be minor or repetitive in nature.

Motor neuropathy leads to an acquired deformity due to exaggeration of the plantar arch and clawing, altered gait with abnormal loading.

Autonomic Neuropathy

Autonomic dysfunction leads to an increased blood flow and bone resorption, both of which propagate the development of Charcot foot. The increased blood flow, vasodilatation, and arteriovenous shunting occur secondary to sympathetic denervation.

Calcitonin gene-related peptide (CGRP) is a calcitonin secretogogue, which is widely distributed in the sensory afferents of the spinal cord. It has been shown to antagonize the inflammatory actions of RANKL by augmenting the release of IL-10 (an anti-inflammatory cytokine) by monocytes. In diabetic neuropathy, with impending nerve damage, there is depletion in CGRP stores, leading to unopposed effects of RANKL and subsequent joint disintegration.

Mechanical Stress

Any form of sheer stress can prove detrimental to the insensitive foot. This induces soft tissue damage along with trabecular microfractures in the subchondral cancellous bone. Defective healing of these microfractures results in diminished subchondral bone pliability to withstand shock.

Furthermore, elevated peak plantar pressures tend to occur over a reduced plantar surface area or bony deformity (as in an equinus deformity) compared with an increased body mass.[20]

Trauma

Trauma may be evident in the form of a fracture or an overlying ulcer. CN may even develop after a first ray amputation or other surgical procedures. Regardless of the manifestation, any injury to an insensate foot triggers a cascade of inflammatory events.[21]

Osteopenia

A generalized loss of bone mineral density (BMD) is evident in diabetes. In the foot, the changes may be severe enough to result in insufficiency fractures around the ankle or in the metatarsals. Reduction in BMD is more pronounced in type 1 DM compared with type 2 DM.[22] In type 1 DM, this is mostly due to loss of islet peptides, such as insulin and amylin, both of which act as growth factors for bone. Other factors contributing to an increased incidence of osteopenia in diabetes include associated vitamin D deficiency, secondary hyperparathyroidism, and the use of steroids as immunosuppressants in recipients of pancreatic or renal transplants.[23] The role of CGRP in preserving bone density should also be considered. As discussed previously, CGRP indirectly curtails osteoclastogenesis by primarily inducing apoptosis of monocytes. In diabetic neuropathy, there is a depletion of CGRP at the nerve endings, leading to a loss of the inhibitory influence on monocytes and further unrestrained local osteolysis.

Ankle Equinus

An equinus deformity also contributes to the development of CN with collapse of the midfoot or avulsion fracture of the posterior process of the calcaneus. This faulty posture results from the combined effects of hypotonic ankle dorsiflexors and the unopposed action of the triceps surae. This joint contracture may be consequent to advanced glycation end products (AGEs)-related modification of collagen, resulting in stiffness of the tendons.[24]

Role of Advanced Glycation End Products

Formation of AGEs, the pathologic hallmark of uncontrolled diabetes, is known to induce apoptosis of mesenchymal stem cells and osteoblasts.[25,26] This mechanism is mediated through receptor for AGEs. Moreover, there is defective collagen formation due to the effect of AGEs.[27,28] The cumulative effects of apoptosis and AGEs-modified collagen results in osteopenia.

ANATOMIC PATTERNS OF BONE AND JOINT DESTRUCTION

Five characteristic anatomic patterns of bone and joint destruction have been described in diabetic individuals with CN (from data compiled by Sanders and Mrdjenovich[29] and Sanders and Frykberg[30]).

Pattern I (Forefoot)

Pattern I (forefoot) involves the interphalangeal joints, phalanges, metatarsophalangeal joints, or distal metatarsal bones, thereby predisposing to plantar ulceration. Radiologic findings include concentric resorption of bone that may be seen as a characteristic hourglass appearance of the phalangeal diaphyses. The bases of the proximal phalanges broaden to form a cup around the metatarsal head. A characteristic x-ray finding is the pencil-like tapering of the metatarsal bones with a sucked candy stick appearance attributed to the resorption of the distal metatarsal bones and phalanges.

Pattern II (Tarsometatarsal Joints)

Pattern II (tarsometatarsal [TMT] joints) is characterized by involvement of the TMT, or Lisfranc, joints and is often associated with plantar ulceration over the deformed area. Normally, the second metatarsal base is securely recessed in the intercuneiform mortise and this framework is responsible for stabilizing the midfoot. Any disruption of this architecture weakens the foot and causes malalignment of the metatarsals over the tarsals resulting in collapse of the affected joint.

Pattern III (Naviculocuneiform, Talonavicular, and Calcaneocuboid Joints)

Pattern III (naviculocuneiform, talonavicular, and calcaneocuboid joints) is characterized by dislocation of the navicular bone or by disintegration of the naviculocuneiform joints, ultimately leading to collapse of the midfoot.

Pattern IV (Ankle and Subtalar Joints)

Pattern IV (ankle and subtalar joints) involves the ankle joint with or without subtalar joint involvement, which may be associated with medial or lateral malleolar fractures. Continued weight bearing on the affected limb stretches and weakens the collateral ligaments with ultimate collapse of the joint.

Pattern V (Calcaneus)

Pattern V (calcaneus) is the least common anatomic presentation (approximately 2%) and is characterized by an extra-articular avulsion fracture of the posterior tubercle of the calcaneus. There is a high occurrence in those who have undergone renal transplantation.

These anatomic patterns may occur singly or in combination in any given individual. The most frequent joint involvement is seen in patterns I, II, and III, and the most severe structural deformity and functional instability are seen in patterns II and IV. A combination of patterns II and III constitutes the classical rocker bottom foot deformity.

It is valuable to use imaging modalities to detect changes of the susceptible foot, before any inflammatory process takes its toll. Radiographs, although the initial imaging modality for CN,[31] do not predict the risk of acquiring CN. In such instances, dual-energy x-ray absorptiometry can detect a diminished BMD in high-risk diabetic patients.[32] An MRI is efficient in detecting trivial changes, such as bone edema or microfractures, during the early stages of CN and this correlates with signs of CN.[33]

NONPHARMACOLOGIC MANAGEMENT

As emphasized previously, a fracture of the insensate foot acts as a harbinger for the development of CN. In order to prevent repetitive trauma, various interventional strategies have been used that could hinder the inflammatory process and prolong the healing period. Immobilization and reduction of weight-bearing stress (offloading) are key objectives when considering the following therapeutic options. Staging of CN is mandated in order to select the appropriate treatment. The Eichenholtz classification was developed in 1966, in an attempt to demonstrate the clinical progression of CN.[34] It initially included 3 stages; however, an additional stage (ie, stage 0) has been included (modified Eichenholtz classification).[35]

Stage 0 (Prodromal Period)

Stage 0 (prodromal period) describes a patient with peripheral neuropathy who has sustained an acute sprain or fracture in the ankle or foot but does not have stage 1 disease. The foot appears erythematous, warm, and swollen with prominent peripheral pulses. In addition, there is associated joint instability with worsening deformity. Radiographs may be normal at this stage but subtle changes, like bone marrow edema, subchondral cysts, and microfractures, can be detected on MRI scans.

Stage 1 (Acute or Developmental Phase)

In stage 1 (acute or developmental phase), the inflammatory response is exaggerated with worsening of the underlying deformity. Radiographs show joint effusion, bone fragmentation, and joint subluxation.

Stage 2 (Subacute or Coalescent Phase)

Stage 2 (subacute or coalescent phase) is characterized by a decrease in warmth, redness, and swelling. Radiographs show sclerotic bone surrounding the joint, resorption of debris, and fusion of larger bony fragments.

Stage 3 (Reconstructive Phase)

In stage 3 (reconstructive phase), there is continued resolution of the inflammation. Radiographs show remodeling of bone and some reformation of the joint architecture.

Secondary prevention during stage 0 is imperative, because clinical deterioration can be restrained during this stage.

Total contact cast

Total contact cast (TCC) is regarded as the gold standard technique for immobilization, especially during stage 1, which has been highlighted by a recent consensus statement.[1] The TCC was devised with an objective to provide a cushioning effect to the entire plantar surface with simultaneous redistribution of elevated plantar pressures. Earlier studies have shown that TCC is the ideal method to achieve plantar pressure redistribution.[36] Evidence from a study by Kimmerle and Chantelau proved that early intervention with TCC enables better healing rates without deformities.[37] A longitudinal study on CN patients, conducted by Armstrong and colleagues,[2] also highlighted the need and effectiveness of reduction in weight bearing stress with the help of a TCC.

Here the affected limb is immobilized in an irremovable TCC, with an objective of dampening the inflammatory process in order to achieve a quiescent stage. Initially, the TCC is replaced at 3 days, and then checked each week. The TCC consists of a well-molded, minimally padded cast that maintains a close contact with the entire plantar aspect of the foot and the lower leg as well. The cast should be changed frequently to avoid pistoning as the edema subsides. The decision to continue casting depends on the resolution of superficial inflammatory signs (ie, until the swelling has subsided and the temperature of the affected foot is within 2°C of the contralateral foot).[38] Although the TCC has disadvantages, such as the lack of expertise to apply a TCC, impaired routine activities, increased instability, and so forth, it is still considered the best option for achieving adequate resolution of bone destruction.

Removable cast walkers
Although they afford immediate offloading, removable cast walkers (RCWs) are associated with poor healing rates because patients have a tendency to take them off frequently. They are usually used during stage 2 as the superficial signs of inflammation subside.[38]

Extradepth shoes
Extradepth shoes with custom-molded insoles are typically used in stage 3 along with custom-molded orthoses, to prevent the occurrence of ulcers over a deformed foot. They are generally used once the skeletal remodeling process has resolved, with an intention to protect the high-risk areas, like the midfoot, from ulceration.[39]

Ankle-foot orthosis
This custom device, the ankle-foot orthosis, is intended primarily for those patients with large infected wounds or severe bony deformity. Healing rates, however, are poor due to continued weight bearing.

Charcot restraint orthotic walker
The Charcot restraint orthotic walker is another indication for severe foot deformities. It is a bivalved total-contact device, which externally fixates the ankle. It is applied as part of the transition process between a TCC and bespoke footwear, as skeletal remodeling eventually settles down.

Both ankle-foot orthosis and Charcot restraint orthotic walkers are reserved for hind foot CN.[40]

MEDICAL MANAGEMENT OF CHARCOT FOOT

Antiresorptive agents, like bisphosphonates (BPPs) and calcitonin, have gained popularity after their use in conditions characterized by excessive bone turnover. Their use in the treatment of CN has also been suggested as having some benefit based on data obtained from small human clinical trials, although larger trials are required to confirm their place in the medical management of acute CN.

Bisphosphonates
The unique role of BPPs as antiresorptive agents came into being with the concept that its naturally occurring analog (ie, inorganic pyrophosphate [PPi]) had the ability to inhibit ectopic calcification. The basic structure of BPPs is composed of 2 phosphonate groups bound to a central carbon atom instead of an oxygen atom (PPi). This renders the PCP molecule more stable and resistant to enzymatic hydrolysis. The 2 phosphonate groups are responsible for binding to bone mineral and for antiresorptive potency. In order to amplify its range of activity, additional structural modifications (like the addition of R1 and R2 side chains to the central carbon atom and esterification of the phosphonate groups) have been made, which are thereby responsible for the variability in potency among different classes of BPPs.[41]

General mechanism of action

Once absorbed, BPP dissipates rapidly to the bone, owing to their high affinity for hydroxyapatite crystals, and gets deposited beneath the osteoclasts, at sites of active remodeling, especially the trabeculae. An acidic milieu is created during the process of bone resorption, which facilitates the dissociation of BPPs from hydroxyapatite crystals and its uptake by osteoclasts by fluid-phase endocytosis.

First-generation BPPs

First-generation BPPs possess minimally modified side chains and are non-nitrogenous in nature. These include medronate, clodronate, etidronate, and tiludronate and are the least potent among the BPPs. They act by producing cytotoxic β,γ-methylene analogs of ATP that bear a close resemblance to PPi. High intracellular concentrations of these analogs (AppCp-type nucleotides) inhibit key ATP-dependent mitochondrial enzymes, such as adenine nucleotide translocase, which affects mitochondrial membrane permeability. The resulting caspase activation leads to irreversible apoptosis of osteoclasts.[42]

Second-generation BPPs (Aminobisphosphonates)

Second-generation BPPs (aminobisphosphonates) include agents, such as alendronate, ibandronate, and pamidronate, and are 10 to 100 times more potent than first-generation BPPs, depending on the presence of an amino group in the side chain or addition of other groups to the nitrogen atom. They inhibit farnesyl pyrophosphate synthase, a key enzyme in the mevalonate pathway of cholesterol synthesis that is required for osteoclast survival. Blockade of farnesyl pyrophosphate synthase results in decreased amounts of geranyl pyrophosphate and farnesyl pyrophosphate. Farnesyl pyrophosphate and geranyl pyrophosphate are required for prenylation of small GTPases, which participate in cellular events, including cell division, vesicle transport, nuclear assembly, and control of the cytoskeleton.[43] Hence, prevention of prenylation of small GTPases due to inhibition of farnesyl pyrophosphate synthase by BPPs leads to an interruption of the cytoskeletal reorganization of the osteoclast, with loss of the ruffled border and sealing zone and osteoclast apoptosis.[44]

Third-generation BPPs

Risedronate and zoledronate belong to this subcategory of BPPs and are 10,000 times more potent than the first-generation BPPs. Their extreme potency is explained by the presence of a nitrogen atom within a heterocyclic ring. In addition to blocking farnesyl pyrophosphate synthase, they block the subsequent enzymatic reaction in the mevalonate pathway.

Pharmacokinetics

BPPs have a poor oral bioavailability, ranging from 5% to 10%, which is due to their low lipophilicity and their high negative charge.[45] For certain BPPs that can be administered parenterally, however, an increased bioavailability of approximately 50% to 75% can be achieved. They are not metabolized and are thus excreted unaltered by the kidney. Caution is exercised especially in patients with renal insufficiency and is usually not recommended if the glomerular filtration rate is less than 30 mL/min.

Adverse effects

Predominant side effects are gastrointestinal related and include nausea, vomiting, dyspepsia, esophageal irritation or esophagitis, ulceration, and even diarrhea. Transient flu-like symptoms occur after intravenous administration and are attributed to the release of cytokines (IL-6 and TNF-α) after stimulation of macrophages.[46] They do not recur during subsequent administrations. Large intravenous doses should be administered slowly to avoid the risk of nephrotoxicity. Osteonecrosis of the jaw rarely occurs with high doses of aminobisphosphonates and is further exacerbated by risk factors that involve concomitant use of corticosteroids, prior dental surgery, and comorbid illness, such as diabetes and anemia. No conclusive data with regards to the pathogenesis have been established.[47]

Bisphosphonates in Charcot foot clinical trials

The efficacy of BPPs in the treatment of CN has been investigated in a few randomized controlled trials (RCTs). In 1994, Selby and colleagues,[48] in a single labeled non-randomized trial, instituted a course of pamidronate infusions to patients with CN over 10 weeks and demonstrated improvement of symptoms, reduced foot temperatures, and a significant reduction in alkaline phosphatase levels. Their therapeutic effect was further studied by Jude and colleagues,[49] in a larger trial conducted across 4 centers in the United Kingdom. In this double-blinded, placebo-controlled trial, patients with CN were randomized to receive pamidronate (90 mg) versus normal saline infusion as placebo (single dose). In both groups, additional conservative measures with immobilization and bed rest were instituted as part of standard therapy. The treated group experienced a greater (but not significant) fall in temperature of the affected foot after 2 weeks and improvement in reported symptoms. Measures of bone turnover were also reduced in the treatment group.

Anderson and colleagues[50] retrospectively analyzed the short-term effects of variable doses of pamidronate infusions on acute CN in 13 patients compared with 10 control patients without BPP therapy. Again, a significant reduction in foot temperatures and bone alkaline phosphatase levels was observed. Another randomized control trial with oral alendronate (70 mg weekly for 6 months) also demonstrated a significant reduction in bone resorption markers along with a significant improvement in BMD.[51]

According to recommendations of the American Diabetes Association (ADA) consensus report,[1] there is limited evidence to support the use of BPP therapy in acute CN. Therefore, additional prospective, larger, well-powered RCTs are required to attest the role of BPPs in the acute management of CN.

Calcitonin

Calcitonin is a 32–amino acid peptide secreted by the parafollicular cells (C-cells) of the thyroid gland embryonically derived from the ultimobranchial bodies. This hormone contains an intrachain disulphide bond between the cysteine residues at positions 1 and 7 along with a proline amide group, which accounts for the hormone's functional activity. Its secretion depends on the prevailing serum calcium levels.

Mechanism of action

Calcitonin binds to calcitonin receptor, which is situated on osteoclasts and neural and renal cells. The calcitonin receptor is a G protein–coupled cell surface receptor, which mediates its activity through adenylate cyclase and phospholipase C. It impairs osteoclastic mediated bone resorption by a direct inhibitory effect on osteoclasts, which constitutes an impairment of cytoplasmic motility, secretory activity, and a reduction in the number of osteoclasts.[52] This occurs through loss of ruffled borders of osteoclasts and reduction in the secretion of lysosomal enzymes. Besides its inhibitory effects on osteoclasts, calcitonin exerts antiapoptotic effects on osteocytes and osteoblasts. Other effects include inhibition of calcium reabsorption from the renal tubules and regulation of renal vitamin D_3 production.

It has also been proposed that calcitonin may exert anabolic effects on bone via CGRP. CGRP is a 37–amino acid derivative obtained from splicing of the calcitonin gene at exon 4. CGRP is located at nerve endings in close proximity to leptinergic neurons. Leptin seems to regulate bone formation via the sympathetic nervous system through adrenergic receptors situated on osteoblasts.

Pharmacokinetics
Human calcitonin has a half-life of approximately 10 minutes. Salmon calcitonin has a longer half-life and is more potent than human calcitonin, making it more attractive as a therapeutic agent. Its affinity for the human calcitonin receptor is 40 times more than that of human calcitonin.[53] Although less superior than BPPs, it has a safer therapeutic profile in patients with renal insufficiency. Calcitonin undergoes hepatic and renal metabolism.

Adverse effects
Adverse effects include nausea, vomiting, flushing, hand swelling, urticaria, and, rarely, intestinal cramping. These effects are minimal, however, with intranasal administration.

Role of calcitonin in clinical trials
Calcitonin's use in CN was first demonstrated by Bem and colleagues[54] in an RCT that used intranasal calcitonin (200 IU daily) and oral calcium versus oral calcium alone in 32 diabetic patients with acute CN in addition to standard care of CN. By 3 months, there was a significant reduction in bone resorption markers (namely, 1 carboxy-terminal telopeptide domain of type 1 collagen) and bone-specific alkaline phosphatase levels.

NOVEL TARGETS FOR FUTURE TRIALS

Given the established evidence of inflammatory pathways involved in the causation of Charcot foot, several studies have been conducted that have explored the potential role of agents that hinder the damaging effects of these inflammatory mediators. Therefore, it is imperative to exploit the benefits of these agents as future candidates in managing CN.

The role of proinflammatory cytokines in the pathogenesis of CN has been investigated in a few studies.[8,55] Targeting the mediators of the inflammatory pathway, such as TNF-α, IL-1, and RANKL, would be an innovative step in the future.

TNF-α Inhibitors

TNF-α is the central instigator in the cytokine system, which stimulates the production of additional cytokines that promote joint destruction. TNF-α binds to 2 receptors, type 1 TNF receptor (p55) and type 2 TNF receptor (p75), which are found on immune, inflammatory, and endothelial cells. Various clinical trials have evaluated the use of agents that target TNF-α, especially in chronic inflammatory polyarthritic conditions, such as rheumatoid arthritis (RA), because it is highly expressed at sites of joint destruction.[56]

So far, 3 of such agents have been Food and Drug Administration approved for the management of RA in combination with methotrexate and in refractory cases. Adalimumab is a recombinant human IgG1 monoclonal antibody that binds to human TNF-α with high affinity. Etanercept is a recombinant-soluble p75 TNF receptor:Fc fusion protein composed of a ligand-binding portion of a human TNF-α receptor fused to the Fc portion of human IgG1. Infliximab is a chimeric anti–TNF-α IgG1 monoclonal antibody that consists of a human constant region and a murine variable region.[57] They bind to TNF-α and prevent interaction with its corresponding receptor.

These trials have successfully demonstrated an improvement in signs and symptoms, reduction in disability, and retardation of radiographic evidence of joint destruction.[58–60]

IL-1β Blockers

IL-1 is another proinflammatory cytokine, which, like TNF-α, plays a critical role in bone destruction in RA. Anakinra is a nonglycosylated, recombinant form of the naturally occurring IL-1 receptor antagonist, whose use has been recommended for the management of RA.[61] A 6-month RCT led by Cohen and colleagues[62] has also proved a significant improvement in clinical, laboratory, and radiologic parameters in RA patients receiving subcutaneous injections of anakinra (100 mg per day) versus placebo with background methotrexate therapy.

RANKL Inhibitors

Denosumab (DMB), a human monoclonal antibody (IgG2) to RANKL, has proved its ability to prevent bone resorption in healthy postmenopausal women, men, and patients with multiple myeloma or metastatic breast cancer. Formerly known as AMG 162 (Amgen), DMB binds specifically to human RANKL and thus prevents the interaction of RANKL with RANK. Its use has been well established in human studies. A phase II, randomized, double-blinded, placebo-controlled study demonstrated that the addition of twice-yearly injections of DMB to ongoing treatment with methotrexate inhibited structural damage, improved BMD, and suppressed bone turnover in RA patients, without increasing the rate of adverse events compared with placebo treatment.[63] Another study in postmenopausal women showed that when DMB was administered subcutaneously at 3-month or 6-month intervals over a period of 12 months, a sustained decrease in bone turnover and a rapid increase in BMD were observed.[64] Given the evidence of its potential benefits, DMB may prove an ideal agent for CN.

Because CN and RA share a similar pathogenesis (ie, RANKL/OPG signaling pathways, with involvement of similar triggering factors [IL-1β and TNF-α]),[8,55] the role of immunomodulators in targeting the RANKL/OPG pathway can be explored in future trials.

THE ADA CONSENSUS REPORT

A recent ADA consensus report[1] provides an overview of CN, from pathogenesis to management. It states that CN commonly occurs as a complication of diabetic neuropathy, which is confounded by other minor predisposing factors, resulting in the classical rocker-bottom midfoot deformity. In an insensate foot, minor traumatic events trigger an inflammatory cascade, which is governed by the RANKL/OPG pathway mediated through proinflammatory cytokines, namely TNF-α and IL-1β. Repetitive trauma further accentuates the effects of proinflammatory cytokines, leading to localized osteolysis at the affected site.

To facilitate early diagnosis of CN, the report has provided an algorithm, which illustrates the ideal approach in the management of such patients (**Fig. 1**). This approach is further influenced by the interpretation of various imaging modalities that aid in the diagnosis of CN. Offloading and immobilization indefinitely remain the mainstay of therapy. The role of available antiresorptive agents is currently debatable and, therefore, larger trials are required to justify its use in the management of CN.

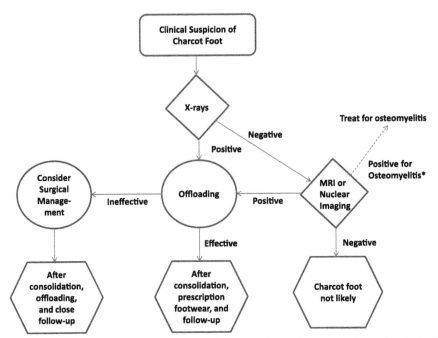

Fig. 1. Basic approach to the management of Charcot foot. *Osteomyelitis can be difficult to distinguish from the Charcot foot. (*From* Rogers LC, Frykberg RG, Armstrong DG, et al. The charcot foot in diabetes. Diabetes Care 2011;34:212; with permission.)

SUMMARY

The Charcot foot is a problematic clinical entity that worsens in the absence of timely intervention. As of now, based on the ADA consensus report, offloading with TCC continues to remain the mainstay of therapy for CN.[1] A standardized approach to the management of CN is depicted in **Fig. 1**. Furthermore, ongoing inflammatory activity can be controlled with antiresorptive agents, like BPPs and calcitonin; however, data acquired from larger trials with these agents are awaited. Newer agents that target the inflammatory cascade have been identified and applied in limited clinical trials in non-Charcot conditions. Their potential role in the future management of CN has yet to be established.

REFERENCES

1. Rogers LC, Frykberg RG, Armstrong DG, et al. The Charcot foot in diabetes. Diabetes Care 2011;34:2123–9.
2. Armstrong DG, Todd WF, Lavery LA, et al. The natural history of acute Charcot's arthropathy in a diabetic foot specialty clinic. Diabet Med 1997;14:357–63.
3. Sanders LJ, Frykberg RG. Charcot neuroarthropathy of the foot. Levin and O'Neal's the diabetic foot. 6th edition. St Louis (MO): Mosby; 2001. p. 439–65.
4. Franklin RB, Marie BD, Henry MK. Hormones and disorders of mineral metabolism. Williams textbook of endocrinology. 12th edition. Philadelphia: Elsevier; 2011. p. 1246.
5. Joseph AL, Ernesto C, Lawrence GR. Metabolic bone disease. Williams textbook of endocrinology. 12th edition. Philadelphia: Elsevier; 2011. p. 1310.

6. Mangan DF, Welch GR, Wahl SM. Lipopolysaccharide, tumor necrosis factor-α and IL-1β prevent programmed cell death (apoptosis) in human peripheral blood monocytes. J Immunol 1991;146:1541-6.

7. McConkey DJ, Hartzell P, Amador-Perez JF, et al. Calcium-dependent killing of immature thymocytes by stimulation via the CD3/T cell receptor complex. J Immunol 1989;143:1801-6.

8. Jeffcoate W. The role of proinflammatory cytokines in the cause of neuropathic osteoarthropathy (acute Charcot foot) in diabetes. Lancet 2005;366:2058-61.

9. Hofbauer LC, Schoppet M. Clinical implications of the osteoprotegerin/RANKL/RANK system for bone and vascular diseases. JAMA 2004;292:490-5.

10. Demer L, Abedin M. Skeleton key to vascular disease. J Am Coll Cardiol 2004;44:1977-9.

11. Sinha S, Munichoodappa C, Kozak GP. Neuro-arthropathy (Charcot joints) in diabetes mellitus: a clinical study of 101 cases. Medicine (Baltimore) 1972;51:191-210.

12. Offley SC, Guo TZ, Wei T, et al. Capsaicin-sensitive sensory neurons contribute to the maintenance of trabecular bone integrity. J Bone Miner Res 2005;20:257-67.

13. Collin-Osdoby P, Rothe L, Bekker S, et al. Decreased nitric oxide levels stimulate osteoclastogenesis and bone resorption both in vitro and in vivo on the chick chorioallantoic membrane in association with neoangiogenesis. J Bone Miner Res 2000;15:474-88.

14. Turner CH, Pavalko FM. Mechanotransduction and functional response of the skeleton to physical stress: the mechanisms and mechanics of bone adaptation. J Orthop Sci 1998;3:346-55.

15. Feng Y, Tang Y, Guo J, et al. Inhibition of LPS-induced TNF-α production by calcitonin gene-related peptide (CGRP) in cultured mouse peritoneal macrophages. Life Sci 1997;61:281-7.

16. Gough A, Abraha H, Li F, et al. Measurement of markers of osteoclast and osteoblast activity in patients with acute and chronic diabetic Charcot neuroarthropathy. Diabet Med 1997;14:527-31.

17. Trepman E, Nihal A, Pinzur MS. Current topics review: Charcot neuroarthropathy of the foot and ankle. Foot Ankle Int 2005;26:46-63.

18. Pinzur MS. Current concepts review: Charcot arthropathy of the foot and ankle. Foot Ankle Int 2007;28:952-9.

19. Chantelau E, Onvlee GJ. Charcot foot in diabetes: farewell to the neurotrophic theory. Horm Metab Res 2006;38:361-7.

20. Cavanagh PR, Sims DS Jr, Sanders LJ. Body mass is a poor predictor of peak plantar pressure in diabetic men. Diabetes Care 1991;14:750-5.

21. Foltz KD, Fallat LM, Schwartz S. Usefulness of a brief assessment battery for early detection of Charcot foot deformity in patients with diabetes. J Foot Ankle Surg 2004;43:87-92.

22. Hofbauer LC, Brueck CC, Singh SK, et al. Osteoporosis in patients with diabetes mellitus. J Bone Miner Res 2007;22:1317-28.

23. Matricali GA, Bammens B, Kuypers D, et al. High rate of Charcot foot attacks early after simultaneous pancreas-kidney transplantation. Transplantation 2007;83:245-6.

24. Grant WP, Sullivan R, Sonenshine DE, et al. Electron microscopic investigation of the effects of diabetes mellitus on the Achilles tendon. J Foot Ankle Surg 1997;36:272-8 [discussion: 330].

25. Kume S, Kato S, Yamagishi S, et al. Advanced glycation end-products attenuate human mesenchymal stem cells and prevent cognate differentiation into adipose tissue, cartilage, and bone. J Bone Miner Res 2005;20:1647–58.
26. Alikhani M, Alikhani Z, Boyd C, et al. Advanced glycation end products stimulate osteoblast apoptosis via the MAP kinase and cytosolic apoptotic pathways. Bone 2007;40:345–53.
27. Brownlee M, Cerami A, Vlassara H. Advanced glycosylation end products in tissue and the biochemical basis of diabetic complications. N Engl J Med 1998;318:1315–21.
28. Monnier VM, Glomb M, Elgawish A, et al. The mechanism of collagen cross-linking in diabetes: a puzzle nearing resolution. Diabetes 1996;45:67–72.
29. Sanders LJ, Mrdjenovich D. Anatomical patterns of bone and joint destruction in neuropathic diabetics. Diabetes 1991;40:529A.
30. Sanders LJ, Frykberg RG. Diabetic neuropathic osteoarthropathy: Charcot foot. In: Levin ME, O'Neal LW, Bowker JH, editors. The high risk foot in diabetes mellitus. New York: Churchill Livingstone; 1991. p. 297–338.
31. Frykberg RG, Eneroth M. Principles of conservative management. In: Frykberg RG, editor. The diabetic charcot foot: principles and management. Brooklandville (MD): Data Trace Publishing Company; 2010. p. 93–116.
32. Jirkovska AP, Kasalicky P, Boucek P, et al. Calcaneal ultrasonomentry in patients with Charcot osteoarthropathy and its relationship with densitometry in the lumbar spine and femoral neck and with markers of bone turnover. Diabet Med 2001;18:495–500.
33. Schlossbauer T, Mioc T, Sommerey S, et al. Magnetic resonance imaging in early stage charcot arthropathy; correlation of imaging findings and clinical symptoms. Eur J Med Res 2008;13:409–14.
34. Thomas CC, Eichenholtz SN. Charcot joints. Springfield (IL):1966.
35. Johnson JE. Operative treatment of neuropathic arthropathy of the foot and ankle. J Bone Joint Surg Am 1998;80:1700–9.
36. Armstrong DG, Lavery LA. Elevated peak plantar pressures in patients who have Charcot arthropathy. J Bone Joint Surg Am 1998;80:365–9.
37. Kimmerle R, Chantelau E. Weight-bearing intensity produces charcot deformity in injured neuropathic feet in diabetes. Exp Clin Endocrinol Diabetes 2007;115:360–4.
38. Armstrong DG, Lavery LA. Monitoring healing of acute Charcot's arthropathy with infrared dermal thermometry. J Rehabil Res Dev 1997;34:317–21.
39. Giurini JM. Applications and use of in-shoe orthoses in the conservative management of Charcot foot deformity. Clin Podiatr Med Surg 1994;11:271–8.
40. Frykberg RG, Zgonis T, Armstrong DG, et al. Diabetic foot disorders. A clinical practice guideline (2006 revision). J Foot Ankle Surg 2006;45:1–66.
41. Russell RG, Watts NB, Ebetino FH, et al. Mechanisms of action of bisphosphonates: similarities and differences and their potential influence on clinical efficacy. Osteoporos Int 2008;19:733–59.
42. Lehenkari PP, Kellinsalmi M, Napankangas JP, et al. Further insight into mechanism of action of clodronate: inhibition of mitochondrial ADP/ATP translocase by a nonhydrolyzable, adenine-containing metabolite. Mol Pharmacol 2002;61:1255–62.
43. Itzstein C, Coxon FP, Rogers MJ. The regulation of osteoclast function and bone resorption by small GTPases. Small GTPases 2011;2:117–30.
44. Green JR. Bisphosphonates: preclinical review. Oncologist 2004;9:3–13.
45. Fleisch H. Bisphosphonates: mechanisms of action. Endocr Rev 1998;19:80–100.

46. Schweitzer DH, Oostendorp-van de Ruit M, Van der Pluijm G, et al. Interleukin-6 and the acute phase response during treatment of patients with Paget's disease with the nitrogen-containing bisphosphonate dimethylaminohydroxypropylidene bisphosphonate. J Bone Miner Res 1995;10:956–62.

47. Hoff AO, Toth BB, Altundag K, et al. Osteonecrosis of the jaw in patients receiving intravenous bisphosphonate therapy. J Clin Oncol 2006;24:8528.

48. Selby PL, Young MJ, Boulton AJ. Bisphosphonates: a new treatment for diabetic Charcot neuroarthropathy? Diabet Med 1994;11:28–31.

49. Jude EB, Selby PL, Burgess J, et al. Bisphosphonates in the treatment of Charcot neuroarthropathy: a double-blind randomised controlled trial. Diabetologia 2001;44:2032–7.

50. Anderson JJ, Woelffer KE, Holtzman JJ, et al. Bisphosphonates for the treatment of Charcot neuroarthropathy. J Foot Ankle Surg 2004;43:285–9.

51. Pitocco D, Ruotolo V, Caputo S, et al. Six-month treatment with alendronate in acute Charcot neuroarthropathy: a randomized controlled trial. Diabetes Care 2005;28:1214–5.

52. Zaidi M, Inzerillo AM, Moonga BS, et al. Forty years of calcitonin—where are we now? A tribute to the work of Iain Macintyre, FRS. Bone 2002;30:655–63.

53. Kapurniato A, Taylor JW. Structural and conformational requirements for human calcitonin activity. Design, synthesis and study of lactam bridge analogs. J Med Chem 1995;38:836–47.

54. Bem R, Jirkovska A, Fejfarova V, et al. Intranasal calcitonin in the treatment of acute Charcot neuroosteoarthropathy: a randomized controlled trial. Diabetes Care 2006;29:1392–4.

55. Baumhauer JF, O'Keefe RJ, Schon LC, et al. Cytokine-induced osteoclastic bone resorption in Charcot arthropathy: an immunohistochemical study. Foot Ankle Int 2006;27:797–800.

56. Hetland ML, Christensen IJ, Tarp U, et al. Direct comparison of treatment responses, remission rates, and drug adherence in patients with rheumatoid arthritis treated with adalimumab, etanercept, or infliximab: results from eight years of surveillance of clinical practice in the nationwide Danish DANBIO registry. Arthritis Rheum 2010;62:22–32.

57. Scott DL, Kingsley GH. Tumor necrosis factor inhibitors for rheumatoid arthritis. N Engl J Med 2006;355:704–12.

58. Keystone EC, Kavanaugh AF, Sharp JT, et al. Radiographic, clinical, and functional outcomes of treatment with adalimumab (a human anti-tumor necrosis factor monoclonal antibody) in patients with active rheumatoid arthritis receiving concomitant methotrexate therapy: a randomized, placebo-controlled, 52-week trial. Arthritis Rheum 2004;50:1400–11.

59. van der Heijde D, Klareskog L, Rodriguez-Valverde V, et al. Comparison of etanercept and methotrexate, alone and combined, in the treatment of rheumatoid arthritis: two-year clinical and radiographic results from the TEMPO study, a double-blind, randomized trial. Arthritis Rheum 2006;54:1063–74.

60. Lipsky PE, van der Heijde DM, St Clair EW, et al. Infliximab and methotrexate in the treatment of rheumatoid arthritis. Anti-Tumor Necrosis Factor Trial in Rheumatoid Arthritis with Concomitant Therapy Study Group. N Engl J Med 2000;343:1594–602.

61. Dinarello CA. Blocking interleukin-1β in acute and chronic autoinflammatory diseases. J Intern Med 2011;269:16–28.

62. Cohen SB, Moreland LW, Cush JJ, et al. A multicentre, double blind, randomised, placebo controlled trial of anakinra (Kineret), a recombinant interleukin 1

receptor antagonist, in patients with rheumatoid arthritis treated with background methotrexate. Ann Rheum Dis 2004;63:1062–8.

63. Cohen SB, Dore RK, Lane NE, et al. Denosumab treatment effects on structural damage, bone mineral density, and bone turnover in rheumatoid arthritis: a twelve-month, multicenter, randomized, double-blind, placebo-controlled, phase II clinical trial. Arthritis Rheum 2008;58:1299–309.

64. McClung MR, Lewiecki EM, Cohen SB, et al. Denosumab in postmenopausal women with low bone mineral density. N Engl J Med 2006;354:821–31.

Orthopaedic Surgery and the Diabetic Charcot Foot

Wei Shen, MD, PhD, Dane Wukich, MD*

KEYWORDS

• Diabetes • Foot • Charcot • Orthopaedic surgery

KEY POINTS

- Due to the systemic manifestations of diabetes mellitus and complex presentations in the foot and ankle with osteoporotic bone, potentially impaired blood supply, and profound peripheral neuropathy, a multidisciplinary team care approach is optimal.
- Foot and ankle surgeons must work in concert with specialists from other disciplines, such as endocrinology, vascular surgery, orthotics, infectious disease, and nursing.
- Modern advanced diagnostic and imaging techniques have improved the knowledge regarding the biomechanics, biology, and pathophysiology of Charcot neuroarthropathy.

INTRODUCTION

Charcot neuroarthropathy (CN) is a progressive degeneration of a weight-bearing joint, a process marked by bony destruction, bone resorption, and eventual deformity that can be limb-threatening. Historically, syphilis and leprosy were the most common causes of CN; however, diabetes mellitus (DM) has emerged as the most common cause of CN over the past several decades. The surgical management of CN is a challenging problem for reconstructive surgeons. Because of the systemic manifestations of DM and complex presentations in the foot and ankle with osteoporotic bone, potentially impaired blood supply, and profound peripheral neuropathy, a multidisciplinary team care approach is optimal. The exact composition of the team may vary from region to region; however, foot and ankle surgeons must work in concert with specialists from other disciplines, such as endocrinology, vascular surgery, orthotics, infectious disease, and nursing.

PATHOANATOMY

The natural history of the Charcot foot is one of gradual healing over many months and up to even a year. As the acute inflammation and swelling subside, new bone forms,

University of Pittsburgh Medical Center Comprehensive Foot and Ankle Center, Pittsburgh, PA, USA
* Corresponding author.
E-mail address: wukichdk@upmc.edu

Med Clin N Am 97 (2013) 873–882
http://dx.doi.org/10.1016/j.mcna.2013.03.013
0025-7125/13/$ – see front matter © 2013 Elsevier Inc. All rights reserved.

optimally leading to consolidation and stability of the foot. Regardless of which anatomic classification system is used, the midfoot is most commonly affected, representing approximately 60% of all cases.[1] The typical foot deformity involves the tarsometatarsal joint, creating forefoot abduction, secondary hindfoot valgus, and a contracted gastrocnemius-soleus muscle, which ultimately results in the classic rocker bottom deformity (**Figs. 1** and **2**). Pinzur[2] has reported that 60% of midfoot CN can be successfully managed with nonsurgical means. Although involvement of the ankle and hindfoot is less common, these proximal deformities are less well tolerated and more likely to require surgery.[1] CN has a major negative influence on the quality of life in patients with diabetes.[3,4] A study of 41 consecutive patients with CN reported lower Medical Outcome Study Short Form 36-item health survey (SF-36) component scores in physical functioning, social functioning, and general health perceptions compared with the general population and chronically ill control subjects, although the mental component scores did not seem to differ significantly.[3]

Brodsky and Rouse[5] proposed an anatomic classification of CN and described the following 4 types:

- Type 1 involves the tarsometatarsal and naviculocuneiform joints (60%)
- Type 2 involves the hindfoot (25%)
  - Subtalar joint
  - Talonavicular joint
  - Calcaneocuboid joint
- Type 3A involves the ankle (10%)
- Type 3B is a pathologic fracture of the calcaneal tuberosity (5%)

Another popular classification system by Sanders and Frykberg[6] is based on 5 anatomic sites of involvement and includes the following:

- Lisfranc (tarsometatarsal) joints (40%)
- Chopart (talonavicular and calcaneocuboid joints) and naviculocuneiform joint (30%)
- Forefoot (15%)
- Ankle joint (10%)
- Calcaneus (5%).

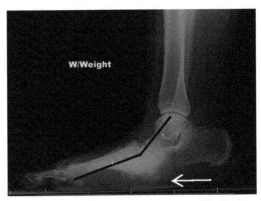

Fig. 1. Weight-bearing lateral foot radiograph of a patient with midfoot CN of the right foot. This radiograph demonstrates a typical "rocker bottom" deformity. The patient's heel is not touching the ground and his lateral talar first metatarsal angle is −38° (normal 0°). (*white arrow*) Plantar exostosis of the midfoot.

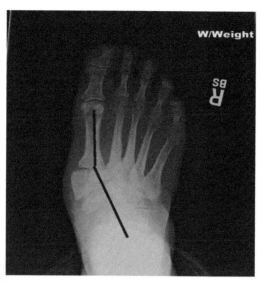

Fig. 2. Weight-bearing anterior/posterior radiograph of the patient in **Fig. 1**, demonstrating abduction of the forefoot in relationship to the midfoot and hindfoot. The AP talar first metatarsal demonstrates an abduction angle of 32° (normal 0°).

Eichenholtz[7] described a classification and staging system that is also commonly used to monitor the phases of healing by assessing radiographic and clinical signs of inflammation (**Table 1**). Proper staging and anatomic classification are used to guide the nonsurgical and surgical treatment algorithm of CN. The goals of treatment are to maintain a plantigrade foot that will allow weight-bearing, maintain ambulation, and remain free of ulceration. The treatment of stage 1 CN (destruction and inflammation) primarily involves offloading with a total contact cast, which helps to maintain alignment during the healing phase. As radiologic evidence of healing progresses and inflammation subsides, patients are transitioned into a removable prefabricated brace or a bivalved custom-molded polypropylene ankle-foot orthosis.[8] When radiographic evidence of healing is present and all signs of inflammation have resolved, the patient is transitioned to an accommodative shoe with a molded insole. Despite intensive treatment, up to 50% of patients may develop a deformity that requires some type of surgical treatment.

Table 1
Eichenholtz classification

	Skin Appearances	Bone (Radiographic)
Stage 0	Unilateral edema, erythema, and warm, intact skin	No or local osteoporosis
Stage I	Unilateral edema, erythema, and warmth	Osseous destruction, joint dislocation, or subluxation
Stage II	Decreased edema, erythema, and warmth	Coalescence of small fracture fragments and absorption of fine bone debris
Stage III	No edema, erythema, and warmth	Consolidation and remodeling of fracture fragments

Surgical treatment of CN should not be taken lightly despite the temptation to intervene early with the goal being to hasten the healing phase. Most surgeons prefer to delay surgery until inflammation subsides, although 2 small series have reported successful outcomes in patients with stage 1 CN.[9,10] The bone quality during the acute phase of CN often can be suboptimal due to osteoclastic resorption, making it difficult to obtain secure fixation and facilitation of bone healing. The rate of surgical complications is high due to comorbidities of DM, such as neuropathy, peripheral artery disease, and vitamin D deficiency.

No comparative studies have been performed evaluating the types of surgery, type of fixation, or whether surgery provides better outcomes than nonoperative treatment.[11] The decision to proceed with surgery is multifactorial and is typically influenced by patient comorbidities and compliance, deformity location and severity, and the presence of infection, ulcers, or instability. Lowery and colleagues[11] performed a systemic review that has summarized the literature of the past 50 years in a comprehensive manner. The authors noted that the literature on surgical management of CN comprises noncontrolled retrospective cases series, case reports, and expert opinion articles.

Lowery and colleagues[11] identified 96 papers that met the criteria for their review. The surgical procedures performed included drainage of infections, debridement of ulcers, exostectomy, arthrodesis, amputation, and a case report of total ankle replacement. Based on the systemic review, the authors made the following conclusions:

1. Surgical intervention during the acute phase of CN (stage 1) is encouraging, but the literature lacks controlled studies to support this. Therefore, the evidence for acute phase surgical intervention is inconclusive at this time.
2. The most common location requiring surgical intervention for Charcot patients is the midfoot (59%), and the second most common location is the ankle (29%).
3. Exostectomy is useful to relieve bony pressure that cannot be accommodated with orthotics and prosthetic means.
4. Lengthening of the Achilles tendon or gastrocnemius muscle reduces forefoot pressure and improves the alignment of the ankle and hindfoot relative to the midfoot and forefoot.
5. Forty-three of 54 studies included joint arthrodesis as a treatment option, either alone or in conjunction with another procedure. Arthrodesis is useful in patients with instability, pain, or recurrent ulcerations who fail nonoperative treatment. The literature demonstrates satisfactory results using arthrodesis despite a high rate of incomplete bony union.
6. Inconclusive data exist to recommend one form of fixation over another (ie, internal vs external) in the surgical reconstruction of the foot and ankle in patients who are not infected.

Future prospective randomized controlled studies or prospective series would constitute important contributions to the literature regarding the surgical management of Charcot foot. Although surgeons who reconstruct Charcot deformities may think that surgery is beneficial, no definitive conclusions can be made at this time with regard to the benefit of surgery, the timing of surgery, and the choice of surgical procedures.

STRATEGIES OF SURGICAL MANAGEMENT

Historically, foot and ankle surgery in patients with DM was only performed for infected foot ulcers and amputations. Surgeons who treat patients with DM have long recognized that these patients are more likely to experience wound-healing problems, surgical site infections, and nonunions than patients without DM, and many surgeons have avoided performing elective surgery in this high-risk group.[12–15] Over the past 15 years surgical management of CN has become more popular because of improved methods of fixation, aggressive vascular surgery, and better glycemic management. The decision for surgical intervention is multifactorial and is typically influenced by patient comorbidities and compliance, deformity location and severity, and the presence of infection, pain, or instability (**Box 1**). Proponents of surgical intervention cite lower risk of infection, less deconditioning of the patients, and lowering amputation rates, although these reasons are not supported by controlled studies.[16,17]

Surgical procedures can be categorized as ablative, curative, and prophylactic/reconstructive. Ablative procedures include amputation, drainage, and debridement of nonviable bone and soft tissue. Curative procedures mainly consist of exostectomy, which may be necessary when ulceration is caused by a bony prominence such a rocker bottom deformity of the midfoot. Prophylactic/reconstructive procedures include realignment osteotomies, tendon balancing procedures, and arthrodesis, often performed in combination. The primary goals of surgical treatment of neuropathic diabetic patients are to prevent ulceration, infection, and amputation by reducing pressure, re-creating anatomic alignment, and restoring foot stability.

TYPES OF SURGERY
Exostectomy

Total contact cast, total contact orthosis, and accommodative shoe wear have been used as nonsurgical measures to treat diabetic CN. When nonsurgical treatment fails to achieve ulcer healing, removal of bony prominences (exostectomy) can be useful. These prominences most commonly affect the midfoot and develop when the tarsal bones dislocate during stage 1 (see **Fig. 1**). Foot ulceration results when increased plantar pressure is applied to areas of the skin that do not customarily bear weight. Although both medial and lateral column exostectomy can be successful, medial column exostectomy may be more predictable.[16] Care must be taken to remove enough bone without causing iatrogenic instability. Limb-salvage rates of 90% have been reported with this technique, although revision surgery may be required in up to 25% of patients.[5,16,18] Exostectomy is usually most effective for Brodsky type 1 deformities, which involve the tarsometatarsal joints.[5] Soft tissue procedures including Achilles tendon lengthening should be combined with exostectomy for those patients who have concomitant recurrent plantar ulceration and equinus contracture.[19,20]

Arthrodesis

In deformities associated with instability and marked malalignment, arthrodesis and/or corrective osteotomy typically is necessary to achieve limb salvage. The selection of

Box 1
Indications for surgical management of CN
Pain not successfully managed by nonoperative therapy
Recurrent ulcer even initially healed with nonoperative treatment
Chronic deformity with increased plantar pressure and risk of ulceration
Significant deformity with secondary ulcer that failed nonoperative treatment
Significant chronic instability not amenable to brace or cast treatment

specific arthrodesis procedure depends on the location of the involved joints and surgeon preference. Deformities may be corrected acutely in a single stage or gradually over time using multiplane external fixation. In general, internal fixation devices (screws, plates, and intramedullary nails) are used in noninfected patients. Patients with active soft tissue or bone infection typically are treated with external fixation. In selected cases, internal and external fixation can be combined to increase stability of the construct. Although the specific duration of non-weight-bearing may vary based on surgeon preference, 3 months of non-weight-bearing is a reasonable timeframe to allow osseous healing and minimize hardware failure. The exact time to initiate weight-bearing should be guided by clinical signs of healing. Despite the tremendous advances achieved over the past decade, the complication rate of Charcot reconstruction remains relatively high.[12,14,15] Common complications include infection, recurrent ulceration, hardware failure, nonunion, and malunion.[12] Although bony union is desirable, a stable, fibrous union may result in patient satisfaction due to the absence of pain and the ability to brace the deformity. In the systematic review by Lowery and colleagues[11] an overall fusion rate of 76% was reported.

Amputation

Amputation is typically the last resort for patients who fail surgical reconstruction, particularly if infection cannot be eradicated. Saltzman and colleagues[21] reported a 2.7% annual rate of amputation in patients followed in a structured program, and nearly one-third of patients with CN who presented with a foot ulcer ultimately required a major amputation. Major amputations are associated increased mortality and impaired function, and despite advances in limb salvage techniques, some patients will ultimately require major amputation. Although amputation is often perceived as failure and associated with reduced quality of life, selected patients with infected, non-reconstructable deformities may benefit from major amputation.[22] Thirteen patients who underwent transtibial amputation for non-reconstructable CN were evaluated using the SF-36 and the Foot and Ankle Ability Measure.[22] The authors found significant improvement after transtibial amputation in the SF-36 Physical Component Summary score and the Foot and Ankle Ability Measurement (mean follow-up of 79 weeks). Although the SF-36 Mental Component Summary score improved, the improvement did not achieve statistical significance. Twelve of the 13 patients were satisfied with the amputation and had no reservations. Although loss of a limb is a devastating complication in patients with DM, this study provides some evidence for optimism in these high-risk patients. Preservation of limb length is preferable to reduce energy expenditure with future prosthesis usage and every attempt should be made to avoid a transfemoral amputation.

CONTROVERSIES REGARDING SURGICAL TREATMENT
Internal Versus External Fixation

Internal fixation devices, including plates, screws, and intramedullary nail constructs, have been widely used for osteotomies and arthrodesis with success. Over the past 10 to 15 years, external fixation has gained popularity as a less invasive surgical method in patients with foot deformity associated with CN. A distinct advance of external fixation is that it permits concurrent treatment of infection and deformity. Deformities can be acutely corrected during a single stage, allowing easy access to soft tissue wounds. Patients who have compromised soft tissue envelopes, poor bone quality, and morbid obesity may also benefit from the use of external fixation with limb salvage rates approaching 90%.[23–25] In the largest study of external fixation, 83 patients with

CN of the midfoot and hindfoot were definitively managed with external fixation achieving a limb salvage rate of 96%.[23] Three of the 83 patients required transtibial amputation because of uncontrolled infection or unstable pseudarthrosis. The use of external fixation in patients with diabetes is not without complications, and pin tract infections occur in nearly 100% of patients.[26]

Acute or Chronic Intervention

Traditionally, nonoperative treatment is regarded as the primary option of treatment, whereas surgery is reserved for those who fail nonoperative treatment. Surgical intervention during the acute stage to prevent further deformity remains controversial. Simon and colleagues[10] reported promising results with fusion during the stage I, although this study was small (14 patients) and lacked a control group. Another noncontrolled study retrospectively reviewed 22 patients (26 feet) who underwent primary surgical reconstruction and reorientation arthrodesis with encouraging results.[9]

CHALLENGES OF SURGERY
Surgical Site Infection

Patients with DM, particularly whose disease is poorly controlled, may have associated comorbid conditions that place them at increased risk for postoperative infections. A retrospective series of 1000 consecutive foot and ankle surgical cases compared the infection rate between patients with and without DM.[14] Significantly more infections occurred in individuals with DM (13.2%) than those without DM (2.8%). The findings of this retrospective study were validated in a prospective series that demonstrated a 2.4 times higher rate of surgical site infection rate in patients with CN.[15]

Vitamin D Deficiency

The importance of Vitamin D in bone metabolism is well known. In patients with DM, a lack of vitamin D may play an important role in the development of Charcot foot, as well as the bone healing and remodeling after surgical treatment of the Charcot foot. Yoho and colleagues[27] reported that serum 25-hydroxyvitamin D levels were significantly lower in patients with DM compared with patients without DM. Greenhagen and colleagues[28] found that the calcaneal bone mineral density of patients with diabetes and CN was significantly lower than a control group of patients without diabetes. Lumbar scores did not differ between these 2 groups, suggesting that patients with DM and CN have a regional reduction in bone mineral density as opposed to a systemic deficiency. Based on these studies, assessment of vitamin D levels and bone mineral density may provide additional input in planning reconstructive surgery in diabetic patients with CN.

Nonunion and Malunion

Nonunion and malunion are common complications associated with impaired bone and fracture healing in patients with DM.[12,13,29–31] Patients undergoing ankle fracture repair with complications of DM (neuropathy, peripheral artery disease, or renal disease) had a 3.4 times increased risk of a noninfectious complication (malunion, nonunion, or CN) and 5 times higher likelihood of needing revision surgery/arthrodesis when compared with patients with uncomplicated DM.[13] Patients with DM who undergo major arthrodesis have higher rates of nonunion than patients without DM, and both long-term and short-term glycemic control are important in avoiding noninfectious complications.[12]

Surgical repair of nonunions or malunions is indicated when those resultant deformities are unstable and unbraceable. Elective surgical repair in diabetic patients with peripheral artery disease should be delayed until evaluation and clearance by a vascular surgeon. Ideally, surgery should be performed after eradication of infection; however, in some cases this is not possible. When surgery is performed in patients with active infection, the use of external fixation is preferable and large internal fixation devices, such as plates and rods, should be avoided. The use of external fixation provides osseous stability while permitting access to wounds. External fixation can be used as a definitive or staged technique, allowing for concurrent treatment of bone deformity and infection. Regardless of what method of fixation is used, the goals of surgery are to restore stability and anatomic alignment, eradicate infection, improve pain, heal ulcers, and reduce abnormal pressures.

Despite advances in surgical techniques, nonunion and malunion remain difficult problems for surgeons who treat CN. At a mean follow-up of 52 months, Sammarco and colleagues[32] achieved complete osseous union in 16 of the 22 patients (73%), whereas 6 patients (27%) had incomplete or no healing. This small series is consistent with the results of the systematic review, which found a union rate of 76%.[11] A retrospective study of 154 arthrodesis patients that compared patients with and without DM found that patients with DM had significantly higher rates of noninfectious complications.[12]

SUMMARY

Many surgical and nonsurgical options exist with the aim of improving quality of life and preventing amputation in patients with CN. A multidisciplinary approach is necessary to achieve the best outcomes in this high-risk group. Modern advanced diagnostic and imaging techniques have improved knowledge regarding the biomechanics, biology, and pathophysiology of CN. Despite these advances, surgical management has lagged behind and is based largely on retrospective case series and expert opinion. Although the surgeons of today are better equipped to manage CN, the optimal timing and specific method of surgical treatment have yet to be defined. Multicenter, prospective studies may be the best way to study this relatively uncommon problem.

REFERENCES

1. Rogers LC, Frykberg RG, Armstrong DG, et al. The Charcot foot in diabetes. Diabetes Care 2011;34(9):2123–9.
2. Pinzur M. Surgical versus accommodative treatment for Charcot arthropathy of the midfoot. Foot Ankle Int 2004;25(8):545–9.
3. Pakarinen TK, Laine HJ, Maenpaa H, et al. Long-term outcome and quality of life in patients with Charcot foot. Foot Ankle Surg 2009;15(4):187–91.
4. Sochocki MP, Verity S, Atherton PJ, et al. Health related quality of life in patients with Charcot arthropathy of the foot and ankle. Foot Ankle Surg 2008;14(1):11–5.
5. Brodsky JW, Rouse AM. Exostectomy for symptomatic bony prominences in diabetic charcot feet. Clin Orthop Relat Res 1993;(296):21–6.
6. Sanders LI, Frykberg RG. The Charcot foot. In: Bowker JH, Pfeifer MA, editors. Levin and O'Neal's the diabetic foot. 7th edition. Philadelphia: Mosby Elsevier; 2007. p. 258.
7. Eichenholtz S. Charcot joints. Springfield: CC Thomas; 1966.
8. Verity S, Sochocki M, Embil JM, et al. Treatment of Charcot foot and ankle with a prefabricated removable walker brace and custom insole. Foot Ankle Surg 2008; 14(1):26–31.

9. Mittlmeier T, Klaue K, Haar P, et al. Should one consider primary surgical reconstruction in charcot arthropathy of the feet? Clin Orthop Relat Res 2010;468(4): 1002–11.
10. Simon SR, Tejwani SG, Wilson DL, et al. Arthrodesis as an early alternative to nonoperative management of charcot arthropathy of the diabetic foot. J Bone Joint Surg Am 2000;82(7):939–50.
11. Lowery NJ, Woods JB, Armstrong DG, et al. Surgical management of Charcot neuroarthropathy of the foot and ankle: a systematic review. Foot Ankle Int 2012;33(2):113–21.
12. Myers TG, Lowery NJ, Frykberg RG, et al. Ankle and hindfoot fusions: comparison of outcomes in patients with and without diabetes. Foot Ankle Int 2012;33(1): 20–8.
13. Wukich DK, Joseph A, Ryan M, et al. Outcomes of ankle fractures in patients with uncomplicated versus complicated diabetes. Foot Ankle Int 2011;32(2):120–30.
14. Wukich DK, Lowery NJ, McMillen RL, et al. Postoperative infection rates in foot and ankle surgery: a comparison of patients with and without diabetes mellitus. J Bone Joint Surg Am 2010;92(2):287–95.
15. Wukich DK, McMillen RL, Lowery NJ, et al. Surgical site infections after foot and ankle surgery: a comparison of patients with and without diabetes. Diabetes Care 2011;34(10):2211–3.
16. Catanzariti AR, Mendicino R, Haverstock B. Ostectomy for diabetic neuroarthropathy involving the midfoot. J Foot Ankle Surg 2000;39(5):291–300.
17. Henke PK, Blackburn SA, Wainess RW, et al. Osteomyelitis of the foot and toe in adults is a surgical disease: conservative management worsens lower extremity salvage. Ann Surg 2005;241(6):885–92 [discussion: 892–4].
18. Rosenblum BI, Giurini JM, Miller LB, et al. Neuropathic ulcerations plantar to the lateral column in patients with Charcot foot deformity: a flexible approach to limb salvage. J Foot Ankle Surg 1997;36(5):360–3.
19. Armstrong DG, Stacpoole-Shea S, Nguyen H, et al. Lengthening of the Achilles tendon in diabetic patients who are at high risk for ulceration of the foot. J Bone Joint Surg Am 1999;81(4):535–8.
20. Mueller MJ, Sinacore DR, Hastings MK, et al. Effect of Achilles tendon lengthening on neuropathic plantar ulcers. A randomized clinical trial. J Bone Joint Surg Am 2003;85(8):1436–45.
21. Saltzman CL, Hagy ML, Zimmerman B, et al. How effective is intensive nonoperative initial treatment of patients with diabetes and Charcot arthropathy of the feet? Clin Orthop Relat Res 2005;(435):185–90.
22. Wukich DK, Pearson KT. Self-reported outcomes of trans-tibial amputations for non-reconstructable Charcot neuroarthropathy in patients with diabetes: a preliminary report. Diabet Med 2013;30(3):e87–90.
23. Cooper PS. Application of external fixators for management of Charcot deformities of the foot and ankle. Foot Ankle Clin 2002;7(1):207–54.
24. Fabrin J, Larsen K, Holstein PE. Arthrodesis with external fixation in the unstable or misaligned Charcot ankle in patients with diabetes mellitus. Int J Low Extrem Wounds 2007;6(2):102–7.
25. Farber DC, Juliano PJ, Cavanagh PR, et al. Single stage correction with external fixation of the ulcerated foot in individuals with Charcot neuroarthropathy. Foot Ankle Int 2002;23(2):130–4.
26. Wukich DK, Belczyk RJ, Burns PR, et al. Complications encountered with circular ring fixation in persons with diabetes mellitus. Foot Ankle Int 2008;29(10): 994–1000.

27. Yoho RM, Frerichs J, Dodson NB, et al. A comparison of vitamin D levels in nondiabetic and diabetic patient populations. J Am Podiatr Med Assoc 2009;99(1):35–41.
28. Greenhagen RM, Wukich DK, Jung RH, et al. Peripheral and central bone mineral density in Charcot's neuroarthropathy compared in diabetic and nondiabetic populations. J Am Podiatr Med Assoc 2012;102(3):213–22.
29. Prisk VR, Wukich DK. Ankle fractures in diabetics. Foot Ankle Clin 2006;11(4):849–63.
30. Wukich DK, Kline AJ. The management of ankle fractures in patients with diabetes. J Bone Joint Surg Am 2008;90(7):1570–8.
31. Wukich DK, Shen JY, Ramirez CP, et al. Retrograde ankle arthrodesis using an intramedullary nail: a comparison of patients with and without diabetes mellitus. Foot Ankle Surg 2011;50(3):299–306.
32. Sammarco VJ, Sammarco GJ, Walker EW Jr, et al. Midtarsal arthrodesis in the treatment of Charcot midfoot arthropathy. J Bone Joint Surg Am 2009;91(1):80–91.

Topical and Biologic Therapies for Diabetic Foot Ulcers

Nicholas A. Richmond, BS, Alejandra C. Vivas, MD,
Robert S. Kirsner, MD, PhD*

KEYWORDS

- Diabetic foot ulcers • Wound care • Topical antiseptics • Biologic therapies

KEY POINTS

- Cadexomer iodine and silver-based dressings have broad-spectrum antimicrobial activity and have been shown to be effective in reducing bacterial bioburden with decreased rates of bacterial resistance and contact sensitivity.
- Advanced dressings containing extracellular matrix components reduce inflammatory cytokines and proteolytic enzymes while increasing the presence of growth factors, leading to decreased degradation of existing matrix and increased formation of new collagen and granulation tissue.
- Advanced biologic therapies should be considered for recalcitrant diabetic ulcers that fail to improve with standard of care over a period of 4 weeks. Combination of these therapies with standard of care is superior to standard of care alone.

INTRODUCTION

Healing of neuropathic diabetic foot ulcers (DFUs) is a challenge and in control groups of randomized control trials in which standard-of-care treatment alone is performed, healing rates remain low, approximately 30% at 20 weeks of care.[1] For this reason management of DFUs requires a systematic approach to achieve more successful outcomes and ultimately avoid amputations.

The foundation of the treatment of DFUs includes restitution of skin perfusion if peripheral arterial disease is coexistent, offloading of the affected foot, infection control, and good wound care. Most importantly, assuring adequate blood flow and providing offloading are critical as they provide for proper oxygen delivery and redistribution of the pressure in the plantar aspect of the foot.

Good wound care includes debridement, use of appropriate dressings, and topical antimicrobials when needed. Dressings should aim to achieve a moist wound

Department of Dermatology and Cutaneous Surgery, University of Miami Miller School of Medicine, Miami, FL, USA
* Corresponding author. University of Miami Miller School of Medicine, 1600 Northwest 10th Avenue, RMSB, Room 2023-A, Miami, FL 33136.
E-mail address: rkirsner@med.miami.edu

Med Clin N Am 97 (2013) 883–898
http://dx.doi.org/10.1016/j.mcna.2013.03.014
0025-7125/13/$ – see front matter © 2013 Elsevier Inc. All rights reserved.

environment that promotes healing and reduces excessive bacterial bioburden. Wound type, location, amount of exudate, and history of allergic reaction should be considered when choosing a dressing. For large exudative wounds, dressings with high absorbency properties may be more appropriate but dry wounds may need the addition of moisture through hydrogels, hydrocolloids, or nonabsorbent dressings. More advanced dressings containing collagen and other extracellular matrix proteins are sometimes required to reduce the effects of an exaggerated inflammatory state that has been associated with chronic wounds.

Despite good wound care and the use of sophisticated dressings, many DFUs remain difficult to heal; therefore, the need for progressive adjuvant therapies, including growth factors and cellular therapies in addition to standard of care practices, exists. Several recent advancements in this field have been reported to improve healing rates. Herein, the topical and biologic therapies for DFUs are reviewed (**Table 1**).

TREATMENT OF DFUS WITH TOPICAL ANTISEPTICS

DFUs are particularly prone to infection, often resulting in severe complications. In addition to overt infection, it is thought that in some cases even lower levels of bacteria may impede wound healing as well. Although all DFUs are colonized by bacteria, it is not until they reach a "critical mass" that delayed healing is thought to occur. Several studies have shown high bacterial loads, ranging from 10^5 to 10^6 CFU/mL of wound fluid, are predictive of poor healing.[2–5] Polymicrobial colonization of chronic wounds may have a negative impact as well, with studies suggesting the presence of 4 or more bacterial species is associated with nonhealing.[6,7] Current DFU guidelines recommend the prompt use of systemic antibiotics for the treatment of acute infection and suggest the use of topical antimicrobial agents to combat heavy colonization.

As a result of the concern related to wound bioburden, topical treatments aimed at reducing the bacterial load of DFUs have gained favor. Although various products are currently on the market, there is a paucity of high-quality evidence supporting their use. Antiseptics may be preferable to topical antibiotics because of decreased rates of bacterial resistance and contact sensitivity.[8] Two of the most commonly used products include cadexomer iodine and silver-based dressings.

Cadexomer Iodine

Cadexomer iodine consists of 0.9% iodine coupled to a water-soluble polysaccharide complex, commercially available as gel or dressing designed to absorb wound exudate, while simultaneously releasing iodine in a delayed manner. The slow release of iodine is intended to kill bacteria without causing harm to the wound bed. Although previous investigations of iodine-containing solutions showed in vitro and in vivo toxicity to skin cells,[9,10] a study specifically evaluating cadexomer iodine found it to be nontoxic in vitro to human fibroblasts.[11] Cadexomer iodine has been associated with lower treatment costs than standard care[12] and its antimicrobial effects have been well demonstrated. In a pig model, daily application of cadexomer iodine significantly reduced methicillin-resistant *Staphylococcus aureus* and total bacteria colonization of acute partial thickness wounds.[13] In addition, in a recent 6-week prospective, noncomparative, multicenter study evaluating the effect of cadexomer iodine on the diabetic foot ulcers, Schwartz and colleagues[14] found a significant reduction in bacterial counts at weeks 3 and 6, in addition to a 53.6% median reduction in wound surface area. Although no randomized controlled trials (RTC) have shown improved rates of DFU healing, accelerated rates of epithelialization in venous leg ulcers (VLU) and pressure ulcers have been reported.[15–18]

Table 1
Level of evidence supporting topical and advanced biologic therapies for DFUs

Therapy	Reference	Study Type	Clinical Outcomes
Cadexomer iodine	Mertz et al,[13] 1999	Pig model (acute partial thickness wounds)	Daily application significantly reduced MRSA and total bacteria colonization at 24, 48, and 72 h as compared with both air-exposed control and cadexomer (vehicle) dressing ($P<.004$, $P<.003$).
	Schwartz et al,[14] 2013	Prospective, noncomparative, multicenter study	Significant reduction in bacterial counts at weeks 3 and 6, in addition to a 53.6% median reduction in wound surface area over 6 wk.
Silver containing dressings	Rayman et al,[21] 2005	Prospective, noncomparative study	18 DFU were treated for 4 wk. The mean relative ulcer area reduction was 56%, which translates into weekly healing rate of 3.6% and weekly ulcer area reduction of 14% silver-containing nonadhesive dressing showed good exudates control. Only 2 infections occurred among study ulcers compared with all 6 nonstudy ulcers that became infected.
	Jude et al,[22] 2007	Prospective, multicenter, RCT	Mean time to healing was not statistically different between groups. However, silver-containing hydrofiber dressing–treated ulcers had significantly greater reduction in depth as compared with calcium alginate treated ulcers (0.25 cm vs 0.13 cm; $P = .04$).
Collagen/oxidize regenerated cellulose dressing	Veves et al,[24] 2002	Prospective, multicenter, RCT	In patients with ulcers of less than 6-mo duration, 45% of treatment patients achieved complete healing compared with 33% of controls (standard of care) at 12 wk ($P = .056$). Patients' rating of collagen/oxidized regenerated cellulose dressing was significantly higher ($P = .01$).
	Kakagia et al,[25] 2007	Prospective randomized trial	51 patients were randomized to receive collagen/oxidized regenerated cellulose dressing, autologous growth factors, or both. At 8 weeks, the group receiving the combination of treatments had significantly greater reduction in ulcer size than either treatment alone ($P<.001$).
SIS wound matrix	Niezgoda et al,[28] 2005	Prospective, multicenter, randomized trial	At 12 wk of treatment, 49% of SIS wound matrix-treated patients had achieved complete wound closure compared with 28% of rhPDGF-treated patients ($P = .055$).

(continued on next page)

Table 1
(continued)

Therapy	Reference	Study Type	Clinical Outcomes
Bovine bilayer acellular matrix	Iorio et al,[30] 2011	Retrospective review	Of the 59 diabetic wounds that were identified as being at low risk for amputation, 49 (83%) resulted in healing and preservation of limb length. Of the 28 diabetic wounds that were deemed as high risk for amputation, only 13 (46%) resulted in healing and preservation of limb length.
	Clerici et al,[31] 2010	Prospective, noncomparative study	30 patients with surgical DFUs with exposed tendon/bone received bilayer acellular matrix before skin grafting instead of primary wound closure with proximal amputation. Complete wound healing occurred in 26 (86.7%) of patients and the amputation level was significantly more distal (P<.003) than otherwise indicated.
Human acellular dermal regenerative tissue matrix	Winters et al,[32] 2008	Retrospective, noncomparative, multicenter study	Healing rate of 90% was achieved after a single application of the human acellular dermal regenerative tissue matrix. The median time to complete healing was 11 wk.
	Reyzelman et al,[33] 2009	Prospective, multicenter, RCT	At 12 wk, Graftjacket achieved a higher rate of complete healing and a shorter mean time to healing than standard of care (69.6%/5.7 wk and 46.2%/6.8 wk, respectively). After adjusting for initial ulcer size, rate of healing was superior to control (P = .0233).
HYAFF 11-based autologous dermal and epidermal grafts	Caravaggi et al,[34] 2003	Prospective, multicenter, RCT	At 11 wk, the dorsal diabetic foot ulcer healing rate was significantly higher in the treatment group (67% vs 31%, P = .049). However, plantar ulcers failed to show a statistically significant difference.
	Uccioli et al,[35] 2011	Prospective, multicenter, RCT	At 12 wk, complete ulcer healing was not statistically significantly different (24% of treated vs 21% controls). However, time to achieve 50% reduction in ulcer area was significantly faster in the treatment group (P = .018). At 20 wk, dorsal ulcers had a 2-fold better chance of wound healing per unit time following autograft treatment (P = .047). In a subgroup of dorsal hard-to-heal ulcers, there was a 3.65-fold better chance of wound healing following autograft treatment of dorsal ulcers (P = .035).
Bilayered human skin equivalent	Veves et al,[40] 2001	Prospective, multicenter, RCT	At 12 wk, 56% (63/112) of treatment group patients achieved complete wound healing compared with 38% (36/96) of the control group (P = .0042). The Kaplan-Meier median time to complete healing was significantly less in the treatment group as well (65 vs 90 d, P = .0026).
	Edmonds et al,[41] 2009	Prospective, multicenter, RCT	At 12 wk, 51.5% (17/33) of subjects receiving the bilayered human skin equivalent had achieved complete wound closure compared with 26.3% (10/38) of the control group (P = .049). The median time to healing for the treatment group was 84 d, however was indeterminate for the control group.

	Study	Study type	Findings
Dermal skin substitute	Marston et al,[44] 2003	Prospective, multicenter, RCT	At 12 wk, weekly application of the dermal skin substitute produced significantly higher healing rates than control in patients with DFUs >6 wk duration (30% vs 18%, $P = .023$). The treatment group also achieved a significantly faster time to complete wound healing ($P = .04$) and registered a higher median percent wound closure at week 12 (91% vs 78%, $P = .044$).
Recombinant human platelet-derived growth factor (rhPDGF)	Bhansali et al,[48] 2009	Prospective RCT	Patients (n = 20) were randomized to receive either daily application of 0.01% rhPDGF-BB or moist saline dressings, in addition to offloading using a modified total contact cast. By 20 wk, both groups had achieved 100% wound closure. The mean time to complete healing was significantly faster in the treatment group (50.1 vs 86.1 d, $P = .02$).
	Wieman et al,[49] 1998	Prospective, multicenter, double-blind RCT	By 20 wk, Becaplermin gel (100 μg/g) significantly increased the incidence of complete wound closure (50 vs 35%, $P = .007$) and decreased the time to achieve complete wound closure (86 vs 127 d, $P = .013$) as compared with placebo gel.
	Steed et al,[36] 2006	Prospective, multicenter, RCT	Over 20 wk, 48% (29/61) of patients randomized to the rhPDGF-BB group achieved complete wound healing compared with only 25% (14/57) of placebo group patients ($P = .01$). The median reduction in wound area was not statistically different between the groups.
	Margolis et al,[51] 2005	Retrospective cohort study	In a review of 24,898 patients with DFUs, 9.6% were noted to have received rhPDGF. rhPDGF was found to be effective with respect to wound healing (RR = 1.32) and the prevention of amputation (RR = 0.65).
Platelet-rich plasma derivatives	Driver et al,[62] 2006	Prospective, multicenter, randomized, double-blind RCT	In a per protocol analysis, after adjusting for wound size, the group receiving platelet-rich plasma gel yielded a significantly higher wound healing rate (81.3%, 13/16 vs 42.1%, 8/19) than the group receiving control gel ($P = .036$). Time-to-healing was significantly faster for the treatment group as well ($P = .0177$).
	Saad Setta et al,[63] 2011	Prospective, RCT	The mean time to healing was significantly faster for the platelet-rich plasma group than the platelet-poor plasma group (11.5 vs 17.1 wk, $P<.005$). The number of patients achieving complete healing by 20 wk did not significantly differ between the groups (12/12, PRP; 9/12, PPP).
	de Leon et al,[64] 2011	Prospective case series	In 285 chronic wounds receiving PRP gel, a positive response (decrease in wound area, volume, or length of undermining, sinus tracts, or tunneling) occurred in 96.5% of wounds in a mean time of 2.2 wk and mean of 2.8 treatments.
	Margolis et al,[37] 2001	Retrospective cohort study	Patients treated with platelet releasate were more likely to heal than those receiving standard care at a wound care center (RR 1.14-1.59). The effect was even more pronounced in patients with severe wounds.

Abbreviations: MRSA, methicillin-resistant *Staphylococcus aureus*; PPP, platelet-poor plasma.

Silver-Containing Dressings

Silver has long been used as a topical agent for the treatment of both acute and chronic wounds. Silver-based antiseptics have demonstrated broad-spectrum activity and have been shown to be effective at killing antibiotic-resistant bacteria.[19,20] Dressings designed to maintain a moist wound environment and absorb large amounts of exudate, while providing the antimicrobial properties of silver, may be particularly useful for DFUs. Although the intended use of the silver within dressings is to reduce bioburden in the dressing, a benefit to the wound bed is also expected. Recently, a silver-releasing foam dressing was evaluated for the treatment of DFUs and found to be safe and supportive of healing.[21] An RCT found hydrofiber dressing containing ionic silver to be significantly better at reducing DFU depth than calcium alginate dressings.[22]

USE OF ADVANCED ACELLULAR DRESSINGS

The extracellular matrix (ECM) plays a critical role in tissue repair. During the normal wound-healing process, ECM serves as a scaffold that facilitates cell migration and interaction, with the capability of modulating cellular behavior.[23] In chronic wounds, often because of high wound proteases, ECM is damaged or deficient. In the wake of research stressing its importance, multiple products have been developed to mimic the structure and composition of ECM. Advanced dressings made of collagen, glycosaminoglycans, oxidized regenerated cellulose, and hyaluronic acid among others provide matrices and scaffolds and may decrease the chronic inflammatory state of the wound by absorbing excess proteolytic enzymes, such as matrix metalloproteinases, leading to decreased degradation and increased formation of new collagen and granulation tissue. In addition, reduction of proteolytic enzymes may increase the presence of growth factors, conceivably leading to an improved pro-healing state.[24]

Collagen/Oxidized Regenerated Cellulose Dressing

Collagen/oxidized regenerated cellulose dressing (*Promogran*; Systagenix Wound Management, Quincy, MA, USA), a composite of a sterile, freeze-dried oxidized regenerated cellulose (ORC) and collagen, is indicated for the management of exudating wounds. Although an RCT evaluating its use for DFUs concluded that while higher rates of complete healing were achieved in ulcers of less than 6 months' duration, the difference was not statistically significant. However, greater patient satisfaction was noted.[24] In addition, collagen/ORC dressing may act synergistically with autologous growth factors to accelerate DFU healing.[25] The collagen/ORC dressing can also be with impregnated silver (Prisma; Systagenix Wound Management), which has been reported to reduce both wound size and inflammatory cytokine and protease levels significantly.[26]

Small Intestine Submucosa

Small intestine submucosa (SIS; Oasis Wound Matrix; Healthpoint Biotherapeutics, Fort Worth, TX, USA) wound matrix is an acellular biomaterial derived from porcine small intestine submucosa, consisting mainly of type I, III, IV, and V collagen.[27] Results from a randomized, prospective, controlled multicenter trial found SIS wound matrix noninferior to Becaplermin (rhPDGF) at healing diabetic foot ulcers by 12 weeks.[28]

Bilayer Acellular Matrix

Bilayer acellular matrix (Integra; Integra LifeSciences, Plainsboro, NJ, USA) was United States Food and Drug Administration (FDA) approved in 1996 for the treatment of life-threatening burn injuries. More recently the FDA has approved its use for a wide range of reconstructive applications including VLU, degloving injuries, and scar contractures. The bilayer, acellular matrix is a dermal replacement layer composed of cross-linked collagen and glycosaminoglycans, such as chondroitin sulfate, that act as a scaffold for regenerating dermal skin cells and inducing the signaling cascade that prompts angiogenesis, cellular migration, and collagen remodeling. The top layer is a temporary epidermal substitute that is made of silicone and functions to control fluid loss and serve as a bacterial barrier. Once dermal skin has regenerated, the silicone outer layer is removed and for larger wounds it can be replaced with an epidermal skin graft.[29] Recent case reports of the use of dermal substitutes to cover the exposed tendons and bones in diabetic feet have been reported with good healing and preservation of stump length.

A retrospective review of 105 patients who underwent application of Integra for DFUs reported its successful use in limb salvage in patients at low risk for amputation. In patients at higher risk for amputation, 46% of limbs were salvaged.[30] In another study, surgical debridement of acutely infected diabetic foot ulcers with exposed tendon/bone was followed by coverage with the bilayer acellular matrix. After 21 days, a skin graft was performed. Complete wound healing occurred in 86.7% of patients. In these patients, the amputation level was significantly more distal ($P<.003$) than what would have otherwise been required for immediate wound closure.[31]

Integra in the management of exposed tendon and bone tissues following treatment of deep wound infections in patients with diabetes allowed timely wound healing and preserved maximal foot length. This collagen bilayer matrix seems to offer stable coverage in the appropriately selected DFUs, promoting healing over exposed tendon/bone, and may be beneficial in preventing further patient morbidity or limb loss.

Human Acellular Dermal Regenerative Tissue Matrix

Human Acellular Dermal Regenerative Tissue Matrix (GraftJacket; Wright Medical Technology, Inc, Arlington, TN, USA), a dermal tissue matrix derived from processed decellularized cadaveric dermis, is intended to provide scaffolding for epidermal migration and revascularization of chronic wounds. Full-thickness debridement before suturing or stapling the product to the wound bed is generally recommended. Clinical trials have demonstrated human acellular dermal regenerative tissue matrix is well-tolerated and have supported its use for DFUs. In an open-label experience, for chronic, full-thickness, diabetic lower extremity wounds for which conservative treatment had failed, the use of human acellular dermal matrix resulted in a healing rate of 90% with only a single application.[32] The median time to complete healing was 11 weeks. In a 12-week, prospective, multicenter RCT of DFUs, Graftjacket achieved a higher rate of complete healing and a shorter mean time to healing than standard of care (69.6%/5.7 weeks and 46.2%/6.8 weeks, respectively). After adjusting for initial ulcer size, rate of healing was superior to control ($P = .0233$).[33]

Hyaff-11

Hyaff-11 (VLA Health Care, Berkshire, UK) is a novel hyaluronan-based biomaterial composed of a benzyl ester of hyaluronic acid. Following degradation, the dressing releases a high concentration of hyaluronic acid into the wound. Obtained in several different morphologies (ie, sponges, fibers, threads, and microfibers), Hyaff is biodegradable and bioabsorbable. It serves as a biologic scaffold for many cellular transplants, including human vascular endothelial cells, autologous chondrocytes, mesenchymal stem cells, fibroblasts, and keratinocytes. Hyalomatrix (Anika Therapeutics, Bedford, MA, USA), which is a tridimensional Hyaff matrix, is currently being used for the management of chronic wounds, including DFUs. Hyaff has also been recently used as a scaffold to grow cultured expanded autologous fibroblasts (Hyalograft 3D autograft; Anika Therapeutics) and cultured expanded autologous keratinocytes (Laserskin autograft; Anika Therapeutics) for the treatment of wounds. Cells are obtained from the individual's skin through a biopsy specimen.

An RCT conducted by Caravaggi and colleagues[34] compared treatment with Hyalograft-3D autograft followed by Laserskin autograft with standard care in 82 patients with DFUs. The study demonstrated a significantly higher rate of healing for dorsal ulcers; however, it failed to do so for plantar ulcers. Adverse events were equally distributed between the study groups and determined to be unrelated to the treatment.

In a larger scale study with long-term follow-up of patients with plantar and dorsal DFUs, subjects were randomized to control, consisting of nonadherent paraffin gauze, or dermal tissue engineered autografts followed by an epidermal autograft 2 weeks later. Standard of care was provided to both groups. At 12 weeks, complete ulcer healing was not statistically significantly different (24% of treated vs 21% controls).[35] However, time to achieve 50% reduction in ulcer area was significantly faster in the treatment group ($P = .018$). Similar to conclusions drawn by Caravaggi and colleagues, dorsal ulcers benefitted from treatment as well. At 20 weeks, dorsal ulcers had a 2-fold better chance of wound healing per unit time following autograft treatment ($P = .047$). In a subgroup of dorsal hard-to-heal ulcers, there was a 3.65-fold better chance of wound healing following autograft treatment of dorsal ulcers ($P = .035$). This study suggested that the dermal/epidermal autografting using the Hyaff scaffold is potentially useful in patients with hard-to-heal diabetic dorsal ulcers.

ADVANCED BIOLOGIC THERAPIES

The use of advanced adjuvant therapies is currently included in treatment algorithms for DFUs.[36] Among DFUs receiving standard care only for a period of 4 weeks, those wounds that did not reduce in size by more than 53% were found to have decreased likelihood of healing at 12 weeks. The Wound Healing Society recommends changing the therapy and/or adding adjuvant treatments if the wound size reduction is not significant (<50%) over that timeframe (4 weeks) using standard of care[36] because the longer a wound is open, the greater the risk of wound infection, osteomyelitis, and ultimately, amputation. For these recalcitrant ulcers, the use of topical therapies including biologic treatments, such as bioengineered cell-based therapies, recombinant growth factors, and platelet-rich plasma, among others, may be necessary to stimulate healing, prevent limb loss, and improve quality of life for patients.

The gold standards of the biologic therapies for DFUs are 2 cell-based therapy products (bioengineered skin equivalent and dermal substitute) and the recombinant platelet-derived growth factor given the high level of evidence that support their use.

Randomized controlled trials have demonstrated that advanced biologic therapies in combination with standard care including offloading and debridement lead to improved healing of DFUs compared with standard care alone.[37]

It has been shown that regardless of the advanced biologic therapy used, larger wounds, more severe wound grades, longer duration, and prolonged time to treatment with advanced biologic therapies were significantly associated with longer time to healing.[38]

Allogeneic Bilayered Human Skin Equivalent

Approved by the FDA for VLU and neuropathic DFUs in 2000, allogeneic bilayered human skin equivalent (Apligraf; Organogenesis Inc, Canton, MA, USA), a bilayered tissue-engineered product, consists of a bovine collagen matrix with neonatal fibroblasts, overlaid by a stratified epithelium containing living keratinocytes. It is devoid of blood vessels, hair follicles, sweat glands, or other cell types, such as Langerhan cells, melanocytes, macrophages, or lymphocytes.[39] It has been shown that the fibroblasts produce matrix proteins and all cytokines and growth factors that are produced by autologous skin during the healing process.

In an RTC of up to 5 weekly applications of bilayered human skin equivalent in patients with chronic plantar DFUs, the treatment group achieved a significantly higher healing rate ($P = .0042$) and shorter time to complete closure ($P = .0026$) than those receiving standard of care.[40]

In another RCT comparing the efficacy of this product plus standard of care versus standard care alone in the treatment of neuropathic DFUs, results showed higher incidence of wound closure by 12 weeks ($P = .049$) and shorter time to complete wound healing in the Apligraf group compared with the standard therapy group ($P = .059$).[41]

The persistence of the bilayered cultured skin equivalent is limited as its DNA is present only in a minority of wounds at week 4. Therefore it is thought that the positive effect on wound healing is related to the expression of growth factors and cytokines provided by the transient presence of the allogeneic cells and interact with the host cells.[42]

Based on the hypothesis that cells in chronic wounds are "stalled" or inactive and incapable of entering into an activation cycle, researchers think that Apligraf can reverse this process.

Ongoing research is using microarray technology to identify and characterize the molecular mechanisms through which Apligraf promotes healing of VLU. Understanding molecular impairments in nonhealing wounds and the mechanism through which Apligraf successfully promotes healing will promote and expand its clinical use, bringing cell-based therapy to a different level.

Dermal Skin Substitute

Approved by the FDA in 2001 for the treatment of DFUs, dermal skin substitute (Dermagraft Advanced Tissue Sciences, La Jolla, CA, USA), a human fibroblast-derived dermal substitute overlies a bioabsorbable polyglactin mesh scaffold. The mesh material is biodegradable and the human cells produce human dermal collagen, matrix proteins, growth factors, and cytokines, which help rebuild the damaged tissue. Dermagraft does not contain macrophages, lymphocytes, blood vessels, or hair follicles. It is indicated for full-thickness DFUs that have been present for longer than 6 weeks, not involving tendon, muscle, joint capsule, or bone.[43]

In a large, phase 3 RCT, weekly application of the dermal skin substitute produced significantly higher healing rates than control in patients with DFUs of greater than 6 weeks' duration (30% vs 18%, $P = .023$). The treatment group also achieved a significantly faster time to complete wound healing ($P = .04$) and registered a higher median percentage wound closure at week 12 (91% vs 78%, $P = .044$). Dermagraft-treated patients were 1.7 times more likely to have complete wound closure at any given time than were the control patients, respectively.[44] Ulcer-related adverse events were significantly lower in the Dermagraft-treated group.

Before application with human fibroblast–derived dermal substitute, wounds must be extensively debrided to arrive at healthy tissue.[45]

rhPDGF

In chronic DFUs, the healing process is impaired in part because of an abnormal expression and release of growth factors, which may be sequestered and unable to perform their metabolic roles, or excessively degraded by cellular or bacterial proteases. Becaplermin (Regranex; Healthpoint Biotherapeutics) is a recombinant PDGF that is produced by incorporation of the gene for the B-chain of human PDGF into the yeast *Saccharomyces cerevisiae*.[46] The resultant product is a protein composed of 2 identical polypeptide chains that has biologic activities similar to endogenous PDGF, which promotes wound healing by chemotactic recruitment and proliferation of cells, including fibroblasts, smooth muscle cells, and endothelial cells, and also induces angiogenesis and production of fibronectin and hyaluronic acid.[47] Becaplermin is commercially available as a gel and is the only FDA-approved and European Medicines Agency–approved growth factor for use in the management of DFUs that extend through the dermis into subcutaneous tissue in patients with adequate arterial perfusion.

RCTs have provided evidence for the efficacy of becaplermin, indicating increased rates of complete healing and faster times to complete closure of DFUs. Cost analyses have repeatedly shown a favorable cost-effectiveness ratio as well.[48–50]

Pivotal trials have shown that at week 20, 35% more ulcers healed in the group receiving rhPDGF than in the group receiving standard of care. Effectiveness data support its benefit as well. In a retrospective cohort study, of 24,898 individuals with a DFU, 9.6% received rhPDGF. The relative risk for undergoing amputation after receiving rhPDGF was 0.65 (0.54, 0.78) as compared with those who did not receive rhPDGF. This research suggests rhPDGF to be more effective than standard therapy in healing and preventing amputation.[51]

The formulation of Becaplermin is a preserved gel for topical use that contains 100 μg becaplermin per gram of gel. Of concern, endogenous PDGF has been found to stimulate tumor-infiltrating fibroblasts found in human melanoma cells[52] and is overexpressed in all stages of human astrocytoma growth.[53] This information led to the hypothesis that, although systemic absorption is minimal, it would be biologically possible that topical administration of recombinant PDGF could promote cancer.[54] In addition, based on the results of 2 studies that reported an overall increase in incidence of new cancer and mortality rate secondary to malignancy in becaplermin-exposed patients, the FDA added a black box warning in 2008 to its safety label stating that the risk of death from cancer in patients who used 3 or more tubes of Regranex was 5 times higher compared with nonusers. However, this was not supported by longer term follow-up of becaplermin users matched to a cohort of nonusers, indicating no elevated cancer mortality risk overall, which suggested that Becaplermin does not seem to increase the risk of cancer or cancer mortality.[55,56]

Autologous Platelet-Rich Plasma

Autologous platelet-rich plasma (PRP) is a biologic therapy that has a lower level of evidence. It is defined as a portion of the plasma fraction of autologous blood having a platelet concentration above baseline. PRP is also referred to as platelet-enriched plasma, platelet-rich concentrate, autologous platelet gel, and platelet releasate. Platelet gels and releasates are prepared from PRP. The gelatinlike malleable product results by adding thrombin and calcium to PRP, cleaving fibrinogen, to form fibrin, which polymerizes, producing a gluelike gel.

The term "releasate" was introduced to describe a liquid product that is prepared either by platelet activation using thrombin or by platelet destruction by freeze-thawing. Platelet releasate functions by principles similar to those of recombinant human platelet–derived growth factor BB, but is not standardized in its production. Although the term "releasate" is functionally appropriated for thrombin-activated products, the term "lysate" is more appropriate for products prepared by freeze-thawing.[57]

Platelet concentrates have been used successfully in repairing artificial bone defects and inducing bone mineralization in animal and human in vivo studies and also in Ophthalmology, especially for macular holes and corneal epithelial defects.[58]

Platelets initiate wound repair by releasing locally acting growth factors via α-granules degranulation. The secretory proteins contained in the α-granules of platelets include platelet-derived growth factor, insulinlike growth factor, vascular endothelial cell growth factor, platelet-derived angiogenic factor, and transforming growth factor-β, cytokines, and chemokines. In addition, PRP may suppress cytokine release and limit the inflammatory phase, interacting with macrophages to improve tissue healing, and regeneration promotes new capillary growth and accelerates epithelialization.[59] It has been found that the expression of multiple growth factors is increased in granulation tissue of refractory diabetic dermal ulcers after the treatment of PRP.[60]

A simple process of centrifugation of autologous whole blood (20 mL of the patient's blood spun for 60 seconds) separates it into 3 layers: red blood cells (bottom layer), platelet-poor plasma (top layer), and platelet concentrate that contains leukocytes (PRP) (middle layer). PRP fraction is combined with ascorbic acid and calcified thrombin in a standardized ratio to activate the platelets and form a gel containing a fibrin matrix.[61] Platelets trapped in the gel are activated and release bioactive molecules slowly over 7 to 10 days. Clinically valuable PRP contains at least one million platelets per microliter. Autologous blood is preferred to homologous blood as a source of PRP to avoid concern about transmittable diseases and antibody formation, effectively preventing the risk of graft-versus-host disease.

There is evidence that PRP favors the healing process and has favorable outcomes on the treatment of DFUs. The first reported prospective, double-blind, multicenter RCT of 72 diabetic foot ulcer patients demonstrated using a per protocol analysis that common-size ulcers treated with PRP gel healed significantly more (81.3% vs 42.1%) than their control gel matching group ($P = .036$), concluding that when used with good wound care, most nonhealing DFUs treated with autologous PRP gel can be expected to heal.[62]

In another smaller RCT, application of PRP led to a statistically significant shorter mean healing time compared with platelet-poor plasma.[63] In a large, observational case series PRP gel intervention demonstrated a clinical relevance response rate of 96.5% of all wounds within 2.2 weeks and 2.8 treatments, suggesting that this treatment can possibly reverse the nonhealing state of chronic DFUs.[64]

In a retrospective cohort study by Margolis and colleagues,[37] the effect of platelet releasate was greatest in those with the most severe wounds, such as those affecting deeper anatomic structures.

Based on a cost-effectiveness analysis, the use of PRP gel can result in improved quality of life and lower cost of care over a 5-year period compared with other treatment modalities for nonhealing DFUs.[65]

It can also be used as an adjuvant therapy in diabetic foot surgeries because the formation of a platelet plug provides both hemostasis and secretion of biologically active proteins that accelerate postoperative wound healing.[66]

COMPARING ADVANCED BIOLOGIC THERAPIES

A retrospective cohort study by Kirsner and colleagues[67] of 2517 patients with refractory DFUs aimed to determine potential differences in effects of bilayered cultured skin equivalent, topical recombinant growth factor, and platelet releasate on healing outcomes. They found superior effectiveness of the engineered skin construct with an overall median time to healing of 100 days. In a cost-effectiveness analysis of DFU treatment options, both platelet releasate and rhPDGF yielded better healing rates than standard care. In a cost-effectiveness analysis of DFU treatment options, both platelet releasate and rhPDGF yielded better healing rates than standard care.[68] When compared head-to-head, rhPDGF was less costly and more effective than platelet releasate at 20 weeks of therapy (**Table 1**).

> "Wounds treated with engineered skin as the first advanced biologic therapy were 31% more likely to heal than wounds first treated with topical recombinant growth factor (*P*<.001), and 40% more likely to heal than those first treated with platelet releasate (*P* = .01)."[38]

SUMMARY

Chronic DFUs are a growing global health concern due to the implied high rates of morbidity and mortality. Standard-of-care modalities sometimes are not sufficient for some recalcitrant ulcers. The use of adjuvant topical therapies including advanced dressings and biologic therapies should be considered in patients whose DFU did not reduce in size after receiving standard care for a period of 4 weeks. These advanced treatments must be used in combination with standard care measures, including debridement, moist wound healing, offloading, and infection control.

REFERENCES

1. Margolis DJ, Kantor J, Berlin JA. Healing of diabetic neuropathic foot ulcers receiving standard treatment. A meta-analysis. Diabetes Care 1999;22:692–5.
2. Elek SD. Experimental staphylococcal infections in the skin of man. Ann NY Acad Sci 1956;65:85–90.
3. Krizek TJ, Pobson MD, Kho E. Bacterial growth and skin graft survival. Surg Forum 1967;18:518.
4. Lookingbill DP, Miller SM, Knowles RC. Bacteriology of chronic leg ulcers. Arch Dermatol 1978;114:1765–8.
5. Bendy RH, Nuccio PA, Wolfe E, et al. Relationship of quantitative wound bacterial counts to healing of decubiti: effect of topical gentamicin. Antimicrobial Agents Chemother 1964;10:147–55.
6. Trengrove NJ, Stacey MC, McGechie D, et al. Qualitative bacteriology and leg ulcer healing. J Wound Care 1996;5:277–80.
7. Davies CE, Hill KE, Newcombe RG, et al. A prospective study of the microbiology of chronic venous leg ulcers to reevaluate the clinical predictive value of tissue biopsies and swabs. Wound Repair Regen 2007;15:17–22.
8. Drosou A, Falabella A, Kirsner RS. Antiseptics on wounds: an area of controversy. Wounds 2003;15:149–66.

9. Balin AK, Pratt L. Dilute povidone-iodine solutions inhibit human skin fibroblast growth. Dermatol Surg 2002;28:210–4.

10. Damour O, Hua SZ, Lasne F, et al. Cytotoxicity evaluation of antiseptics and antibiotics on cultured human fibroblasts and keratinocytes. Burns 1992;18:479–85.

11. Zhou LH, Nahm WK, Badiavas E, et al. Slow release iodine preparation and wound healing: in vitro effects consistent with lack of in vivo toxicity in human chronic wounds. Br J Dermatol 2002;146:365–74.

12. Apelqvist J, Ragnarson Tennvall G. Cavity foot ulcers in diabetic patients: a comparative study of cadexomer iodine and standard treatment. An economic analysis alongside a clinical trial. Acta Derm Venereol 1996;76:231–5.

13. Mertz PM, Oliveira-Gandia MF, Davis SC. The evaluation of a cadexomer iodine wound dressing on methicillin resistant Staphylococcus aureus in acute wounds. Dermatol Surg 1999;25:89–93.

14. Schwartz JA, Lantis JC 2nd, Gendics C, et al. A prospective, non comparative, multicenter study to investigate the effect of cadexomer iodine on bioburden load and other wound characteristics in diabetic foot ulcers. Int Wound J 2013;10(2):193–9.

15. Hansson C. The effects of cadexomer iodine paste in the treatment of venous leg ulcers compared with hydrocolloid dressing and paraffin gauze dressing. Int J Dermatol 1998;37:390–6.

16. Floyer C, Wilkinson JD. Treatment of venous leg ulcers with cadexomer iodine with particular reference to iodine sensitivity. Acta Chir Scand Suppl 1988;544:60–1.

17. Harcup JW, Saul PA. A study of the effect of cadexomer iodine in the treatment of venous leg ulcers. Br J Clin Pract 1986;40:360–4.

18. Moberg S, Hoffman L, Grennert ML, et al. A randomized trial of cadexomer iodine in decubitus ulcers. J Am Geriatr Soc 1983;31:462–5.

19. Lansdown AB. Silver 1: its antimicrobial properties and mechanism of action. J Wound Care 2002;11:125–30.

20. Wright JB, Lam K, Burrell RE. Wound management in an era of increasing bacterial antibiotic resistance: a role for topical silver treatment. Am J Infect Control 1998;26:572–7.

21. Rayman G, Rayman A, Baker NR, et al. Sustained silver-releasing dressing in the treatment of diabetic foot ulcers. Br J Nurs 2005;14:109–14.

22. Jude EB, Apelqvist J, Spraul M, et al. Prospective randomized controlled study of Hydrofiber dressing containing ionic silver or calcium alginate dressings in non-ischaemic diabetic foot ulcers. Diabet Med 2007;24:280–8.

23. Raghow R. The role of extracellular matrix in postinflammatory wound healing and fibrosis. FASEB J 1994;8:823–31.

24. Veves A, Sheehan P, Pham HT. A randomized, controlled trial of Promogran (a collagen/oxidized regenerated cellulose dressing) vs standard treatment in the management of diabetic foot ulcers. Arch Surg 2002;137:822–7.

25. Kakagia DD, Kazakos KJ, Xarchas KC, et al. Synergistic action of protease-modulating matrix and autologous growth factors in healing of diabetic foot ulcers. A prospective randomized trial. J Diabet Complications 2007;21:387–91.

26. Cullen B, Boyle C, Rennison T, et al. ORC/Collagen Matrix Containing Silver Controls Bacterial Bioburden while Retaining Dermal Cell Viability. Poster presented at EWMA Prague. May 2006.

27. Demling RH, Niezgoda JA, Haraway GD, et al. Small intestinal submucosa wound matrix and full-thickness venous ulcers: preliminary results. Wounds 2004;16:18–22.

28. Niezgoda JA, Van Gils CC, Frykberg RG, et al. Randomized clinical trial comparing OASIS Wound Matrix to Regranex Gel for diabetic ulcers. Adv Skin Wound Care 2005;18(5 Pt 1):258–66.

29. Stern R, McPherson M, Longaker MT. Histologic study of artificial skin used in the treatment of full-thickness thermal injury. J Burn Care Rehabil 1990;11(1):7–13.

30. Iorio ML, Goldstein J, Adams M, et al. Functional limb salvage in the diabetic patient: the use of a collagen bilayer matrix and risk factors for amputation. Plast Reconstr Surg 2011;127:260–7.

31. Clerici G, Caminiti M, Curci V, et al. The use of a dermal substitute to preserve maximal foot length in diabetic foot wounds with tendon and bone exposure following urgent surgical debridement for acute infection. Int Wound J 2010;7: 176–83.

32. Winters CL, Brigido SA, Liden BA, et al. A multicenter study involving the use of a human acellular dermal regenerative tissue matrix for the treatment of diabetic lower extremity wounds. Adv Skin Wound Care 2008;21:375–81.

33. Reyzelman A, Crews RT, Moore JC, et al. Clinical effectiveness of an acellular dermal regenerative tissue matrix compared to standard wound management in healing diabetic foot ulcers: a prospective, randomised, multicentre study. Int Wound J 2009;6:196–208.

34. Caravaggi C, De Giglio R, Pritelli C, et al. HYAFF 11-based autologous dermal and epidermal grafts in the treatment of noninfected diabetic plantar and dorsal foot ulcers: a prospective, multicenter, controlled, randomized clinical trial. Diabetes Care 2003;26:2853–9.

35. Uccioli L, Giurato L, Ruotolo V, et al. Two-step autologous grafting using HYAFF scaffolds in treating difficult diabetic foot ulcers: results of a multicenter, randomized controlled clinical trial with long-term follow-up. Int J Low Extrem Wounds 2011;10:80–5.

36. Steed DL, Attinger C, Colaizzi T, et al. Guidelines for the treatment of diabetic ulcers. Wound Repair Regen 2006;14:680–92.

37. Margolis DJ, Kantor J, Santanna J, et al. Effectiveness of platelet releasate for the treatment of diabetic neuropathic foot ulcers. Diabetes Care 2001; 24:483–8.

38. Kirsner RS, Warriner R, Michela M, et al. Advanced biological therapies for diabetic foot ulcers. Arch Dermatol 2010;146:857–62.

39. Apligraf. 2010 Organogenesis. Available at: http://www.apligraf.com/professional/what_is_apligraf/index.html. Accessed January 22, 2013.

40. Veves A, Falanga V, Armstrong DG, et al, Apligraf Diabetic Foot Ulcer Study. Graftskin, a human skin equivalent, is effective in the management of noninfected neuropathic diabetic foot ulcers: a prospective randomized multicenter clinical trial. Diabetes Care 2001;24:290–5.

41. Edmonds M, European and Australian Apligraf Diabetic Foot Ulcer Study Group. Apligraf in the treatment of neuropathic diabetic foot ulcers. Int J Low Extrem Wounds 2009;8:11–8.

42. Hu S, Kirsner RS, Falanga V, et al. Evaluation of Apligraf persistence and basement membrane restoration in donor site wounds: a pilot study. Wound Repair Regen 2006;14:427–33.

43. Advanced biohealing, dermagraft. Advanced BioHealing, Inc; 2007. Available at: http://www2.dermagraft.com/wp-content/uploads/2012/11/DG-1001-05_Dermagraft-Directions-for-Use.pdf. Accessed on January 22, 2013.

44. Marston WA, Hanft J, Norwood P, et al, Dermagraft Diabetic Foot Ulcer Study Group. The efficacy and safety of Dermagraft in improving the healing of chronic

diabetic foot ulcers: results of a prospective randomized trial. Diabetes Care 2003;26:1701–5.

45. Marston WA. Dermagraft, a bioengineered human dermal equivalent for the treatment of chronic nonhealing diabetic foot ulcer. Expert Rev Med Devices 2004;1:21–31.

46. Nagai MK, Embil JM. Becaplermin: recombinant platelet derived growth factor, a new treatment for healing diabetic foot ulcers. Expert Opin Biol Ther 2002;2: 211–8.

47. Papanas N, Maltezos E. Becaplermin gel in the treatment of diabetic neuro-pathic foot ulcers. Clin Interv Aging 2008;3:233–40.

48. Bhansali A, Venkatesh S, Dutta P, et al. Which is the better option: recombinant human PDGF-BB 0.01% gel or standard wound care, in diabetic neuropathic large plantar ulcers off-loaded by a customized contact cast? Diabetes Res Clin Pract 2009;83:e13–6.

49. Wieman TJ, Smiell JM, Su Y. Efficacy and safety of a topical gel formulation of recombinant human platelet-derived growth factor-BB (becaplermin) in patients with chronic neuropathic diabetic ulcers. A phase III randomized placebo-controlled double-blind study. Diabetes Care 1998;21:822–7.

50. Steed DL. Clinical evaluation of recombinant human platelet-derived growth factor for the treatment of lower extremity diabetic ulcers. J Vasc Surg 1995; 21:71–8.

51. Margolis DJ, Bartus C, Hoffstad O, et al. Effectiveness of recombinant human platelet-derived growth factor for the treatment of diabetic neuropathic foot ulcers. Wound Repair Regen 2005;13:531–6.

52. Poeschla EM, Buschschacher GL Jr, Wong-Stall F. Etiology of cancer: viruses. In: DeVita VT Jr, Hellman S, Rosenberg SA, editors. Cancer: principles & practice of oncology. 6th edition. Philadelphia: Lippincott Williams & Wilkins; 2001. p. 151.

53. Herlyn M, Satyamoorthy K. Melanoma. In: DeVita VT Jr, Hellman S, Rosenberg SA, editors. Cancer: principles & practice of oncology. 6th edition. Philadelphia: Lippincott Williams & Wilkins; 2001. p. 2010–1.

54. Louis DN, Cavenee WK. Neoplasms of the central nervous system. In: DeVita VT Jr, Hellman S, Rosenberg SA, editors. Cancer: principles & practice of oncology. 6th edition. Philadelphia: Lippincott Williams & Wilkins; 2001. p. 2092.

55. US prescribing information for Regranex [online]. Available at: http://www.regranex.com/Prescribing%20Info.php. Accessed on February 8, 2013.

56. Papanas N, Maltezos E. Benefit-risk assessment of becaplermin in the treatment of diabetic foot ulcers. Drug Saf 2010;33:455–61.

57. Sandri G, Bonferoni MC, Rossi S, et al. Thermosensitive eyedrops contain-ing platelet lysate for the treatment of corneal ulcers. Int J Pharm 2012; 426:1–6.

58. Borzini P, Mazzucco L. Platelet gels and releasates. Curr Opin Hematol 2005; 12(6):473–9.

59. Lacci KM, Dardik A. Platelet-rich plasma: support for its use in wound healing. Yale J Biol Med 2010;83:1–9.

60. Yuan NB, Long Y, Zhang XX, et al. Study on the mechanism of autologous platelet-rich gel to treat the refractory diabetic dermal ulcers. Sichuan Da Xue Xue Bao Yi Xue Ban 2009;40:292–4.

61. Cheong Leong DK, Tan Benedict BC, Loon Chew KT. Autologous growth factors: a biological treatment in sports medicine. Proceedings of Singapore Healthcare 2010;19:229–33.

62. Driver VR, Hanft J, Fylling CP, et al, Autologel Diabetic Foot Ulcer Study Group. A prospective, randomized, controlled trial of autologous platelet-rich plasma gel for the treatment of diabetic foot ulcers. Ostomy Wound Manage 2006;52: 68–70, 72, 74 passim.

63. Saad Setta H, Elshahat A, Elsherbiny K, et al. Platelet-rich plasma versus platelet-poor plasma in the management of chronic diabetic foot ulcers: a comparative study. Int Wound J 2011;8:307–12.

64. de Leon JM, Driver VR, Fylling CP, et al. The clinical relevance of treating chronic wounds with an enhanced near-physiological concentration of platelet-rich plasma gel. Adv Skin Wound Care 2011;24:357–68.

65. Dougherty EJ. An evidence-based model comparing the cost-effectiveness of platelet-rich plasma gel to alternative therapies for patients with nonhealing diabetic foot ulcers. Adv Skin Wound Care 2008;21:568–75.

66. Scimeca CL, Bharara M, Fisher TK, et al. Novel use of platelet-rich plasma to augment curative diabetic foot surgery. J Diabetes Sci Technol 2010;4:1121–6.

67. Kirsner RS, Michela M, Stasik L, et al. Advanced biological therapies for diabetic foot ulcers. Arch Dermatol 2010;146(8):857–62.

68. Kantor J, Margolis DJ. Treatment options for diabetic neuropathic foot ulcers: a cost-effectiveness analysis. Dermatol Surg 2001;27:347–51.

Negative Pressure Wound Therapy and Other New Therapies for Diabetic Foot Ulceration

The Current State of Play

Adam L. Isaac, DPM, David G. Armstrong, DPM, MD, PhD*

KEYWORDS

- Negative pressure wound therapy • Wound chemotherapy • Diabetic foot ulcer
- Theragnostics

KEY POINTS

- An interdisciplinary team approach to limb salvage, combined with a vertical and horizontal strategy for wound healing, may reduce complexity and complications.
- Negative pressure wound therapy (NPWT) continues to be a critical tool in amputation prevention efforts throughout the world, and its indications clearly extend beyond diabetic foot ulcers.
- Fluid instillation with NPWT, otherwise known as "wound chemotherapy," and ultraportable wound care system show tremendous promise.
- Beyond NPWT, the future of wound healing will rely heavily on theragnostics- tools and techniques that can help to quantify key parameters to rapidly direct therapy.

INTRODUCTION

Diabetes now affects more than 371 million people worldwide, with $471 billion spent in 2012 on diabetes-related health care.[1] In 2012, 4.8 million people worldwide died of diabetes, of which half were younger than 60 years.[1] In the United States, 25.8 million people are now living with diabetes, representing 8.3% of the population, and 1.9 million new cases were reported in 2010.[2]

Up to 25% of people with diabetes will develop a foot ulcer at some point during their lifetime,[3] with half developing infection and requiring hospitalization, and 1 in 5

Conflict of Interest Statement: Dr Isaac reports no conflict of interest. Dr Armstrong has received research support from KCI and Spiracur and serves on the scientific advisory board of Spiracur.
Southern Arizona Limb Salvage Alliance (SALSA), Department of Surgery, University of Arizona College of Medicine, 1501 North Campbell Avenue, Tucson, Arizona, AZ 85724, USA
* Corresponding author.
E-mail address: armstrong@usa.net

requiring amputation.[4] Remarkably, care of the lower extremity occupies up to one-third of the total direct costs for diabetes.[5] When compared with funded research and development as a total of overall federal diabetes research and development, this constitutes more than a 600-fold gap.[6]

In 2006, more than 65,700 lower limb amputations were performed in people with diabetes in the United States alone,[2] and people with a history of a diabetic foot ulcer have a 40% greater 10-year mortality rate than patients with diabetes without a foot ulcer.[7] Of the people who undergo a major amputation, 20% to 50% will have their other limb amputated in 1 to 3 years, and greater than 50% will require an amputation in 5 years.[8] After an amputation, the mortality ranges from 13% to 40% at 1 year, 35% to 65% at 3 years, and 39% to 80% at 5 years,[3] which is clearly worse than for most malignancies.[9,10]

When considering the overwhelming statistics, and the rising costs associated with diabetes, the need to develop a standardized protocol for management of the diabetic foot is critical. An interdisciplinary team approach, with members comprising primary care physicians, podiatric surgeons, vascular surgeons, orthopedic surgeons, plastic surgeons, infectious disease specialists, diabetologists, general surgeons, and pedorthist/prosthetists, has been shown to lower rates of amputation and complications in patients with diabetic foot ulcers.[10,11]

Newer, more advanced wound care modalities have also emerged as a critical tool in limb salvage, along with a combined vertical and horizontal approach to wound healing.[12] The vertical strategy for wound healing refers to covering important structures and filling defects with negative pressure wound therapy (NPWT), whereas the horizontal strategy uses skin grafting, bioengineered skin substitutes, and aggressive offloading.

NPWT: MECHANISM OF ACTION

NPWT involves the application of local subatmospheric pressure to a defect. This technique generally involves a wound interface, such as open-celled foam or gauze. This interface is connected to a pump of some type. The factors related to the effectiveness of NPWT are postulated to be multifold. It has been shown to decrease wound margins and promote granulation tissue formation and perfusion.[13–15] It also serves to maintain a moist wound-healing environment. When a wound bed is moist, the lateral voltage gradient is maintained, and a greater potential exists for wound healing.[13] Mechanical stimulation of a wound by NPWT contributes to improved wound healing through macrostrain and microstrain properties.

As NPWT is applied, the wound bed is subjected to a negative, deforming force that stretches individual cells and results in increased cell proliferation, fibroblast migration, and angiogenesis.[16,17] In 2004, Saxena and colleagues[17] reported that the V.A.C. Therapy system (Kinetic Concepts, Inc., San Antonio, TX, USA) was able to produce strains in vitro that were consistent with the levels needed for promoting cellular proliferation. The role of micromechanical forces in the induction of cell proliferation and division have been investigated with respect to the use of tissue expanders for reconstructive plastic surgery and distraction osteogenesis for bone lengthening.[16–18]

The closed negative pressure system created by NPWT also facilitates the removal of exudate and infectious materials in a controlled manner. Wounds with excessive exudate have been shown to contain an increased number of matrix metalloproteinases (MMPs), which degrade the adhesion proteins necessary for wound repair.[19] Furthermore, increased interstitial pressures can occlude the surrounding microvasculature and lymphatics, which deprive tissue of vital nutrients and oxygen.[16,19] Morykwas and colleagues[20] reported a significant reduction in the number of organisms between days 4 (10^8) and 5 (10^5), in wounds undergoing treatment with NPWT. However, in a retrospective review of 25 patients, Weed and colleagues[21] actually found an increase in the bacterial bioburden of 43% of wounds treated with NPWT.

CURRENTLY AVAILABLE NPWT DEVICES

Several devices now exist that allow for the safe and effective delivery of NPWT. The most widely used system is the vacuum-assisted closure device, V.A.C. Therapy, which consists of a reticulated, open-cell foam, covered with a semipermeable adhesive drape, and connected to a negative pressure therapy unit via evacuation tubing. The types of foam used with NPWT have evolved over the years, and are now available in several varieties.[13–15]

The traditional black-colored V.A.C. GranuFoam is made of a porous (400–600 μm), relatively hydrophobic, polyurethane ether, whereas V.A.C. GranuFoam Silver has micro-bonded metallic silver impregnated into the foam. V.A.C. WhiteFoam exists as a white, premoistened, hydrophilic foam made from polyvinyl alcohol, and possesses a high tensile strength. This foam is particularly effective when used as a bolster for skin grafts and when granulation tissue formation is not the desired result, such as in deep space infections. The foam is engineered to apply a uniform pressure throughout the entire wound bed, with the negative pressure unit typically set between 75 to 125 mm Hg on a continuous or intermittent setting (**Fig. 1**).[13–15]

RATIONALE AND OUTCOMES

In an early study on NPWT, Morykwas and colleagues[20] reported a 4-fold increase in blood flow to the subcutaneous tissue and muscle of Chester pigs, when a V.A.C. Therapy system was applied at 125 mm Hg over 15-min intervals. Blood flow values decreased to below baseline at pressures greater than 400 mm Hg. The same authors also found that the increase in local blood flow subsided after a period of 5 to 7 minutes, but that an "off" interval of 2 minutes was sufficient for reestablishing the increase in blood flow.

More recently, in 2005, Timmers and colleagues[22] applied V.A.C. Therapy to the healthy, intact forearm skin of 10 patients, and measured the response of cutaneous blood flow to negative pressure values between 25 and 500 mm Hg. The authors reported a significant increase in cutaneous blood flow at a negative pressure of 300 mm Hg, which is more than double the pressure that was used as the basis for previous studies. These investigators also found no decrease in the baseline blood flow at negative pressures approaching 500 mm Hg.

In 2005, Armstrong and Lavery[23] published the results of one of the first multicenter randomized clinical trials on NPWT, comparing the proportion and rate of wound healing with NPWT versus standard moist wound therapy. The study, which took place over a period of 16 weeks and in 18 study sites, used data from wound healing in 162 patients with diabetes, with wounds secondary to partial foot amputation and evidence of adequate perfusion. The authors found that treatment with NPWT resulted in a higher number of healed wounds (56% vs 39%) and faster healing rates. Furthermore, the rate of granulation tissue formation was increased, and a potential trend toward a reduced risk of reamputation was noted.

In 2008, Blume and colleagues[24] reported the results of a subsequent larger study focusing on NPWT. These investigators found that over a period of 16 weeks, a greater

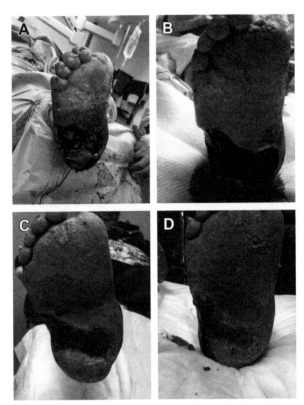

Fig. 1. (*A*) A 51-year-old woman with severe diabetic foot infection, chronic kidney disease stage V, and contralateral below-knee amputation. (*B*) After 4 days of NPWT. (*C*) After application of split-thickness skin graft, 8 weeks postoperative, with use of NPWT as a bolster dressing. (*D*) At 12 weeks postoperative.

proportion of diabetic foot ulcers achieved complete closure with NPWT compared with advanced moist wound therapy (43.2% vs 28.9%). In fact, patients receiving NPWT were noted to require fewer amputations.

NOVEL USES: WOUND "CHEMOTHERAPY"

Fluid instillation therapy, or "wound chemotherapy," is another way in which NPWT can be used as an advanced modality in wound healing and limb salvage. The V.A.C. Ulta Negative Pressure Wound Therapy System, used in conjunction with V.A.C. VeraFlo Therapy, provides a mechanism for delivering and removing fluids across a wound site, while maintaining NPWT.[15] The addition of fluids to a wound undergoing NPWT may be helpful when the wound is contaminated or infected.

Fluids such as Dakin solution (sodium hypochlorite), insulin, doxycycline, biguanide antiseptics, and several others have been reported and investigated in their use with NPWT.[25–27] The instillation of Dakin solution prevents maceration and bacterial colonization within the wound, and the addition of insulin-like growth factor (IGF) has been shown to increase rates of wound healing.[25,27] Furthermore, doxycycline, which is more commonly used for its antimicrobial properties, serves as a competitive inhibitor of MMPs, and tissue necrosis factor-alpha.[26] It may also reduce inflammation in the wound through decreasing nitric oxide synthesis.[26]

The V.A.C. VeraFlo and V.A.C. VeraFlo Cleanse dressings, which are made of polyure-thane ester, are less hydrophobic than V.A.C. GranuFoam, and have a greater tensile strength.[15] An important feature of the V.A.C. Ulta Therapy System is dynamic pressure control, which maintains a minimum negative pressure in between periods of fluid instil-lation. This aids in preventing leaks and accumulating excessive fluid at the wound site.

In a porcine study published in 2011, Lessing and colleagues[28] were able to show a 43% increase in wound fill using V.A.C. VeraFlo Therapy compared with standard NPWT over a course of 7 days. In the study, the investigators used a saline instillation with a 5-minute soak time, followed by 2.5 hours of V.A.C. Therapy. An in vitro study sponsored by Kinetic Concepts, Inc. showed that V.A.C. VeraFlo Therapy combined with polyhexamethylene biguanide was able to reduce *Pseudomonas aeruginosa* bioburden in biofilm by 99.8% (**Fig. 2**).[29]

NOVEL FORM-FACTOR: ULTRA-PORTABLE NPWT

Another advance in NPWT has been the Smart Negative Pressure (SNaP) Wound Care System (Spiracur, Inc., Sunnyvale, CA, USA). SNaP is a novel, non–electrically powered ultra-portable device that uses specialized springs to deliver NPWT. In contrast to other NPWT systems, the SNaP device does not use a battery for its operation and does not require charging. Designed for relatively smaller wounds, the SNaP Wound Care Sys-tem is fully disposable and silent throughout its operation. SNaP is readily available for "off-the-shelf" use, which obviates the need for costly and time-consuming rental agreements that are commonplace with other NPWT devices.[30–32]

Roughly the size and weight of a cell phone, the SNaP device may be worn discreetly around a patient's leg and hidden beneath their clothing. The SNaP system consists of a cartridge, a hydrocolloid dressing layer with integrated nozzle and tubing, and a foam interface. The application process is simple and quick, and the cartridge, which doubles as the storage canister (60 mL capacity), can deliver negative pres-sures of 75, 100, and 125 mm Hg.[30–32]

In a prospective, multicenter, randomized controlled comparative effectiveness study, Armstrong and colleagues[33] treated 115 patients with noninfected, nonische-mic, nonplantar lower extremity diabetic and venous wounds using either the SNaP Wound Care System or V.A.C. Therapy. Over a period of 16 weeks, and in 17 study centers, the authors reported that at 4, 8, 12, and 16 weeks, the SNaP-treated patients demonstrated noninferiority compared with the V.A.C.–treated patients with respect to percent decrease in wound area. In terms of promoting complete wound closure, the authors found that the SNaP Wound Care System was not significantly different than the V.A.C. System. The mean application time for the SNaP was significantly shorter than for the V.A.C., and patients treated with the SNaP Wound Care System reported improved activities of daily living and less interruption in sleep. They also noted an improvement in the noise level, with better levels of comfort in social situa-tions, and overall wearability (**Fig. 3**).

BEYOND DIABETIC FOOT ULCERATION WITH NPWT

Certainly the indications for NPWT extend beyond the treatment of diabetic foot and venous leg ulcers. For example, NPWT can be used as an adjunctive treatment after the application of split-thickness skin grafts. NPWT can serve as a bolster dressing by preventing the accumulation of fluid beneath the graft site, which is a common cause of graft failure.[20] In 2004, Moisidis and colleagues[34] noted a qualitative improvement (50%) in the take of split-thickness skin grafts that underwent postoperative treatment with NPWT.

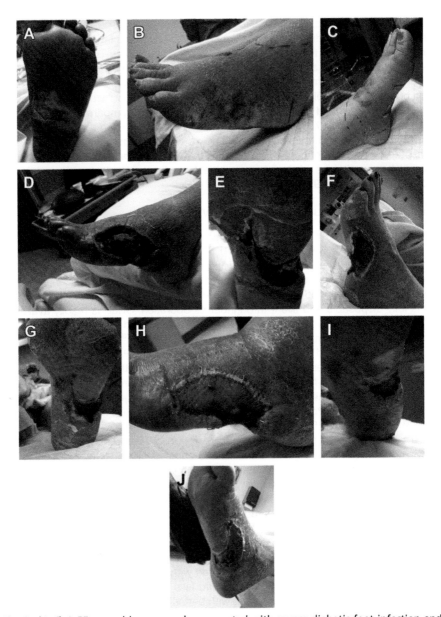

Fig. 2. (*A–C*) A 55-year-old woman who presented with severe diabetic foot infection and septic shock. (*D, E*) After emergent debridement with application of NPWT for 10 days. (*F, G*) After 7 weeks of NPWT. (*H, I*) After application of split-thickness skin graft. Immediately after graft application, NPWT with white foam dressing was applied for 4 days. (*J*) Three months post operative.

NPWT has also been shown to improve outcomes in the management of traumatic open fractures. In 2009, Stannard and colleagues[35] published a prospective randomized study examining 58 patients with 62 open fractures who were treated with either standard wet-to-dry dressings or NPWT, and found that the group treated with NPWT was one-fifth as likely to develop an infection as the control group. The application of

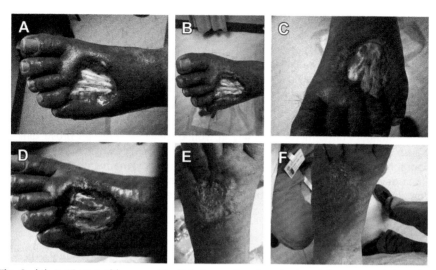

Fig. 3. (*A*) A 46-year-old man with diabetes and a chronic dorsal foot wound, for which treatment with a split-thickness skin graft failed. (*B*) After application of acetic acid 3% for 3 weeks. (*C*) After 1 week of NPWT with a non–electrically powered ultra-portable device. (*D*) Four weeks after NPWT with a non–electrically powered device. (*E*) Four weeks after application of split-thickness skin graft, in which a non–electrically powered NPWT device was used as a postoperative bolster. (*F*) 8 weeks after skin grafting.

NPWT over closed-incision sites has also gained popularity recently. Through applying NPWT over a clean closed incision, the surrounding soft tissue is splinted and the wound bed is protected.[36] Furthermore, the need for frequent dressing changes, especially on high-risk incision sites, is minimized, which has been shown in some cases to lower the incidence of dehiscence and infection.[37,38]

The use of NPWT over closed-incision sites has been reported in cases of coronary artery bypass grafting, abdominal hysterectomy, revisional hip arthroplasty, transmetatarsal amputation, and high-risk fractures of the lower extremity.[36–38] The negative pressure used over a closed incision is typically set between 75 and 125 mm Hg, and a nonadherent dressing is usually applied between the incision site and the foam layer.

The Prevena Incision Management System (Kinetic Concepts, Inc.) is a device specifically designed for applying NPWT over closed-incision sites. The system is compact, with a 45-mL canister, and includes a semipermeable incision dressing, impregnated with ionic silver.[39] In 2012, Stannard and colleagues[38] published the results of a prospective, randomized, multicenter clinical trial investigating the treatment of postoperative tibial plateau, pilon, and calcaneal fractures with closed-incision NPWT. The authors were able to demonstrate a decreased incidence of wound dehiscence and infection in 249 patients, with an even distribution of 263 tibial plateau, pilon, and calcaneal fractures. They found that the relative risk of developing an infection was 1.9 times higher in patients treated with standard postoperative dressings compared with those receiving closed-incision NPWT.

THERAGNOSTICS

Beyond NPWT, the future of wound care and limb salvage will rely heavily on the organization and integration of care, with an emphasis placed on identifying key points in healing and warning signs for recurrence.[40] Technology that is portable, durable, automated, intelligent, ubiquitous, integrable, and affordable will have a significant impact on wound diagnostics and what is referred to as *theragnostics*. Improvements in wound measurement and inflammation and infection detection have the potential to greatly impact wound healing and limb preservation.

It is widely understood that the prognostic value of wound measurement correlates strongly with wound healing. However, the assessment of wound size is often overlooked because of the limited human and economic resources found in most clinical settings. Furthermore, accuracy in wound measurement can prove difficult because of the complex geometry of many wounds. Recently, advances in intelligent topographic recognition technology, as demonstrated by the handheld Aranz and Eykona devices, and improvements in metric reconstruction have addressed many of the current issues involving accurate and consistent wound measurement.[40]

PROTEASES

Another way technology may pave the way for improved outcomes in wound care is in the assessment of inflammation, particularly the role of proteases in wound diagnostics. Proteases, which participate in the normal wound healing process through breaking down damaged extracellular matrix and connective tissue proteins, play a critical role in wound healing. If the level of protease activity is too high, the balance between tissue breakdown and repair can be disrupted. If this occurs, the inflammatory phase is prolonged and wound healing may be delayed.[41]

MMPs represent a major group of proteases involved in custodial aspects of the dermal matrix in wound healing. A registry focused on markers of protease activity, in different types of wounds and at different stages of healing, could prove extremely useful in predicting wound healing. However, clinical signs do not always correlate with the presence of high protease activity. Thus, a point-of-care protease test could help guide clinicians select the most appropriate treatment for a difficult-to-treat wound.[41] The bacterial colonization of wounds is yet another factor that contributes to delayed wound healing. Colonies of bacteria have been shown to be unique to the individual from whom they are taken, and genomic sequencing, which is rapid and affordable, could allow for individually tailored pharmacotherapy.[40]

THE FUTURE

Advances in diagnostic equipment and computer-automated appliances will continue to change wound care. One example is a device capable of measuring peak plantar pressures during the stance phase of gait, which can be built into a shoe or sock and provide real-time feedback. This device could serve as an early warning system for high-risk patients. Another innovation could be pneumatic compression devices outfitted with accelerometry, which would allow dynamic changes in pressure, depending on the activity level of the patient.[40]

The sharing of information between patients in Web-based communities is another way in which technology can transform health care.[40] Many times patients find solace in knowing that they are not alone in their struggle, and that help is just a click away. Furthermore, the ability to track patients using a wound electronic medical record (WEMR) could increase patient safety and quality of care for years to come. A standardized database of clinically relevant variables, such as age, baseline laboratory values, wound area, narrative data, and culture and pathology reports, has the potential to identify wounds at risk for delayed healing. The WEMR has the potential to change the current landscape of wound care through promoting research and enabling collaborative efforts between wound and limb salvage centers worldwide.[42]

SUMMARY

As of 2012, the number of people with diabetes is increasing in every country, and half of the people with diabetes do not know they are afflicted with the malady.[1] Furthermore, it is believed that every 20 seconds a lower limb is lost around the world because of complications related to diabetes.[6] In a short period, NPWT has transformed wound care across the globe, and other technologies are beginning to emerge that may provide clinicians with the tools necessary for identifying wounds at risk for delayed healing and recurrence. The future of diabetic limb salvage will rely heavily on these and other advances.

REFERENCES

1. International Diabetes Federation. IDF diabetes atlas. 5th edition. Brussels (Belgium): International Diabetes Federation; 2011. Available at: http://www.idf.org/diabetesatlas. Accessed on January 5, 2013.
2. Centers for Disease Control and Prevention. National diabetes fact sheet: national estimates and general information on diabetes and prediabetes in the United States, 2011. Atlanta (GA): U.S. Department of Health and Human Services, Centers for Disease Control and Prevention; 2011.
3. Singh N, Armstrong DG, Lipsky BA. Preventing foot ulcers in patients with diabetes. JAMA 2005;293(2):217–28.
4. Lavery LA, Armstrong DG, Wunderlich RP, et al. Risk factors for foot infections in individuals with diabetes. Diabetes Care 2006;29(6):1288–93.
5. Driver VR, Fabbi M, Lavery LA, et al. The costs of diabetic foot: the economic case for the limb salvage team. J Vasc Surg 2010;52(Suppl 3):17S–22S.
6. Armstrong DG, Kanda VA, Lavery LA, et al. Mind the gap: the disparity between research funding and costs of care for diabetic foot ulcers. Diabetes Care, in press.
7. Iversen MM, Tell GS, Riise T, et al. History of foot ulcer increases mortality among individuals with diabetes: ten-year follow-up of the Nord-Trøndelag Health Study, Norway. Diabetes Care 2009;32(12):2193–9.
8. Van Gils CC, Wheeler LA, Mellstrom M, et al. Amputation prevention by vascular surgery and podiatry collaboration in high-risk diabetic and nondiabetic patients. The Operation Desert Foot experience. Diabetes Care 1999;22(5):678–83.
9. Armstrong DG, Wrobel J, Robbins JM. Guest editorial: are diabetes-related wounds and amputations worse than cancer? Int Wound J 2007;4(4):286–7.
10. Armstrong DG, Mills JL. Toward a change in syntax in diabetic foot care: prevention equals remission. J Am Podiatr Med Assoc 2013;103(2):161–2.
11. Rogers LC, Andros G, Caporusso J, et al. Toe and flow: essential components and structure of the amputation prevention team. J Am Podiatr Med Assoc 2010;100(5):342–8.
12. Armstrong DG, Andros G. Use of negative pressure wound therapy to help facilitate limb preservation. Int Wound J 2012;9(Suppl 1):1–7.
13. Armstrong DG, Attinger CE, Boulton AJ, et al. Guidelines regarding negative wound therapy (NPWT) in the diabetic foot. Ostomy/wound management 50: (4B Suppl),3S.
14. Blitz NM. Vacuum assisted closure in lower extremity reconstruction. In: Dockery GL, Crawford ME, editors. Lower extremity soft tissue and cutaneous plastic surgery. Edinburgh (United Kingdom): Saunders; 2006. p. 343–58.

15. V.A.C. Ulta™ Negative Pressure Wound Therapy System. Available at: http://www.kci1.com/KCI1/vac-ulta. Accessed on January 5, 2013.
16. Andros G, Armstrong DG, Attinger CE, et al, Tucson Expert Consensus Conference. Consensus statement on negative pressure wound therapy (V.A.C. Therapy) for the management of diabetic foot wounds. Ostomy Wound Manage 2006;(Suppl):1–32.
17. Saxena V, Hwang CW, Huang S, et al. Vacuum-assisted closure: microdeformations of wounds and cell proliferation. Plast Reconstr Surg 2004;114(5): 1086–96 [discussion: 1097–8].
18. Olenius M, Dalsgaard CJ, Wickman M. Mitotic activity in expanded human skin. Plast Reconstr Surg 1993;91(2):213–6.
19. Wysocki AB, Staiano-Coico L, Grinnell F. Wound fluid from chronic leg ulcers contains elevated levels of metalloproteinases MMP-2 and MMP-9. J Invest Dermatol 1993;101(1):64–8.
20. Morykwas MJ, Argenta LC, Shelton-Brown EI, et al. Vacuum-assisted closure: a new method for wound control and treatment: animal studies and basic foundation. Ann Plast Surg 1997;38(6):553–62.
21. Weed T, Ratliff C, Drake DB. Quantifying bacterial bioburden during negative pressure wound therapy: does the wound VAC enhance bacterial clearance? Ann Plast Surg 2004;52(3):276–9 [discussion: 279–80].
22. Timmers MS, Le Cessie S, Banwell P, et al. The effects of varying degrees of pressure delivered by negative-pressure wound therapy on skin perfusion. Ann Plast Surg 2005;55(6):665–71.
23. Armstrong DG, Lavery LA, Diabetic Foot Study Consortium. Negative pressure wound therapy after partial diabetic foot amputation: a multicentre, randomized controlled trial. Lancet 2005;366(9498):1704–10.
24. Blume PA, Walters J, Payne W, et al. Comparison of negative pressure wound therapy using vacuum-assisted closure with advanced moist wound therapy in the treatment of diabetic foot ulcers: a multicenter randomized controlled trial. Diabetes Care 2008;31(4):631–6.
25. Giovinco NA, Bui TD, Fisher T, et al. Wound chemotherapy by the use of negative pressure wound therapy and infusion. Eplasty 2010;10:e9.
26. Scimeca CL, Bharara M, Fisher TK, et al. Novel use of doxycycline in continuous-instillation negative pressure wound therapy as "wound chemotherapy". Foot Ankle Spec 2010;3(4):190–3.
27. Scimeca CL, Bharara M, Fisher TK, et al. Novel use of insulin in continuous-instillation negative pressure wound therapy as "wound chemotherapy". J Diabetes Sci Technol 2010;4(4):820–4.
28. Lessing C, Slack P, Hong KZ, et al. Negative pressure wound therapy with controlled saline instillation (NPWTi): dressing properties and granulation response in vivo. Wounds 2011;23:309–19.
29. KCI data on file. V.A.C. VeraFlo™ Therapy. Available at: http://www.kci1.com/KCI1/vac-ulta. Accessed on January 5, 2013.
30. Fong KD, Hu D, Eichstadt S, et al. The SNaP system: biomechanical and animal model testing of a novel ultraportable negative-pressure wound therapy system. Plast Reconstr Surg 2010;125(5):1362–71.
31. Lerman B, Oldenbrook L, Eichstadt SL, et al. Evaluation of chronic wound treatment with the SNaP wound care system versus modern dressing protocols. Plast Reconstr Surg 2010;126(4):1253–61.
32. Lerman B, Oldenbrook L, Ryu J, et al. The SNaP Wound Care System: a case series using a novel ultraportable negative pressure wound therapy device for

the treatment of diabetic lower extremity wounds. J Diabetes Sci Technol 2010; 4(4):825–30.

33. Armstrong DG, Marston WA, Reyzelman AM, et al. Comparative effectiveness of mechanically and electrically powered negative pressure wound therapy devices: a multicenter randomized controlled trial. Wound Repair Regen 2012; 20(3):332–41.

34. Moisidis E, Heath T, Boorer C, et al. A prospective, blinded, randomized, controlled clinical trial of topical negative pressure use in skin grafting. Plast Reconstr Surg 2004;114(4):917–22.

35. Stannard JP, Volgas DA, Stewart R, et al. Negative pressure wound therapy after severe open fractures: a prospective randomized study. J Orthop Trauma 2009; 23(8):552–7.

36. Stannard JP, Atkins BZ, O'Malley D, et al. Use of negative pressure therapy on closed surgical incisions: a case series. Ostomy Wound Manage 2009;55(8): 58–66. Erratum in: Ostomy Wound Manage. 2009;55(9):6.

37. Gomoll AH, Lin A, Harris MB. Incisional vacuum-assisted closure therapy. J Orthop Trauma 2006;20(10):705–9.

38. Stannard JP, Volgas DA, McGwin G 3rd, et al. Incisional negative pressure wound therapy after high-risk lower extremity fractures. J Orthop Trauma 2012;26(1): 37–42.

39. Prevena™ incision management system clinician guide. San Antonio (TX): KCI USA, Inc.; 2010.http://www.kci1.com/KCI1/elabeling. Accessed on February 13, 2013.

40. Armstrong DG, Giovinco NA. Diagnostics, theragnostics, and the personal health server: fundamental milestones in technology with revolutionary changes in diabetic foot and wound care to come. Foot Ankle Spec 2011;4(1):54–60.

41. International consensus. The role of proteases in wound diagnostics. An expert working group review. London: Wounds International; 2011.

42. Golinko MS, Margolis DJ, Tal A, et al. Preliminary development of a diabetic foot ulcer database from a wound electronic medical record: a tool to decrease limb amputations. Wound Repair Regen 2009;17(5):657–65.

Diagnosis and Management of Infection in the Diabetic Foot

Edgar J.G. Peters, MD, PhD*, Benjamin A. Lipsky, MD, FRCP

KEYWORDS

- Diabetic foot • Foot infection • Osteomyelitis • Microbiology • Antibiotic therapy
- Culture techniques

KEY POINTS

- Diagnose foot infections based on the presence of local and systemic clinical signs and symptoms of inflammation and classify the severity based on the Infectious Diseases Society of America/International Working Group on the Diabetic Foot system to help determine proper management.
- Do not culture, or prescribe antibiotics for, clinically uninfected wounds.
- For clinically infected wounds, obtain tissue or an aspirate of purulent secretions for culture.
- Select empirical antibiotic therapy based on the severity of the infection and likely causative pathogens; modify the definitive therapy based on the response to empirical therapy and the wound culture and sensitivity results.
- Aim for the narrowest spectrum and shortest duration of antibiotic therapy that is compatible with the clinical syndrome.

INTRODUCTION

Infections of the foot are common in persons with diabetes mellitus.[1,2] Estimates of the incidence of diabetic foot infections range from a lifetime risk of 4% in persons with diabetes in the community to 7% yearly in patients treated in a tertiary diabetic foot center.[3,4] Most diabetic foot infections occur in a foot wound, especially a neuropathic ulcer, which serves as a point of entry for pathogens. Unchecked, infection can spread contiguously to involve underlying tissues, including bone. Some degree of peripheral arterial disease is present in most patients with a diabetic foot infection and the presence of ischemia can lead to necrosis and further failure of the integrity of the surrounding tissue. A diabetic foot infection is often the pivotal event leading

Department of Internal Medicine, VU University Medical Center, Room ZH4A35, PO Box 7057, Amsterdam NL-1007MB, The Netherlands
* Corresponding author.
E-mail address: ejgpeters@usa.net

Med Clin N Am 97 (2013) 911–946
http://dx.doi.org/10.1016/j.mcna.2013.04.005
0025-7125/13/$ – see front matter © 2013 Elsevier Inc. All rights reserved.

to lower extremity amputation (LEA),[3,5–7] which account for about 60% of all amputations in developed countries.[8] Among patients with a diabetic foot infections, ~50% undergo an amputation, 10% of which are proximal.[9] Most of these amputations are probably avoidable by appropriate care. Given the crucial role that infections play in the cascade toward amputation, all clinicians who see diabetic patients should have at least a basic understanding of how to diagnose and treat this problem. Definitions used in this article are summarized in **Box 1**.

Financial Cost of Diabetic Foot Infections

Based on a study from Sweden published in 1997, the cost of treatment of a diabetic foot infection (corrected for inflation in 2007, calculated from Swedish krona) is US$30,000 without amputation and up to US$58,000 with amputation.[10,11] Of these costs, 95% is related to the prolonged duration of healing and need for surgical procedures, 51% to bandages and topical treatments, and only 4% to antibiotics. Two studies have shown that rationalizing antibiotic protocols based on recommendations of the Infectious Diseases Society of America (IDSA) leads to reduced costs.[12,13]

PATHOPHYSIOLOGY OF INFECTIONS IN DIABETES MELLITUS

Although the evidence is less robust that many believe, people with diabetes seem to be more likely to develop a variety of infections. In a Canadian study of insurance claims for more than 500,000 individuals with diabetes, 50% were admitted to hospital or had a physician claim for an infection, compared with 38% in a matched cohort of individuals without diabetes (risk ratio of 1.2).[17] The risk ratio for osteomyelitis was 4, for sepsis 2 and for death due to any infection 1.84. Furthermore, individuals with

---

Box 1
Definitions

Diabetic foot: infection, ulceration, or destruction of deep tissues of the foot associated with neuropathy and/or peripheral arterial disease in the lower extremity of people with diabetes.[14]

Infection: a pathologic state caused by invasion and multiplication of microorganisms in tissues accompanied by tissue destruction and/or a host inflammatory response.[5,6,14]

Superficial infection: an infection of the skin not extending to any structure below the dermis.[5,15]

Deep infection: an infection deeper than the skin, with evidence of abscess, septic arthritis, osteomyelitis, septic tenosynovitis, or necrotizing fasciitis.[15]

Contamination: external introduction of nonresident bacteria into host tissue. The number and virulence of the organisms and the robustness of the host's immune system determine the next steps.[14] Can also mean contamination of a culture sample after obtaining it from the patient.

Colonization: new bacteria introduced into an ulcer replicate and establish a physiologic state of coexistence without overt tissue damage or host response.[14]

Osteitis: infection of bone cortex, without the involvement of bone marrow.

Osteomyelitis: infection of bone, with involvement of bone marrow.

Acute osteomyelitis: osteomyelitis that is usually of recent onset and characterized by polymorphonuclear infiltrate but without necrosis.[16]

Chronic osteomyelitis: osteomyelitis that has usually been present for at least several weeks and is characterized by round cell infiltrates and necrosis.[16]

Septic arthritis: infection of a joint.

diabetes had an 80% increased risk for cellulitis. Another 12-month cohort study in 7417 patients with diabetes, conducted as part of the Second Dutch National Survey of General Practice, also suggested that patients with diabetes had a higher incidence of pneumonia, urinary tract infection, and skin infections.[18] Although 2 landmark studies linked better survival in surgical patients in intensive care units with better glucose control,[19,20] later meta-analyses could not support this finding in medical patients.[21,22]

It is not well understood what is happening on a physiologic level to increase the risk or severity of infections in persons with diabetes. Several in vitro studies have demonstrated some adverse effects of hyperglycemia and other metabolic disturbances on the immune system. Diabetes seems to have multifactorial effects on various parts of the immune system (**Box 2**).

The humoral innate immune response consists of local vasoactive cytokines, the complement system, and proinflammatory cytokines. Local vasoactive cytokines, such as bradykinin, lead to vasodilatation through a nitric oxide (NO) response. In hyperglycemia, however, the dysregulation can lead to vasoconstriction instead, resulting in hypoxia, and to impaired influx of phagocytes.[23,24] Complement activation occurs more often in patients with type 2 diabetes who use insulin than in patients with type 1 diabetes and non–insulin-treated patients.[25] More recent studies have shown that increased glucose concentrations can inhibit complement-mediated immune

---

Box 2
Immune systems affected by diabetes mellitus

Humoral innate system

- Dysfunction of endothelial nitric oxide synthase/nitric oxide system leading to vasoconstriction
  - Ischemia
  - Impaired polymorphonuclear cell (PMN) influx
- Complement cascade disturbances
  - General complement cascade activation
  - Inhibition of specific complement responses
  - Decrease of complement-mediated phagocytosis
- Increased proinflammatory cytokine production
  - Increased inflammatory state
  - Decreased insulin sensitivity

Cellular innate system

- PMN function impairment
  - Decreased chemotaxis
  - Decreased adherence
  - Decreased phagocytosis
  - Decreased superoxide formation leading to diminished intracellular killing capacity

Adaptive immune system

- T-cell and B-cell function
  - Possibly impaired vaccination response

activities.[26,27] Proinflammatory cytokine levels are increased in hyperglycemia, which can lead to increased insulin resistance through a couple of pathways. This, in turn, can cause more hyperglycemia, further increased levels of proinflammatory cytokines, and insulin resistance.[28]

Phagocytes or polymorphonuclear cells (PMNs) form the cellular innate immune system. PMNs and monocytes in patients with diabetes show impaired chemotaxis, adherence, phagocytosis, and intracellular killing,[29–34] which seem to be normalized by insulin treatment.[35] Accumulation of advanced glycation end products (AGE) leads to impaired PMN transendothelial migration.[36] Studies of the effectiveness of various agents that might improve PMN function, such as granulocyte colony-stimulating factor (G-CSF) in diabetic foot infections,[37,38] have provided conflicting results. A systematic review of controlled trials on the effectiveness of G-CSF in diabetic foot infections published in 2009 reported no apparent effect on resolution of infection or healing of the foot ulcer, but a reduced need for surgical interventions, especially amputations, and a shorter duration of hospitalization.[39,40]

The influence of diabetes on the adaptive immune system (ie, T cells and immuno-globulins) is less well characterized. Protection after vaccination against influenza, *Streptococcus pneumoniae*, and hepatitis B has been found to be adequate in clinical studies.[41–44] Nevertheless, vaccination studies have demonstrated some specific defects in the cellular adaptive immune system in patients with type 1 diabetes regardless of glycemic control.[45–47] At least 1 study suggested that improved metabolic control helps to optimize the adaptive immune system.[48]

RISK FACTORS FOR INFECTION

Only a few studies have specifically assessed risk factors for diabetic foot infection. A prospective multicenter study of persons with diabetes compared 150 patients with a foot infection (complicated by osteomyelitis in 20% of cases) with 97 patients who did not develop a foot infection.[49] Factors significantly associated with developing a foot infection included having a wound that extended to bone (based on a positive probe to bone test, odds ratio [OR] of 6.7), a foot ulcer with a duration >30 days (OR 4.7), a history of recurrent foot ulcers (OR 2.4), a wound of traumatic cause (OR 2.4), and the presence of peripheral vascular disease (defined as absent peripheral pulses or an ankle-brachial index [ABI] <0.9 [OR 1.9]). Only 1 infection occurred in a patient without a previous or concomitant foot ulcer. Another retrospective review of 112 patients with a severe diabetic foot infection found that, by multivariate analysis, factors associated with developing an infection were having a previous amputation (OR 19.9); peripheral vascular disease (OR 5.5); or peripheral sensory neuropathy (OR 3.4).[50] Other noncontrolled studies have identified renal insufficiency and renal transplantation[51–53] and walking barefoot as risk factor for diabetic foot infection.[54] The identified risk factors are summarized in **Box 3**.

CLINICAL SIGNS AND SYMPTOMS

The diagnosis of diabetic foot infection is based on clinical findings. Although the classic clinical signs and symptoms of inflammation (ie, redness, warmth, induration, pain/tenderness, and loss of function) are somewhat subjective, there is general consensus and some published data supporting their usefulness (**Table 1**).[55,56] The presence of neuropathy or ischemia may alter these signs of inflammation and infection, making them less obvious.[57] Pain may be mitigated by (or attributed to) peripheral neuropathy. Peripheral arterial disease, as well as autonomic neuropathy and diminished skin blood flow, may reduce erythema or induration. The improper functioning

Box 3
Risk factors for developing a diabetic foot infection

- Palpable bone test (positive probe to bone test)
- Foot ulcer present for more than 30 days
- History of recurrent foot ulcers
- Traumatic cause of foot ulcer
- Previous lower extremity amputation
- Peripheral sensory neuropathy
- Renal insufficiency and renal transplantation
- Walking barefoot

of leukocytes (see earlier) can also contribute to the absence of signs of inflammation. These features have led some to accept alternative signs (eg, purulent and nonpurulent discharge, fetid odor, necrosis, undermining of wound edges, poor granulation tissue and lack of wound healing) as evidence of infection.[58–60]

Table 1
Infectious Diseases Society of America (IDSA) and PEDIS classification on diabetic foot infection

Clinical Manifestation of Infection	PEDIS Grade	IDSA Infection Severity
No symptoms or signs of infection	1	Uninfected
Infection involving the skin and the subcutaneous tissue only (without involvement of deeper tissues and without systemic signs as described below). At least 2 of the following items are present: • Local swelling or induration • Erythema >0.5–2 cm around the ulcer • Local tenderness or pain • Local warmth • Purulent discharge (thick, opaque to white, or sanguineous secretion) Other causes of an inflammatory response of the skin are excluded (eg, trauma, gout, acute Charcot neuro-osteoarthropathy, fracture, thrombosis, venous stasis)	2	Mild
Erythema >2 cm plus 1 of the items described above (swelling, tenderness, warmth, discharge) or Infection involving structures deeper than skin and subcutaneous tissues such as abscess, osteomyelitis, septic arthritis, fasciitis No systemic inflammatory response signs, as described below	3	Moderate
Any foot infection with the following signs of a systemic inflammatory response syndrome. This response is manifested by 2 or more of the following conditions: • Temperature >38°C or <36°C • Heart rate >90 beats/min • Respiratory rate >20 breaths/min or $Paco_2$ <32 mm Hg • White blood cell count >12,000 or <4000/mm^3 or 10% immature (band) forms	4	Severe

PEDIS stands for perfusion, extent (size), depth (tissue loss), infection, and sensation (neuropathy).
Data from Refs.[14,55,56,83]

Systemic inflammatory signs, such as fever, hypotension, delirium, leukocytosis, and increased sedimentation rate and C-reactive protein level, are usually absent, even in severe infections. If these signs are present, however, they define severe infection.[9,61–63] The presence of clinically significant ischemia to the affected foot often increases the severity of the infection. Because all open wounds are at least colonized with bacteria, microbiological data by themselves do not contribute to the diagnosis of infection, but are key for determining the most appropriate therapy. An additional problem is that hospital staff members often do not adequately evaluate the infected diabetic foot. In one 4-year study in a teaching hospital in the United States, only 14% of patients received what was considered to be the minimally acceptable level of evaluation.[61]

CLASSIFICATION

Several classification schemes are available to assess diabetic foot problems, but most are subsections of ulcer classifications. There is no consensus on which classification to use, largely because they have been developed for different purposes. Examples of diabetic foot classification schemes include the Meggit-Wagner,[64,65] PEDIS (an acronym for perfusion, extent (size), depth (tissue loss), infection, and sensation (neuropathy),[14,55] SAD/SAD (an acronym for size, (area, depth), sepsis (infection), arteriopathy, and denervation) and SINBAD (an acronym for site, ischemia, neuropathy, bacterial infection, and death),[66–68] and the UT (University of Texas) classification.[68–70] All are designed as ulcer classifications, but have a separate section to assess the presence of infection. Other schemes were specifically developed as wound scores, such as the USI,[71] the DUSS (Diabetic Ulcer Severity Score) and MAID (palpable pedal pulses [I], wound area [A], ulcer duration [D], and presence of multiple ulcerations [M]),[72,73] and the Diabetic Foot Infection Wound Score.[74–78] The Wound Score devised by Lipsky and colleagues[74] has been shown to be useful for demonstrating improvement in signs of infection and wound healing during treatment, and may also help in comparing the severity of foot wounds in patients in different studies. There is no evidence that one classification system or wound score is better than any other.

PEDIS and IDSA

Specifically assessing infection severity is useful for determining appropriate empirical therapy. The schemes developed by the IDSA and the International Working Group on the Diabetic Foot (IWGDF) are suitable to adequately describe infection and help guide therapy. In general, the other classifications only provide a dichotomous description of infection (absent/present) without further definitions. The PEDIS, IDSA, and S(AD)/SAD provide a semiquantitative 4-point scale to describe infection and may better predict the outcome of a diabetic foot infection. The PEDIS ulcer classification was originally developed by the IWGDF for research purposes.[55] However, it can also be used for clinical practice.[79] It offers a semiquantitative gradation of ulcer severity and the infection part of the classification is almost the same as the IDSA diabetic foot infection classification (see **Table 1**).[56]

The slight differences between the classification systems include the fact that the IDSA describes a moderate infection as a mild infection with more extensive cellulitis, lymphagitic streaks, deep infection, or gangrene, whereas the IWGDF defines it as more extensive cellulitis plus 1 other sign of inflammation or a deep infection. Furthermore, severe foot infection in the IDSA classification is defined as an infection with systemic toxicity or metabolic disturbance, whereas in PEDIS, this is more strictly defined as a patient with a foot infection and 2 or more criteria of the systemic inflammatory response syndrome. A major advantage of both classifications is that the analogy with other infections makes it easier to understand and remember for clinicians with less experience with diabetic foot management. Another advantage is that the system has been validated by being applied to prospective studies of diabetic patients[80–82]; it significantly predicted the need for hospitalization and for limb amputation.[80]

The full PEDIS classification was originally set up to include all types of foot ulcers, which led to a relatively complicated system. As a consequence, the schemes are hard to remember and thus not easy to apply in clinical practice. In a recent study, the system was used for a comparative audit among 14 European diabetic foot centers.[81] In another recent study, it was used to study the usefulness of procalcitonin and C-reactive protein in distinguishing mildly infected from noninfected diabetic foot ulcers.[82]

MICROBIOLOGY

The results of microbiological tests from diabetic foot wound specimens must be interpreted with reference to the clinical situation. Using findings on cultures or Gram stain smears to define infection can be misleading, as all wounds are colonized with bacteria. These may represent resident (colonizing) flora, but may also include potential pathogens. There is no evidence that treating a colonized wound without clinical infection with antimicrobials has any value in either preventing infection or improving ulcer healing.[84–86]

For clinically infected wounds, obtaining appropriate specimens for microbiological analysis is useful to select the optimal antibiotic regimen. Using proper sampling techniques is critically important for obtaining useful results. Vital tissues do not generally have colonizing organisms. Thus, obtaining a sample from deep nonnecrotic tissue taken through noncolonized surroundings or of pus lessens the chance of a false-positive culture due to contamination or colonization. The wound should be sampled after proper debridement of callus and necrotic tissue. Superficial cultures obtained with cotton swabs are easily collected, but less reliable than tissue biopsies or curettings. Most studies have found that swab specimens have more isolates (likely contaminating or colonizing flora) than aseptically obtained deep tissue specimens.[13,87,88] In particular, studies of patients with diabetic foot osteomyelitis have generally found that superficial swab cultures do not correlate well with bone specimens.[89,90]

Most mild infections in patients who have not recently been treated with antibiotics are caused only by aerobic gram-positive cocci, predominantly *Staphylococcus aureus* and/or, to a lesser degree, β-hemolytic streptococci.[14,91–94] Recent studies from developing countries have noted that isolation of *Staphylococcus aureus* in diabetic foot infections is less common than in developed countries (30% vs 75%).[95,96] Cultures of deep wounds with moderate to severe infections, especially in previously treated patients, are usually polymicrobial with mixed gram-positive cocci, gram-negative rods (eg, *Escherichia coli, Proteus, Klebsiella*), sometimes nonfermentative gram-negative rods (eg, *Pseudomonas*), and obligate anaerobes (eg, *Peptostreptococcus, Finegoldia, Bacteroides*).[87,94,97–101] Severe infections may harbor *Pseudomonas aeruginosa*, especially in cases of deep puncture wounds and in patients whose feet are frequently exposed to water.[57,94,102] Anaerobes, often detectable by their feculent odor, are almost always part of a mixed infection with aerobes and typically found in ischemic or necrotic wounds.[103] The most commonly isolated microorganisms in selected clinical circumstances are summarized in **Table 2**.

Diabetic foot wounds may not respond to antibiotic therapy, often because they are infected with unusual and resistant flora.[104–106] Where multidrug-resistant organisms

Table 2
Suggestions for empirical antibiotic regimens based on the IDSA guidelines

Infection Severity	Likely Pathogen	Antimicrobial Agent	Comment
Mild (usually treated with oral antibiotics)	Staphylococcus aureus (MSSA), Streptococcus spp.	Dicloxacillin or flucloxacillin	QID dosing, narrow spectrum, inexpensive
		Clindamycin	Usually active against community acquired MRSA, consider ordering a D-test before using for MRSA. Inhibits protein synthesis of some toxins
		Cephalexin	QID dosing, inexpensive
		Levofloxacin	Once-daily dosing, suboptimal against Staphylococcus aureus
		Amoxicillin/clavulanate	Relatively broad-spectrum oral agent, includes anaerobic coverage
	MRSA	Doxycycline	Active against many MRSA and some gram-negative organisms, uncertain against Streptococcus spp
		Trimethoprim/sulfamethoxazole	Active against MRSA and some gram-negatives Uncertain activity against Streptococcus spp
Moderate (oral or initial parenteral antibiotics) or severe (usually treated with parenteral antibiotics)	MSSA, Streptococcus spp, Enterobacteriaceae, obligate anaerobes	Levofloxacin	Once-daily dosing, suboptimal against Staphylococcus aureus
		Cefoxitin	Second-generation cephalosporin with anaerobic coverage
		Ceftriaxone	Once-daily dosing, third generation cephalosporin
		Ampicillin-sulbactam	Adequate if low suspicion of Pseudomonas aeruginosa
		Moxifloxacin	Once-daily oral dosing. Relatively broad-spectrum, including most obligate anaerobic organisms
		Ertapenem	Once-daily dosing. Relatively broad-spectrum including anaerobes, but not active against Pseudomonas aeruginosa
		Tigecycline	Active against MRSA. Spectrum may be excessively broad. High rates of nausea and vomiting and increased mortality warning
		Levofloxacin or ciprofloxacin with clindamycin	Limited evidence supporting clindamycin for severe Staphylococcus aureus infections; oral and intravenous formulations for both drugs

	Agent	Comments
	Imipenem-cilastatin	Very broad-spectrum (but not against MRSA); use only when this is required. Consider when ESBL-producing pathogens suspected
MRSA	Linezolid	Expensive; increased risk of toxicities when used >2 wk
	Daptomycin	Once-daily dosing. Requires serial monitoring of CPK
	Vancomycin	Vancomycin MICs for MRSA are gradually increasing
Pseudomonas aeruginosa	Piperacillin-tazobactam	TID/QID dosing. Useful for broad-spectrum coverage. Pseudomonas aeruginosa is an uncommon pathogen in diabetic foot infections except in special circumstances
MRSA, Enterobacteriaceae, Pseudomonas, and obligate anaerobes	Vancomycin[a], ceftazidime, cefepime, piperacillin/ tazobactam, aztreonam, or carbapenem	Very broad-spectrum coverage. usually only used for empirical therapy for severe infection. Consider addition of obligate anaerobe coverage if ceftazidime, cefepime, or aztreonam selected

Narrow-spectrum agents (eg, vancomycin, linezolid, daptomycin) should be combined with other agents (eg, a fluoroquinolone) if a polymicrobial infection (especially moderate or severe) is suspected.

Use an agent active against MRSA for patients who have a severe infection, evidence of infection or colonization with this organism elsewhere, or epidemiologic risk factors for MRSA infection.

Select definitive regimens after considering the results of culture and susceptibility tests from wound specimens, as well as the clinical response to the empirical regimen.

Similar agents of the same drug class can probably be substituted for suggested agents.

Some of these regimens do not have FDA approval for complicated skin and skin structure infections.

Abbreviations: CPK, creatine phosphokinase; ESBL, extended-spectrum β-lactamase; FDA, US Food and Drug Administration; MIC, minimum inhibitory concentration; MRSA, methicillin-resistant *Staphylococcus aureus*; MSSA, methicillin-sensitive *Staphylococcus aureus*; QID, 4 times a day; TID, 3 times a day.

[a] Daptomycin or linezolid may be substituted for vancomycin.

Data from Lipsky BA, Berendt AR, Cornia PB, et al. 2012 Infectious Diseases Society of America clinical practice guideline for the diagnosis and treatment of diabetic foot infections. Clin Infect Dis 2012;54(12):e132–73.

(MDROs) are common, the selected antibiotic therapy is often inappropriate.[107] Studies of the outcome of ulcers infected with MDROs, such as methicillin-resistant *Staphylococcus aureus* (MRSA) or vancomycin-resistant *Enterococcus* (VRE), have produced conflicting data. In some studies, patients with MDROs did not have worse outcomes than those without resistant bacteria,[104,108] whereas other studies have suggested that patients infected with MRSA had worse outcomes.[95,109] A potential confounder in these studies is that patients colonized with MRSA might have more often had previous unsuccessful treatments or hospitalizations that led to the colonization with resistant organisms. Another confounder is that most specimens were cultured from superficial swabs, rather than tissue biopsies. This might also explain why most of the patients who did well despite MDROs healed without antimicrobial drugs specifically targeted at these bacteria.[75]

The likelihood of isolating MRSA from a diabetic foot infection has increased over the past decade,[93,105,106,108] but seems to be decreasing more recently. MRSA, especially in the United States, is not only a hospital-associated pathogen, but can also be community acquired.[110] The increase in MRSA isolates with reduced susceptibility to vancomycin is also a concern. More recently, extended-spectrum β-lactamase (ESBL)–producing Enterobacteriaceae are an emerging international problem, including in diabetic foot infections.[95] Identified risk factors for resistant bacteria in foot infections include previous antibiotic therapy, especially of long duration, more frequent hospitalizations for the same ulcer, longer duration of hospital stay, and the presence of underlying osteomyelitis.[104,111]

TREATMENT
Uninfected Wounds

Some favor providing antibiotic treatment for clinically uninfected wounds, believing that high levels of surface colonization (bacterial bioburden) may inhibit healing or that overt signs of infection are obscured in persons with diabetes.[84,86,112] The few available published trials have not found systemic antibiotic treatment of a wound without clinical infection to be effective in either improving healing of ulcers or as prophylaxis against infections.[85,113,114] Given the lack of evidence of efficacy and the known potentially adverse clinical, microbiological, and financial effects of antibiotic therapy, current guidelines discourage prescribing antibiotics for clinically uninfected wounds.[14,56] These wounds do, of course, need other forms of treatment, and if they become clinically infected, they would need antibiotic therapy.

Infected Wounds

General measurements
Treatment of a diabetic foot infection requires a combination of several interventions. Antibiotic therapy is necessary, but not sufficient, to cure most infections, because it must usually be combined with appropriate debridement, pressure offloading, and frequently 1 or more surgical procedures. Surgical management often includes cleansing, removal of callus and necrotic material, and drainage of any purulent collections. Edema should be treated with elevation and compression of the limb. Patients with clinically significant arterial insufficiency may require revascularization to optimize the supply of nutrients, immune cells, and antibiotics. In selected instances, 1 of several adjunctive treatments may be appropriate, as described later.

Antimicrobial therapy
Empirical therapy Most initial antibiotic therapy is empiric, and assessing infection severity is important in determining the most appropriate agents and route of

treatment.[56,115] After the results of appropriately obtained specimens for culture become available, that information, along with consideration of the clinical response to the empirical regimen, can allow the clinician to decide if it is wise to tailor the definitive therapy.

Suggested empirical regimens are summarized in **Table 2**.[56] These recommendations are based predominantly on expert opinion. A meta-analysis published in 2008 found 18 relevant randomized controlled trials that listed factors associated with treatment failure in diabetic foot infections, with a total of 1715 subjects.[115] Use of an antibiotic other than a carbapenem and the presence of MRSA and streptococci were associated with treatment failure in this study. Another systematic review of antimicrobial treatments for diabetic foot ulcers, published in 2006, concluded that the evidence was too weak to recommend any particular antimicrobial agent.[116] Another article critically reviewed randomized controlled trials on the antibiotic treatment of diabetic foot infections published between 1999 and 2009.[117] The investigators noted that discrepancies in study design, inclusion criteria, statistical methodology, and the varying definitions of both clinical and microbiological end points among the studies made it difficult to compare them or to determine which regimen may be the most appropriate.

Comparison of antibiotic agents In 2012, the IWGDF, a consultative section of the International Diabetes Federation, published a systematic review on treatment of diabetic foot infections.[118] The literature search of articles published before August 2010 identified 7517 articles, 33 of which fulfilled predefined criteria for detailed data extraction. Among 12 studies comparing different antibiotic regimens for soft tissue infection, none demonstrated a superior response to the others. Of 7 studies of antibiotic regimens for patients with infection involving both soft tissue and bone, 1 reported a better clinical outcome in those treated with cefoxitin compared with ampicillin/sulbactam, but the others reported no differences between treatment regimens. No published data supported the superiority of any particular route of delivery or the optimal duration of antibiotic therapy in either soft tissue infection or osteomyelitis. Results from 2 studies suggested that early surgical intervention was associated with a significant reduction in major amputation, but the methodological quality of each study was low. The conclusion of each of the reviews is that there have not been many trials, that the methodological quality of the available studies is poor, and there is no strong evidence for specific recommendations of a particular antimicrobial regimen to prevent amputation, resolve infection, or hasten ulcer healing.[115,116,118,119]

Antibiotic penetration Concerns have been raised about how well various antibiotic agents penetrate to the site of infection in the foot. One literature review described studies of serum and tissue levels of antibiotics, which were generally adequate.[119] A study of 26 patients who received intravenous antibiotics for diabetic foot infections found that levels of gentamicin and clindamycin in viable tissues adjacent to the surgical site were low, whereas concentrations of penicillin derivatives were generally higher.[120] Most β-lactam antibiotics achieve relatively high serum levels but lower tissue levels.[121,122] Clindamycin and fluoroquinolones have shown good penetration in bone, biofilm, and necrotic tissue.[123–125] Oral absorption of antibiotics, with exception of some oral β-lactam antibiotics, is usually high enough to make initial oral therapy possible, even in patients with gastropathy caused by autonomic neuropathy.[126]

Antibiotic resistance Because a major recent problem in antibiotic therapy is drug resistance, there have been studies of newer antimicrobial agents. Among the drugs shown to be effective for treating complicated skin and soft tissue infections (often including diabetic foot infections) are linezolid (orally or intravenously) for gram-positive (including MRSA) and anaerobic organisms,[75,127–129] daptomycin (once daily intravenously) for gram-positive organisms (including MRSA),[130] dalbavancin (intravenously) once weekly for gram-positive organisms (including MRSA, not yet licensed),[131,132] telavancin (intravenously) once daily for gram-positive organisms (including MRSA and glycopeptide-resistant strains),[133] tigecycline (intravenously) twice daily for gram-positive and gram-negative bacteria, including anaerobes, VRE, and ESBL producers, but not *Pseudomonas*,[134] ceftobiprole (intravenously) twice daily for gram-positive organisms (including MRSA) and gram-negative organisms,[135,136] moxifloxacin (parenterally or orally) once daily, broad spectrum, but not for MDROs,[137,138] and ertapenem (parenterally) once daily for gram-positive and negative organisms, but not for *Pseudomonas*.[78]

Surgical treatment
Most diabetic foot infections require some surgical intervention. These range from minimal debridement, incision and drainage of purulent collections and resection of devitalized tissue, to bone resections, revascularization, and various levels of amputation. The surgeon must have adequate knowledge of basic anatomic concepts of the foot. Optimally, medical and surgical clinicians should work together to decide when surgery is needed and what type of procedure is most appropriate.[139,140]

Mild infections
Mild infections (PEDIS grade 2) that have not previously been treated with antibiotics are usually caused by staphylococci and sometimes streptococci. Outpatient treatment is safe for most patients, provided they can either care for themselves or have home care available.[56,75,141] Specimens from some mild infections yield gram-negative rods on wound culture, but these are usually secondary colonizers that do not need targeted antibiotic therapy. In situations where MRSA is unlikely to be a pathogen, treatment with a semisynthetic penicillin with antistaphylococcal activity (eg, flucloxacillin or dicloxacillin), a first-generation cephalosporin (eg, cephalexin), or clindamycin for 1 to 2 weeks is appropriate.[56,142,143] Where there is a substantial prevalence of MRSA, wound cultures are especially advisable to ensure adequate antibiotic coverage.[88,119,144] Options for treating MRSA infection include clindamycin (variable susceptibility), trimethoprim-sulfamethoxazole (weak antistreptococcal activity), doxycycline (suboptimal for streptococci), or linezolid (expensive).

Moderate infections
Patients with a moderate infection (PEDIS grade 3), especially of a chronic or previously treated wound, often require broad-spectrum coverage for both gram-positive cocci and gram-negative rods. Anaerobes are not encountered frequently in mild to moderate infections and, when they are present (almost always in a mixed infection), adequate debridement and drainage may be sufficient.[119,142,145] In the presence of necrosis or severe ischemia, however, antibiotic therapy should include coverage for obligate anaerobes. In the IWGDF and IDSA guidelines, the empirical treatment for the group with moderate infection (PEDIS 3) is the same as for severe infection (PEDIS grade 4).[56,142] Options for empirical therapy include combinations of a fluoroquinolone (eg, ciprofloxacin, levofloxacin, moxifloxacin) with clindamycin or a β-lactam antibiotic with anti–β-lactamase activity (eg, amoxicillin-clavulanate or piperacillin/tazobactam).[146] When infection with multiresistant organisms is a concern, a carbapenem (eg, imipenem, meropenem, doripenem) would be an appropriate option.[147]

Hospitalization may be necessary, at least initially, for surgical or diagnostic procedures or parenteral administration of antibiotics. These patients must be observed carefully for their response to treatment, because inappropriate treatment can lead to more proximal amputations in 10% of cases.[5,119,146] The empirical antibiotic regimen should be reconsidered when the results of culture and sensitivity tests are available. Clinicians should aim to cover the most likely pathogens but to target therapy as narrowly as possible. Duration of therapy depends on infection severity, clinical response, and the need for surgical intervention, but rarely needs to be more than 2 to 3 weeks.[56,101,148]

Severe infections

The empirical antibiotic treatment for grade 4 PEDIS infections differs from that for moderate infections mainly in requiring greater consideration for covering resistant bacteria and obligate anaerobes.[56,119,142] Because of the possible high pathogen load, potentially impaired gastrointestinal absorption, and the need for rapid action for these potentially life-threatening infections, broad-spectrum and intravenously administered antibiotics are most appropriate.[56,88,142,145,149] After a few days, most patients who are improving can be switched to oral antibiotic therapy, which is cheaper, safer, less expensive, and easier for patients and medical staff.[126,150]

ADJUNCTIVE TREATMENTS
Topical Treatment

Several studies have assessed the effectiveness of topical antimicrobial treatment in patients with infected diabetic foot ulcers. Most evaluated topical agents (eg, silver dressings, mafenide acetate, povidone and cadexemer-iodine solutions, hypochlorite, peroxide, zinc oxide) as adjuncts to systemic antibiotic treatment. No one of these agents has been proved to offer superior outcomes to others.[151–154] The nonantimicrobial effects of these agents on the process of wound healing are variable.[155] One of the more frequently used topical agents is silver, but 3 recent systematic reviews could not identify any data proving its effectiveness for curing infection or improving wound healing.[151,152,156] A systematic review identified 2 studies on the effect of maggots (larvae) in diabetic foot ulcers.[151,152] In 1 review of patients with vascular disease, the application of larvae was associated with decreased use of antibiotics and need for amputations, suggesting potential antibacterial as well as ulcer-healing effects.[157] Larvae seem to have a direct antimicrobial effect and can perhaps reduce biofilm formation as well.[158,159] Although widely used for wound healing, there are no published studies on the effectiveness of negative pressure or vacuum-assisted therapy on diabetic foot infections including osteomyelitis.[151,152,160]

Revascularization

The combination of infection and ischemia is associated with a particularly bad outcome.[59,81] Revascularization of an ischemic limb, by open surgery or an endovascular procedure, may be beneficial in several ways, including enabling required debridement and minor surgery.[14,161] Restoring the vascular supply also allows delivery of antibiotics and leukocytes, and enhances wound healing. Unfortunately, there are no published studies to clearly define when and what type of vascular surgery should be done in patients with diabetic foot infection.

Hyperbaric Oxygen Therapy

The potential benefits of hyperbaric oxygen therapy for diabetic foot wounds has been much debated.[162–164] A Cochrane analysis published in 2012 concluded that hyperbaric oxygen therapy significantly increased ulcer healing in the short term, but not the long term; furthermore, because the trials had various flaws in design or reporting, they were not confident about the results.[165] Some trials suggest that hyperbaric oxygen decreases the rate of lower extremity amputation in patients with diabetic foot ulcers,[166–168] and might facilitate ulcer healing.[169] However, there are no direct data on the effect of hyperbaric oxygen therapy for infectious aspects of the diabetic foot.[118]

OSTEOMYELITIS
Overview

Osteomyelitis is defined as infection of bone with involvement of bone marrow.[14] In the diabetic foot, these infections usually occur by contiguous spread, usually from a chronic ulcer. Underlying osteomyelitis occurs in up to 15% of patients with a diabetic foot ulcer[170] and about 20% of cases of foot infections in persons with diabetes involve bone.[171] The presence of osteomyelitis has serious consequences: treatment typically involves prolonged antibiotic treatment combined with (sometimes repeated) surgical procedures. Infection of bone greatly increases the likelihood that the patient will require a lower extremity amputation.[49,172]

Microbiology of Osteomyelitis and Biofilm Formation

The most common causative pathogen is *Staphylococcus aureus*, either alone, or in the case of chronically infected wounds, in a polymicrobial infection (usually with gram-negative bacteria).[90,95,173–175] Bone infection, especially in the presence of necrosis, can be persistent because it is associated with impaired immune and inflammatory responses, reduced leukocyte counts, and biofilm formation.[176–179] Biofilm, comprised of colonies of bacteria in a matrix of hydrated polysaccharides, protein, and other molecules, is associated with a slower metabolism and a lower replication rate of bacteria.[180,181] Antimicrobials are therefore less effective and their penetration in the extracellular matrix is impaired.[182–184]

Diagnosis of Osteomyelitis

The diagnosis of osteomyelitis can be difficult. Early infection may be missed because it takes several weeks for the infection to show on plain radiographs. Later infection can be difficult to distinguish from changes caused by noninfectious neuro-osteo (Charcot) arthropathy.[160,185]

Clinical findings

A long-standing nonhealing ulcer overlying a bony prominence, especially in the presence of poor vascular supply, should raise the suspicion of underlying osteomyelitis. The accuracy of a physician's clinical judgment for the presence of osteomyelitis is surprisingly good, with a positive likelihood ratio (+LR) of 5.5 and a negative likelihood ratio (−LR) of 0.54.[171,186,187] Among the clinical diagnostic modalities, fever has a sensitivity of only 19%,[188] the presence of exposed bone has a +LR of 9.2,[171] and an ulcer area greater than 2 cm^2 has a +LR of 7.2.[171]

The probe to bone test, in which a hard gritty structure is palpated with a sterile, blunt, metal probe, is both easy to perform and useful. A negative probe to bone test in a patient in whom the pretest probability of osteomyelitis is low (eg, <20%) can practically rule out the diagnosis, in outpatient and inpatient settings, with a reported negative predictive value of up to 98%. Similarly, in patients with a high pretest probability (eg, >50%), the +LR is 4.3 to 9.4.[189–194]

Laboratory tests

The best of the currently available laboratory tests is the erythrocyte sedimentation rate (ESR).[171,188,195] The pooled LR of osteomyelitis in a patient with an ESR greater than 70 mm/h is 11 (confidence interval [CI] 1.6–79), whereas an ESR greater than 70 mm/h has a pooled −LR of 0.34.[195–197] An increased leukocyte count has a sensitivity of only 14% to 54%.[188] A positive culture from a swab of the surface of an ulcer does not predict underlying osteomyelitis, having a +LR and −LR of 1.0.[188] C-reactive protein and (in limited studies) procalcitonin levels are less useful.

Imaging studies

Plain radiography Characteristic features of osteomyelitis on plain radiographs of the foot are listed in **Box 4**.[171,198–200] The reported sensitivity of plain radiography in osteomyelitis[171,186,187,198,200–213] ranges from 28% to 75%. In a review by Dinh and colleagues,[185] the pooled sensitivity of 4 studies was 0.54, the pooled specificity was 0.68, with a diagnostic odds ratio of 2.84 and a Q statistic of 0.60.[171,198,200,212] In a review by Butalia and colleagues,[196] the summary +LR for plain radiographs in 7 studies was 2.3, whereas the −LR was 0.63.[171,198,200,204,208,209,211] Thus, radiographic results seem to be only marginally predictive if positive. Unfortunately, no studies were identified in these 2 reviews that used sequentially obtained radiographs of the foot over time, which are more likely to predict the presence of osteomyelitis than a single series.

Magnetic resonance imaging Magnetic resonance imaging (MRI) is generally considered the best of the currently available advanced imaging techniques for diagnosing osteomyelitis.[56] The characteristic features of osteomyelitis on MRI are listed in **Box 5**. In 1 recent meta-analysis on the use of MRI in the diabetic foot,[185] in which the prevalence of osteomyelitis ranged from 44% to 86%, the pooled sensitivity was 0.90 and the diagnostic odds ratio was 24.4.[186,187,198,200,206,210,214–224] Nine of the studies evaluated had a prospective setup, and 11 included only subjects with diabetes. In another meta-analysis, the prevalence of criterion-standard defined osteomyelitis was 50% (range 32%–89%), The pooled sensitivity was 77% to 100%, the specificity was 40% to 100%, with a diagnostic OR of 42, the summary +LR was 3.8, and the summary −LR was 0.14.[225]

Box 4
Characteristic features of osteomyelitis on plain radiography

- Periosteal reaction or elevation
- Loss of cortex with bony erosion
- Focal loss of trabecular pattern or marrow radiolucency
- New bone formation
- Bone sclerosis, with or without erosion
- Sequestrum: devitalized bone with radiodense appearance that has become separated from normal bone
- Involucrum: a layer of new bone growth outside existing bone resulting from the stripping off of the periosteum and new bone growing from the periosteum
- Cloaca: opening in an involucrum or the cortex through which sequestra or granulation tissue may be discharged

The bony changes are often accompanied by soft tissue swelling.

Data from Refs.[171,198–200]

Box 5
Characteristic features of osteomyelitis on MRI

- Low focal signal intensity on T1-weighted images
- High focal signal on T2-weighted images
- Increased signal in short tau inversion recovery sequences in bone marrow
- Less specific or secondary changes:
  - Cortical disruption
  - Adjacent cutaneous ulcer
  - Soft tissue mass
  - Sinus tract
  - Adjacent soft tissue inflammation or edema

Data from Refs.[171,186,198,214,219,226]

Nuclear medicine Three recent meta-analyses reviewed nuclear medicine techniques for diagnosing diabetic foot infections.[185,225,227] Several types of nuclear imaging scans are available. Bone scans are usually performed with ^{99m}Tc-methylene diphosphate and osteomyelitis is diagnosed by abnormally increased blood-pool activity and increased intensity localized to the bone.[185] Although bone scans are sensitive, they are nonspecific.[227] A pooled sensitivity of 80% and specificity of 28% was found in studies on 185 subjects.[171,185,198,200,212,228,229] The pooled diagnostic OR was 2.1, indicating poor discriminating ability.[185] The triple phase bone scan was markedly inferior to MRI (diagnostic OR of 3.5 vs 150).[186,200,206,210,218,223–225] The best that can be said for a bone scan is that when negative, it reliably rules out osteomyelitis.

Radiolabeled white blood cells are generally not taken up in healthy bone, making scans with these agents more specific for osteomyelitis (and Charcot osteoarthropathy).[227] The radiopharmacons most commonly used to label leukocytes are technetium (^{99m}Tc) and indium (^{111}In). Two recent meta-analyses found the summary positive predictive values for these agents to be 90% and 72%, respectively, and the negative predictive values were 81% and 83%, respectively.[185,227] Kapoor and colleagues[225] found 3 studies that compared MRI with ^{99m}Tc[224] or ^{111}In[206,210] labeled leukocyte scan. MRI outperformed leukocyte scanning with diagnostic ORs of 120 (CI 62–234) and 3.4 (CI 0.2–62), respectively.[225] Combining labeled leukocytes with bone scan (dual tracer technique) does not improve its diagnostic accuracy.[207]

Other available nuclear medicine techniques include ^{99m}Tc/^{111}In labeled human immunoglobulin G (HIG) and antigranulocyte antigen monoclonal antibodies and their fragments.[227] Because ^{99m}Tc-/^{111}In-HIG uptake is related to vascular permeability and not specific to inflamed tissue, the specificity is lower than radiolabeled leukocytes.[211,230] In a meta-analysis, the pooled positive and negative predictive values calculated from 97 lesions were 72% and 88%, respectively.[227]

Computed tomography/positron emission tomography There have been several studies of computed tomography (CT) and [^{18}F]2-fluoro-2-deoxy-D-glucose (FDG)-positron emission tomography (PET) scans for the diagnosis of osteomyelitis. FDG-PET has a reported sensitivity of 94% to 100% and a specificity of 87% to 100% in osteomyelitis in general.[231–236] In the few studies that have specifically enrolled patients with diabetic foot osteomyelitis, the diagnostic accuracy of FDG-PET was high in most and it was especially helpful for ruling out osteomyelitis.[237–239] One study on diabetic foot patients reported that the combination of FDG-PET and CT had a sensitivity, specificity, and accuracy of 100%, 92%, and 95%, respectively.[240,241]

Bone biopsy

The gold standard for diagnosing osteomyelitis is the combination of microbiological culture and histopathologic examination of bone.[56,142,160] Only culture can identify the responsible pathogens and their antibiotic sensitivities. A bone specimen may be obtained either percutaneously (through uninfected skin) or as part of an operative procedure. Proper technique is important to avoid false-positive results when the biopsy is taken through an area of soft tissue colonization and false-negative results when the area of bone infection is missed.[160] Bone cultures are not needed in every case of diabetic foot osteomyelitis, but they are helpful to guide antibiotic therapy. Senneville and colleagues[89,242] found that cultures of wound swabs were identical to those of bone in only 22.5% of patients; the swabs often yielded a larger number of microorganisms. In 1 study, fine-needle aspiration gave the same result as bone biopsy in only 32% of cases.[242] Where possible, antibiotics should be discontinued (for at least 48 hours and preferably longer) before the biopsy to maximize the yield from cultures.[243,244] Because osteomyelitis, in the absence of soft tissue infection, is usually a chronic low-level infection, it is usually safe to withhold antibiotics.

Diagnostic strategies

In 2008, an IWGDF committee published a consensus progress report on the diagnosis of diabetic foot osteomyelitis.[160] As shown in **Table 3**, using a combination of symptoms, physical examination, laboratory tests, and imaging studies, patients can be placed in 1 of 4 categories. Over time, the diagnosis can become more or less likely, depending on changing clinical and laboratory findings, but this is not taken into account in the scheme. Furthermore, the scheme has not yet been validated by any study.

Treatment of Osteomyelitis

Treatment of diabetic foot osteomyelitis is difficult because of the frequent presence of necrotic bone and biofilm and perhaps by the limited presence of leukocytes and insufficient levels of antibiotics. Several recent reviews have provided guidance.[118,160]

Role of surgery

It has long been held that treating diabetic foot osteomyelitis requires surgical debridement of necrotic and infected bone, but there have been hundreds of reports of apparently successful remission without surgery.[245] Recent systematic reviews concluded that, based on several observational studies, there is little evidence to help choose between primarily medical and primarily surgical treatment.[118,160] Tan and colleagues[246] found that, in 112 patients with a high proportion of deep infections, amputation and death were less common in patients receiving early surgical intervention. Ha Van and colleagues[247] found that healing rates were higher and more rapid for 32 patients treated with conservative orthopedic surgery compared with historical controls who received only antibiotics. Pittet and colleagues[248] reported that, among 50 patients with deep foot infection and suspected osteomyelitis, the healing rate was 70% in patients treated without surgery. Simpson and colleagues[249] found that, in 50 patients with chronic osteomyelitis, surgical resection was associated with a significantly lower relapse rate. In a noncontrolled study on 237 patients, Henke and colleagues[250] found that patients treated with surgery had a nonsignificantly different rate of proximal amputations compared with patients treated with antibiotics only

Table 3
Scheme for the diagnosis of osteomyelitis

Category	Posttest Probability of Osteomyelitis	Management Advice	Criteria	Comments
Definite (beyond reasonable doubt)	>90%	Treat for osteomyelitis	Bone sample with positive culture *AND* positive histology *OR* Purulence in bone found at surgery *OR* Atraumatically detached bone fragment removed from ulcer by podiatrist/surgeon *OR* Intraosseous abscess found on MRI *OR* Any 2 probable criteria *OR* One probable and 2 possible criteria *OR* Any 4 possible criteria below	Sample must be obtained at surgery or through uninvolved skin Definite purulence identified by experienced surgeon Definite bone fragment identified by experienced surgeon/podiatrist
Probable (more likely than not)	51%–90%	Consider treating, but further investigation may be needed	Visible cancellous bone in ulcer *OR* MRI showing bone edema with other signs of osteomyelitis *OR* Bone sample with positive culture but negative or absent histology *OR* Bone sample with positive histology but negative or absent culture *OR* Any 2 possible criteria below	Sinus tract; sequestrum, heel, or metatarsal head involved; cloaca

Possible (but on balance, less rather than more likely)	10%–50%	Treatment may be justifiable, but further investigation usually advised	Plain radiographs show cortical destruction OR MRI shows bone edema OR cloaca, OR Probe to bone positive OR Visible cortical bone OR ESR >70 mm/h with no other plausible explanation OR Nonhealing wound despite adequate offloading and perfusion for >6 wk OR Ulcer of >2 wk duration with clinical evidence of infection
Unlikely	<10%	Usually no need for further investigation or treatment	No signs or symptoms of inflammation AND normal radiographs AND ulcer present for <2 wk or absent AND any ulcer present is superficial OR Normal MRI OR Normal bone scan

Data from Berendt AR, Peters EJ, Bakker K, et al. Diabetic foot osteomyelitis: a progress report on diagnosis and a systematic review of treatment. Diabetes Metab Res Rev 2008;24(Suppl 1):S145–61.

(80% vs 81%). Other noncontrolled studies of outcomes of nonsurgical treatment have reported rates of healing comparable with those after surgery.[150,251,252]

A wide range of surgical interventions have been described, the most frequent including debridement to bleeding bone marrow with epidermal sheet grafting, and 2-stage debridement with secondary closure and limb amputation.[253–256] In 2 studies of diabetic patients with deep foot infections (with and without osteomyelitis), there was a significant reduction of major amputation with early surgery combined with antibiotics versus antibiotics alone (27% to 13% in 1 study,[246] 8% to 0% in another[257]).

There are some potential advantages to surgical therapy, such as shorter duration of treatment and a reduced likelihood of development of bacterial resistance against antibiotics.[247] Disadvantages, however, are the higher likelihood of further foot complications after surgery, such as transfer ulcers and amputations.[258–262] These additional complications are likely caused by changed biomechanical properties of the foot. It is important for clinicians to discuss the options with patients (and their families).

Antimicrobial therapy

In a systematic review published in 2005, Lazzarini and colleagues[263] found 93 studies (17 comparative) on the treatment of osteomyelitis in patients with and without diabetes. They opined that little had been learned from these studies because many did not have the necessary long period of follow-up,[16] the duration of osteomyelitis was often not defined, and there was no distinction between acute and chronic osteomyelitis. Few studies specified the sensitivity of the causing organisms or provided information about surgical procedures or removal of surgical hardware (if present). The systematic review of the IWGDF[118] included 7 studies on antibiotic treatment of diabetic foot infection in which a proportion of the patients ranging from 6% to 81% had osteomyelitis.[75,78,137,145,146,264,265] The specific antibiotic regimen or route of administration did not significantly affect the outcome.

In a more recent systematic review of treatment of chronic osteomyelitis, Spellberg and Lipsky[266] concluded that oral and parenteral therapies achieve similar cure rates; however, oral therapy avoids the risks associated with intravenous catheters and is generally less expensive, making it a reasonable choice for osteomyelitis caused by organisms for which there are appropriate oral agents available. They also noted that the addition of adjunctive rifampin to other antibiotics may improve cure rates. Although the optimal duration of therapy for chronic osteomyelitis remains uncertain, there is no evidence that antibiotic therapy for more than 4 to 6 weeks improves outcomes compared with shorter regimens. Agents with high oral bioavailability and bone penetrations, such as fluoroquinolones and clindamycin, seem to be particularly suitable for treating osteomyelitis.[263] In a retrospective study of 93 patients with diabetic foot osteomyelitis treated with oral antibiotics and limited office debridement,[150] 81% achieved remission after a mean of 40 weeks of therapy. A study that compared oral versus parenteral formulations in 357 patients with diabetic foot infections, of whom 77 had osteomyelitis, reported similar cure rates for oral and parenteral therapy (77% vs 83% for linezolid, and 68% vs 72% for aminopenicillin/β-lactamase inhibitor, respectively).[75]

Antibiotic impregnated beads

Antibiotics can be incorporated into various substances and then inserted into bone infections to elute out over time. The most frequently used product has been gentamicin-containing beads, usually made of polymethylmethacrylate (PMMA). The theoretic advantage of this technique is that a high local dose of aminoglycosides can be given without systemic toxicity. There have been several studies of the effectiveness of these beads in chronic osteomyelitis of various types.[267–270] One FDA-initiated controlled trial of 190 patients treated with intravenous antibiotics, 49 with gentamicin PMMA beads alone, and 145 with a combination of beads and intravenous antibiotics, reported that patients in the combination group were significantly more likely to experience a relapse of infection compared with the patients that were treated with intravenous antibiotics only (43% vs 24%, respectively).[269] The other uncontrolled studies reported resolution rates of 89% to 92%.[267,268,270] A recent systematic review found no prospective study proving gentamicin-containing PMMA beads to be effective in treating orthopedic infections and that these do not show significantly better results when combined with parenteral antibiotics compared with systemic therapy alone. This may be explained partially by reduced aminoglycoside efficacy in the presence of biofilms or gentamicin-resistant bacteria. Moreover, little is known regarding the potential side effects of gentamicin-containing beads.[271]

Duration of treatment

Systematic reviews were unable to determine the optimal duration of antimicrobial therapy in diabetic foot osteomyelitis.[118,160,263,266] In most studies, patients were treated for 6 weeks. In 7 of 93 studies, patients were treated for 6 months.[263] The mean duration of antibiotic treatment found in the 2012 systematic review was short, ranging from 6 days to 28 days.[118] The optimal duration of treatment with antibiotics depends on the amount of debridement or resection provided. Treatment of a few days to a couple of weeks is usually sufficient after aggressive surgical debridement.[49,160,272] Several months may be needed in patients with necrotic and infected bone who undergo limited debridement.[150] The common presumption that osteomyelitis should be treated for 4 to 6 weeks derives from studies of animal models, where bacteria could be cultured from infected bone even after 2 weeks of appropriate treatment.[273]

Adjunctive therapy for osteomyelitis

No studies suggest that the use of larvae, G-CSF, or vacuum-assisted closure is helpful in treating diabetic foot osteomyelitis.[118,160,274]

REFERENCES

1. Boyko EJ, Lipsky BA. Infection and diabetes mellitus. In: Harris IE, editor. Diabetes in America. 2nd edition. Bethesda (MD): National Institutes of Health; 1995. p. 485–96. NIH publication. No. 95-1468.
2. Peleg AY, Weerarathna T, McCarthy JS, et al. Common infections in diabetes: pathogenesis, management and relationship to glycaemic control. Diabetes Metab Res Rev 2007;23(1):3–13.
3. Pecoraro RE, Reiber GE, Burgess EM. Pathways to diabetic limb amputation. Basis for prevention. Diabetes Care 1990;13(5):513–21.
4. Lavery LA, Armstrong DG, Wunderlich RP, et al. Diabetic foot syndrome: evaluating the prevalence and incidence of foot pathology in Mexican Americans and non-Hispanic whites from a diabetes disease management cohort. Diabetes Care 2003;26(5):1435–8.
5. Eneroth M, Larsson J, Apelqvist J. Deep foot infections in patients with diabetes and foot ulcer: an entity with different characteristics, treatments, and prognosis. J Diabetes Complications 1999;13(5–6):254–63.
6. Adler AI, Boyko EJ, Ahroni JH, et al. Lower-extremity amputation in diabetes. The independent effects of peripheral vascular disease, sensory neuropathy, and foot ulcers. Diabetes Care 1999;22(7):1029–35.

7. Nather A, Bee CS, Huak CY, et al. Epidemiology of diabetic foot problems and predictive factors for limb loss. J Diabetes Complications 2008;22(2):77–82.

8. Prompers L, Schaper N, Apelqvist J, et al. Prediction of outcome in individuals with diabetic foot ulcers: focus on the differences between individuals with and without peripheral arterial disease. The EURODIALE Study. Diabetologia 2008; 51(5):747–55.

9. Eneroth M, Apelqvist J, Stenstrom A. Clinical characteristics and outcome in 223 diabetic patients with deep foot infections. Foot Ankle Int 1997;18(11):716–22.

10. Ragnarson Tennvall G, Apelqvist J, Eneroth M. Costs of deep foot infections in patients with diabetes mellitus. Pharmacoeconomics 2000;18(3):225–38.

11. US Census Bureau, Washington, DC. Inflation calculator. 2013. Available at: www.bls.gov/data/inflation_calculator.htm/. Accessed February 2, 2013.

12. Gooday C, Hallam C, Sieber C, et al. An antibiotic formulary for a tertiary care foot clinic: admission avoidance using intramuscular antibiotics for borderline foot infections in people with diabetes. Diabet Med 2013;30(5):581–9.

13. Sotto A, Richard JL, Combescure C, et al. Beneficial effects of implementing guidelines on microbiology and costs of infected diabetic foot ulcers. Diabetologia 2010;53(10):2249–55.

14. International Working Group on the Diabetic Foot. International Consensus on the Diabetic Foot and Supplements, DVD. 2011; Complete IWGDF data DVD guidelines 2011. Available at: http://shop.idf.org. Accessed February 2, 2013.

15. Berendt AR, Lipsky BA. Infection in the diabetic foot. In: Armstrong DG, Lavery LA, editors. Alexandria (VA): American Diabetes Association; 2005. p. 90–8.

16. Mader JT, Shirtliff M, Calhoun JH. Staging and staging application in osteomyelitis. Clin Infect Dis 1997;25(6):1303–9.

17. Shah BR, Hux JE. Quantifying the risk of infectious diseases for people with diabetes. Diabetes Care 2003;26(2):510–3.

18. Muller LM, Gorter KJ, Hak E, et al. Increased risk of common infections in patients with type 1 and type 2 diabetes mellitus. Clin Infect Dis 2005;41(3):281–8.

19. van den Berghe G, Wilmer A, Hermans G, et al. Intensive insulin therapy in the medical ICU. N Engl J Med 2006;354(5):449–61.

20. van den Berghe G, Wouters P, Weekers F, et al. Intensive insulin therapy in the critically ill patients. N Engl J Med 2001;345(19):1359–67.

21. Griesdale DE, de Souza RJ, van Dam RM, et al. Intensive insulin therapy and mortality among critically ill patients: a meta-analysis including NICE-SUGAR study data. CMAJ 2009;180(8):821–7.

22. Van den Berghe G, Mesotten D, Vanhorebeek I. Intensive insulin therapy in the intensive care unit. CMAJ 2009;180(8):799–800.

23. Santilli F, Cipollone F, Mezzetti A, et al. The role of nitric oxide in the development of diabetic angiopathy. Horm Metab Res 2004;36(5):319–35.

24. Kim SH, Park KW, Kim YS, et al. Effects of acute hyperglycemia on endothelium-dependent vasodilation in patients with diabetes mellitus or impaired glucose metabolism. Endothelium 2003;10(2):65–70.

25. Bergamaschini L, Gardinali M, Poli M, et al. Complement activation in diabetes mellitus. J Clin Lab Immunol 1991;35(3):121–7.

26. Saiepour D, Sehlin J, Oldenborg PA. Hyperglycemia-induced protein kinase C activation inhibits phagocytosis of C3b- and immunoglobulin g-opsonized yeast particles in normal human neutrophils. Exp Diabesity Res 2003;4(2):125–32.

27. Saiepour D, Sehlin J, Oldenborg PA. Insulin inhibits phagocytosis in normal human neutrophils via PKCalpha/beta-dependent priming of F-actin assembly. Inflamm Res 2006;55(3):85–91.

28. Turina M, Fry DE, Polk HC Jr. Acute hyperglycemia and the innate immune system: clinical, cellular, and molecular aspects. Crit Care Med 2005;33(7): 1624–33.
29. Delamaire M, Maugendre D, Moreno M, et al. Impaired leucocyte functions in diabetic patients. Diabet Med 1997;14(1):29–34.
30. Perner A, Nielsen SE, Rask-Madsen J. High glucose impairs superoxide production from isolated blood neutrophils. Intensive Care Med 2003;29(4):642–5.
31. Geerlings SE, Hoepelman AI. Immune dysfunction in patients with diabetes mellitus (DM). FEMS Immunol Med Microbiol 1999;26(3–4):259–65.
32. Cavalot F, Anfossi G, Russo I, et al. Insulin, at physiological concentrations, enhances the polymorphonuclear leukocyte chemotactic properties. Horm Metab Res 1992;24(5):225–8.
33. Mowat A, Baum J. Chemotaxis of polymorphonuclear leukocytes from patients with diabetes mellitus. N Engl J Med 1971;284(12):621–7.
34. Hill HR, Augustine NH, Rallison ML, et al. Defective monocyte chemotactic responses in diabetes mellitus. J Clin Immunol 1983;3(1):70–7.
35. Walrand S, Guillet C, Boirie Y, et al. In vivo evidences that insulin regulates human polymorphonuclear neutrophil functions. J Leukoc Biol 2004;76(6): 1104–10.
36. Collison KS, Parhar RS, Saleh SS, et al. RAGE-mediated neutrophil dysfunction is evoked by advanced glycation end products (AGEs). J Leukoc Biol 2002; 71(3):433–44.
37. Gough A, Clapperton M, Rolando N, et al. Randomised placebo-controlled trial of granulocyte-colony stimulating factor in diabetic foot infection. Lancet 1997; 350(9081):855–9.
38. Yönem A, Cakir B, Guler S, et al. Effects of granulocyte-colony stimulating factor in the treatment of diabetic foot infection. Diabetes Obes Metab 2001;3(5): 332–7.
39. Cruciani M, Lipsky BA, Mengoli C, et al. Are granulocyte colony-stimulating factors beneficial in treating diabetic foot infections?: A meta-analysis. Diabetes Care 2005;28(2):454–60.
40. Cruciani M, Lipsky BA, Mengoli C, et al. Granulocyte-colony stimulating factors as adjunctive therapy for diabetic foot infections. Cochrane Database Syst Rev 2009;(3):CD006810.
41. Diepersloot RJ, Bouter KP, van BR, et al. Cytotoxic T-cell response to influenza A subunit vaccine in patients with type 1 diabetes mellitus. Neth J Med 1989; 35(1–2):68–75.
42. el-Madhun AS, Cox RJ, Seime A, et al. Systemic and local immune responses after parenteral influenza vaccination in juvenile diabetic patients and healthy controls: results from a pilot study. Vaccine 1998;16(2–3):156–60.
43. Lederman MM, Schiffman G, Rodman HM. Pneumococcal immunization in adult diabetics. Diabetes 1981;30(2):119–21.
44. Marseglia G, Alibrandi A, d'Annunzio G, et al. Long term persistence of anti-HBs protective levels in young patients with type 1 diabetes after recombinant hepatitis B vaccine. Vaccine 2000;19(7–8):680–3.
45. MacCuish AC, Urbaniak SJ, Campbell CJ, et al. Phytohemagglutinin transformation and circulating lymphocyte subpopulations in insulin-dependent diabetic patients. Diabetes 1974;23(8):708–12.
46. Eibl N, Spatz M, Fischer GF, et al. Impaired primary immune response in type-1 diabetes: results from a controlled vaccination study. Clin Immunol 2002;103(3): 249–59.

47. Spatz M, Eibl N, Hink S, et al. Impaired primary immune response in type-1 diabetes. Functional impairment at the level of APCs and T-cells. Cell Immunol 2003;221(1):15–26.
48. Pozzilli P, Pagani S, Arduini P, et al. In vivo determination of cell mediated immune response in diabetic patients using a multiple intradermal antigen dispenser. Diabetes Res 1987;6(1):5–8.
49. Lavery LA, Armstrong DG, Wunderlich RP, et al. Risk factors for foot infections in individuals with diabetes. Diabetes Care 2006;29(6):1288–93.
50. Peters EJ, Lavery LA, Armstrong DG. Diabetic lower extremity infection: influence of physical, psychological, and social factors. J Diabetes Complications 2005;19(2):107–12.
51. Bartos V, Jirkovska A, Koznarova R. Risk factors for diabetic foot in recipients of renal and pancreatic transplants. Cas Lek Cesk 1997;136(17):527–9 [in Czech].
52. George RK, Verma AK, Agarwal A, et al. An audit of foot infections in patients with diabetes mellitus following renal transplantation. Int J Low Extrem Wounds 2004;3(3):157–60.
53. Hill MN, Feldman HI, Hilton SC, et al. Risk of foot complications in long-term diabetic patients with and without ESRD: a preliminary study. ANNA J 1996;23(4):381–6.
54. Jayasinghe SA, Atukorala I, Gunethilleke B, et al. Is walking barefoot a risk factor for diabetic foot disease in developing countries? Rural Remote Health 2007;7(2):692.
55. Schaper NC. Diabetic foot ulcer classification system for research purposes: a progress report on criteria for including patients in research studies. Diabetes Metab Res Rev 2004;20(Suppl 1):90–5.
56. Lipsky BA, Berendt AR, Cornia PB, et al. 2012 Infectious Diseases Society of America clinical practice guideline for the diagnosis and treatment of diabetic foot infections. Clin Infect Dis 2012;54(12):e132–73.
57. Lavery LA, Walker SC, Harkless LB, et al. Infected puncture wounds in diabetic and nondiabetic adults. Diabetes Care 1995;18(12):1588–91.
58. Williams DT, Hilton JR, Harding KG. Diagnosing foot infection in diabetes. Clin Infect Dis 2004;39(Suppl 2):S83–6.
59. Edmonds M. Double trouble: infection and ischemia in the diabetic foot. Int J Low Extrem Wounds 2009;8(2):62–3.
60. Richard JL, Lavigne JP, Sotto A. Diabetes and foot infection: more than double trouble. Diabetes Metab Res Rev 2012;28(Suppl 1):46–53.
61. Edelson GW, Armstrong DG, Lavery LA, et al. The acutely infected diabetic foot is not adequately evaluated in an inpatient setting. Arch Intern Med 1996;156(20):2373–6.
62. Armstrong DG, Perales TA, Murff RT, et al. Value of white blood cell count with differential in the acute diabetic foot infection. J Am Podiatr Med Assoc 1996;86(5):224–7.
63. Lavery LA, Armstrong DG, Quebedeaux TL, et al. Puncture wounds: normal laboratory values in the face of severe infection in diabetics and non-diabetics. Am J Med 1996;101(5):521–5.
64. Meggitt B. Surgical management of the diabetic foot. Br J Hosp Med 1976;16:227–332.
65. Wagner FW. The dysvascular foot: a system for diagnosis and treatment. Foot Ankle 1981;2:64–122.
66. Macfarlane RM, Jeffcoate WJ. Classification of diabetic foot ulcers: the S(AD) SAD system. Diabet Foot 1999;2(4):123–31.

67. Treece KA, Macfarlane RM, Pound N, et al. Validation of a system of foot ulcer classification in diabetes mellitus. Diabet Med 2004;21(9):987–91.
68. Jeffcoate WJ, Chipchase SY, Ince P, et al. Assessing the outcome of the management of diabetic foot ulcers using ulcer-related and person-related measures. Diabetes Care 2006;29(8):1784–7.
69. Armstrong DG, Lavery LA, Harkless LB. Validation of a diabetic wound classification system. The contribution of depth, infection, and ischemia to risk of amputation. Diabetes Care 1998;21(5):855–9.
70. Oyibo SO, Jude EB, Tarawneh I, et al. A comparison of two diabetic foot ulcer classification systems: the Wagner and the University of Texas wound classification systems. Diabetes Care 2001;24(1):84–8.
71. Knighton DR, Ciresi KF, Fiegel VD, et al. Classification and treatment of chronic nonhealing wounds. Successful treatment with autologous platelet-derived wound healing factors (PDWHF). Ann Surg 1986;204(3):322–30.
72. Beckert S, Witte M, Wicke C, et al. A new wound-based severity score for diabetic foot ulcers: a prospective analysis of 1,000 patients. Diabetes Care 2006; 29(5):988–92.
73. Beckert S, Pietsch AM, Kuper M, et al. M.A.I.D.: a prognostic score estimating probability of healing in chronic lower extremity wounds. Ann Surg 2009;249(4): 677–81.
74. Lipsky BA, Polis AB, Lantz KC, et al. The value of a wound score for diabetic foot infections in predicting treatment outcome: a prospective analysis from the SIDESTEP trial. Wound Repair Regen 2009;17(5):671–7.
75. Lipsky BA, Itani K, Norden C. Treating foot infections in diabetic patients: a randomized, multicenter, open-label trial of linezolid versus ampicillin-sulbactam/ amoxicillin-clavulanate. Clin Infect Dis 2004;38(1):17–24.
76. Ge Y, MacDonald D, Henry MM, et al. In vitro susceptibility to pexiganan of bacteria isolated from infected diabetic foot ulcers. Diagn Microbiol Infect Dis 1999; 35(1):45–53.
77. Lipsky BA, Armstrong DG, Baker NR, et al. Does a diabetic foot infection (DFI) wound score correlate with the clinical response to antibiotic treatment? Data from the SIDESTEP study. Diabetologia 2005;48:A354.
78. Lipsky BA, Armstrong DG, Citron DM, et al. Ertapenem versus piperacillin/ tazobactam for diabetic foot infections (SIDESTEP): prospective, randomised, controlled, double-blinded, multicentre trial. Lancet 2005;366(9498): 1695–703.
79. Widatalla AH, Mahadi SE, Shawer MA, et al. Implementation of diabetic foot ulcer classification system for research purposes to predict lower extremity amputation. Int J Diabetes Dev Ctries 2009;29(1):1–5.
80. Lavery LA, Armstrong DG, Murdoch DP, et al. Validation of the Infectious Diseases Society of America's diabetic foot infection classification system. Clin Infect Dis 2007;44(4):562–5.
81. Prompers L, Huijberts M, Apelqvist J, et al. High prevalence of ischaemia, infection and serious comorbidity in patients with diabetic foot disease in Europe. Baseline results from the Eurodiale study. Diabetologia 2007; 50(1):18–25.
82. Jeandrot A, Richard JL, Combescure C, et al. Serum procalcitonin and C-reactive protein concentrations to distinguish mildly infected from non-infected diabetic foot ulcers: a pilot study. Diabetologia 2008;51(2):347–52.
83. Lipsky BA, Berendt AR, Deery HG, et al. Diagnosis and treatment of diabetic foot infections. Clin Infect Dis 2004;39(7):885–910.

84. Berendt AR, Lipsky BA. Should antibiotics be used in the treatment of the diabetic foot? Diabet Foot 2003;6:18–28.

85. Chantelau E, Tanudjaja T, Altenhofer F, et al. Antibiotic treatment for uncomplicated neuropathic forefoot ulcers in diabetes: a controlled trial. Diabet Med 1996;13(2):156–9.

86. Foster AV, Bates M, Doxford M, et al. Should oral antibiotics be given to "clean" foot ulcers with no cellulitis? [abstract] Noordwijkerhout (The Netherlands): International Working Group on the Diabetic Foot; 1999.

87. Sapico FL, Witte JL, Canawati HN, et al. The infected foot of the diabetic patient: quantitative microbiology and analysis of clinical features. Rev Infect Dis 1984; 6(Suppl 1):S171–6.

88. Lipsky BA, Pecoraro RE, Larson SA, et al. Outpatient management of uncomplicated lower-extremity infections in diabetic patients. Arch Intern Med 1990; 150(4):790–7.

89. Senneville E, Melliez H, Beltrand E, et al. Culture of percutaneous bone biopsy specimens for diagnosis of diabetic foot osteomyelitis: concordance with ulcer swab cultures. Clin Infect Dis 2006;42(1):57–62.

90. Embil JM, Trepman E. Microbiological evaluation of diabetic foot osteomyelitis. Clin Infect Dis 2006;42(1):63–5.

91. Urbancic-Rovan V, Gubina M. Bacteria in superficial diabetic foot ulcers. Diabet Med 2000;17(11):814–5.

92. Lipsky BA, Pecoraro RE, Wheat LJ. The diabetic foot. Soft tissue and bone infection. Infect Dis Clin North Am 1990;4(3):409–32.

93. Goldstein EJ, Citron DM, Nesbit CA. Diabetic foot infections. Bacteriology and activity of 10 oral antimicrobial agents against bacteria isolated from consecutive cases. Diabetes Care 1996;19(6):638–41.

94. Ge Y, MacDonald D, Hait H, et al. Microbiological profile of infected diabetic foot ulcers. Diabet Med 2002;19(12):1032–4.

95. Gadepalli R, Dhawan B, Sreenivas V, et al. A clinico-microbiological study of diabetic foot ulcers in an Indian tertiary care hospital. Diabetes Care 2006;29(8): 1727–32.

96. Abdulrazak A, Bitar ZI, Al-Shamali AA, et al. Bacteriological study of diabetic foot infections. J Diabetes Complications 2005;19(3):138–41.

97. Jones EW, Edwards R, Finch R, et al. A microbiological study of diabetic foot lesions. Diabet Med 1985;2(3):213–5.

98. Hunt JA. Foot infections in diabetes are rarely due to a single microorganism. Diabet Med 1992;9(8):749–52.

99. Louie A, Baltch AL, Smith RP. Gram-negative bacterial surveillance in diabetic patients. Infect Med 1993;10(2):33–45.

100. Candel Gonzalez FJ, Alramadan M, Matesanz M, et al. Infections in diabetic foot ulcers. Eur J Intern Med 2003;14(5):341–3.

101. Wheat LJ, Allen SD, Henry M, et al. Diabetic foot infections. Bacteriologic analysis. Arch Intern Med 1986;146(10):1935–40.

102. Pathare NA, Bal A, Talvalkar GV, et al. Diabetic foot infections: a study of microorganisms associated with the different Wagner grades. Indian J Pathol Microbiol 1998;41(4):437–41.

103. Gerding DN. Foot infections in diabetic patients: the role of anaerobes. Clin Infect Dis 1995;20(Suppl 2):S283–8.

104. Hartemann-Heurtier A, Robert J, Jacqueminet S, et al. Diabetic foot ulcer and multidrug-resistant organisms: risk factors and impact. Diabet Med 2004; 21(7):710–5.

105. Tentolouris N, Jude EB, Smirnof I, et al. Methicillin-resistant *Staphylococcus aureus*: an increasing problem in a diabetic foot clinic. Diabet Med 1999;16(9):767–71.
106. Tentolouris N, Petrikkos G, Vallianou N, et al. Prevalence of methicillin-resistant *Staphylococcus aureus* in infected and uninfected diabetic foot ulcers. Clin Microbiol Infect 2006;12(2):186–9.
107. Mendes JJ, Marques-Costa A, Vilela C, et al. Clinical and bacteriological survey of diabetic foot infections in Lisbon. Diabetes Res Clin Pract 2012; 95(1):153–61.
108. Dang CN, Prasad YD, Boulton AJ, et al. Methicillin-resistant *Staphylococcus aureus* in the diabetic foot clinic: a worsening problem. Diabet Med 2003; 20(2):159–61.
109. Wagner A, Reike H, Angelkort B. Erfahrungen im Umgang mit hochresistenten Keimen bei Patienten mit diabetischem Fuß-Syndrom unter besonderer Berück-sichtigung von MRSA-Infektionen. [Highly resistant pathogens in patients with diabetic foot syndrome with special reference to methicillin-resistant *Staphylococcus aureus* infections]. Dtsch Med Wochenschr 2001;126(48):1353–6 [in German].
110. Moran GJ, Krishnadasan A, Gorwitz RJ, et al. Methicillin-resistant *S. aureus* infections among patients in the emergency department. N Engl J Med 2006; 355(7):666–74.
111. Kandemir O, Akbay E, Sahin E, et al. Risk factors for infection of the diabetic foot with multi-antibiotic resistant microorganisms. J Infect 2007;54(5):439–45.
112. Edmonds M, Foster A. The use of antibiotics in the diabetic foot. Am J Surg 2004;187(5):25S–8S.
113. O'Meara S, Nelson EA, Golder S, et al. Systematic review of methods to diag-nose infection in foot ulcers in diabetes. Diabet Med 2006;23(4):341–7.
114. Hirschl M, Hirschl AM. Bacterial flora in mal perforant and antimicrobial treat-ment with ceftriaxone. Chemotherapy 1992;38(4):275–80.
115. Vardakas KZ, Horianopoulou M, Falagas ME. Factors associated with treatment failure in patients with diabetic foot infections: an analysis of data from random-ized controlled trials. Diabetes Res Clin Pract 2008;80(3):344–51.
116. Nelson EA, O'Meara S, Golder S, et al. Systematic review of antimicrobial treat-ments for diabetic foot ulcers. Diabet Med 2006;23(4):348–59.
117. Crouzet J, Lavigne JP, Richard JL, et al. Diabetic foot infection: a critical review of recent randomized clinical trials on antibiotic therapy. Int J Infect Dis 2011; 15(9):e601–10.
118. Peters EJ, Lipsky BA, Berendt AR, et al. A systematic review of the effectiveness of interventions in the management of infection in the diabetic foot. Diabetes Metab Res Rev 2012;28(Suppl 1):142–62.
119. Lipsky BA. Evidence-based antibiotic therapy of diabetic foot infections. FEMS Immunol Med Microbiol 1999;26(3–4):267–76.
120. Seabrook GR, Edmiston CE, Schmitt DD, et al. Comparison of serum and tissue antibiotic levels in diabetes-related foot infections. Surgery 1991;110(4):671–6.
121. Raymakers JT, Heyden vd JJ, Daemen MJ, et al. Penetration of ceftazidime in ischemic tissues. Proceedings of the Second International Symposium on the Diabetic Foot. Noordwijkerhout (The Netherlands): 1995. [abstract: P-50].
122. Storm AJ, Bouter KP, Diepersloot RJ, et al. Tissue concentrations of an orally administered antibiotic in diabetic patients with foot infections. J Antimicrob Chemother 1994;34(3):449–51.
123. Duckworth C, Fisher JF, Carter SA, et al. Tissue penetration of clindamycin in diabetic foot infections. J Antimicrob Chemother 1993;31(4):581–4.

124. Mueller-Buehl U, Diehm C, Gutzler F, et al. Tissue concentrations of ofloxacin in necrotic foot lesions of diabetic and non-diabetic patients with peripheral arterial occlusive disease. Vasa 1991;20(1):17–21.

125. Kuck EM, Bouter KP, Hoekstra JB, et al. Tissue concentrations after a single-dose, orally administered ofloxacin in patients with diabetic foot infections. Foot Ankle Int 1998;19(1):38–40.

126. Marangos MN, Skoutelis AT, Nightingale CH, et al. Absorption of ciprofloxacin in patients with diabetic gastroparesis. Antimicrob Agents Chemother 1995;39(9):2161–3.

127. Itani KM, Weigelt J, Li JZ, et al. Linezolid reduces length of stay and duration of intravenous treatment compared with vancomycin for complicated skin and soft tissue infections due to suspected or proven methicillin-resistant *Staphylococcus aureus* (MRSA). Int J Antimicrob Agents 2005;26(6):442–8.

128. Weigelt J, Itani K, Stevens D, et al. Linezolid versus vancomycin in treatment of complicated skin and soft tissue infections. Antimicrob Agents Chemother 2005; 49(6):2260–6.

129. Stein GE, Schooley S, Peloquin CA, et al. Linezolid tissue penetration and serum activity against strains of methicillin-resistant *Staphylococcus aureus* with reduced vancomycin susceptibility in diabetic patients with foot infections. J Antimicrob Chemother 2007;60(4):819–23.

130. Lipsky BA, Stoutenburgh U. Daptomycin for treating infected diabetic foot ulcers: evidence from a randomized, controlled trial comparing daptomycin with vancomycin or semi-synthetic penicillins for complicated skin and skin-structure infections. J Antimicrob Chemother 2005;55(2):240–5.

131. Jauregui LE, Babazadeh S, Seltzer E, et al. Randomized, double-blind comparison of once-weekly dalbavancin versus twice-daily linezolid therapy for the treatment of complicated skin and skin structure infections. Clin Infect Dis 2005;41(10):1407–15.

132. Seltzer E, Dorr MB, Goldstein BP, et al. Once-weekly dalbavancin versus standard-of-care antimicrobial regimens for treatment of skin and soft-tissue infections. Clin Infect Dis 2003;37(10):1298–303.

133. Stryjewski ME, O'Riordan WD, Lau WK, et al. Telavancin versus standard therapy for treatment of complicated skin and soft-tissue infections due to gram-positive bacteria. Clin Infect Dis 2005;40(11):1601–7.

134. Doan TL, Fung HB, Mehta D, et al. Tigecycline: a glycylcycline antimicrobial agent. Clin Ther 2006;28(8):1079–106.

135. Noel GJ, Bush K, Bagchi P, et al. A randomized, double-blind trial comparing ceftobiprole medocaril with vancomycin plus ceftazidime for the treatment of patients with complicated skin and skin-structure infections. Clin Infect Dis 2008;46(5):647–55.

136. Noel GJ, Strauss RS, Amsler K, et al. Results of a double-blind, randomized trial of ceftobiprole treatment of complicated skin and skin structure infections caused by gram-positive bacteria. Antimicrob Agents Chemother 2008;52(1):37–44.

137. Lipsky BA, Giordano P, Choudhri S, et al. Treating diabetic foot infections with sequential intravenous to oral moxifloxacin compared with piperacillin-tazobactam/amoxicillin-clavulanate. J Antimicrob Chemother 2007;60(2):370–6.

138. Schaper NC, Dryden M, Kujath P, et al. Efficacy and safety of IV/PO moxifloxacin and IV piperacillin/tazobactam followed by PO amoxicillin/clavulanic acid in the treatment of diabetic foot infections: results of the RELIEF study. Infection 2013; 41(1):175–86.

139. Aragón-Sánchez J. Seminar review: a review of the basis of surgical treatment of diabetic foot infections. Int J Low Extrem Wounds 2011;10(1):33–65.
140. Fisher TK, Scimeca CL, Bharara M, et al. A stepwise approach for surgical management of diabetic foot infections. J Am Podiatr Med Assoc 2010;100(5): 401–5.
141. Lipsky BA, Peters EJ, Berendt AR, et al. Specific guidelines for the treatment of diabetic foot infections 2011. Diabetes Metab Res Rev 2012;28(Suppl 1):234–5.
142. Lipsky BA, Peters EJ, Senneville E, et al. Expert opinion on the management of infections in the diabetic foot. Diabetes Metab Res Rev 2012;28(Suppl 1): 163–78.
143. Senneville E. Antimicrobial interventions for the management of diabetic foot infections. Expert Opin Pharmacother 2005;6(2):263–73.
144. Armstrong DG, Liswood PJ, Todd WF. 1995 William J. Stickel Bronze Award. Prevalence of mixed infections in the diabetic pedal wound. A retrospective review of 112 infections. J Am Podiatr Med Assoc 1995;85(10):533–7.
145. Lipsky BA, Baker PD, Landon GC, et al. Antibiotic therapy for diabetic foot infections: comparison of two parenteral-to-oral regimens. Clin Infect Dis 1997;24(4): 643–8.
146. Grayson ML, Gibbons GW, Habershaw GM, et al. Use of ampicillin/sulbactam versus imipenem/cilastatin in the treatment of limb-threatening foot infections in diabetic patients. Clin Infect Dis 1994;18(5):683–93.
147. Mills JL, Beckett WC, Taylor SM. The diabetic foot: consequences of delayed treatment and referral. South Med J 1991;84(8):970–4.
148. Johnson SW, Drew RH, May DB. How long to treat with antibiotics following amputation in patients with diabetic foot infections? Are the 2012 IDSA DFI guidelines reasonable? J Clin Pharm Ther 2013;38(2):85–8.
149. Peterson LR, Lissack LM, Canter K, et al. Therapy of lower extremity infections with ciprofloxacin in patients with diabetes mellitus, peripheral vascular disease, or both. Am J Med 1989;86(6):801–8.
150. Embil JM, Rose G, Trepman E, et al. Oral antimicrobial therapy for diabetic foot osteomyelitis. Foot Ankle Int 2006;27(10):771–9.
151. Hinchliffe RJ, Valk GD, Apelqvist J, et al. A systematic review of the effectiveness of interventions to enhance the healing of chronic ulcers of the foot in diabetes. Diabetes Metab Res Rev 2008;24(Suppl 1):S119–44.
152. Game FL, Hinchliffe RJ, Apelqvist J, et al. A systematic review of interventions to enhance the healing of chronic ulcers of the foot in diabetes. Diabetes Metab Res Rev 2012;28(Suppl 1):119–41.
153. Apelqvist J, Ragnarson Tennvall G. Cavity foot ulcers in diabetic patients: a comparative study of cadexomer iodine ointment and standard treatment. An economic analysis alongside a clinical trial. Acta Derm Venereol 1996;76(3): 231–5.
154. Apelqvist J, Larsson J, Stenstrom A. Topical treatment of necrotic foot ulcers in diabetic patients: a comparative trial of DuoDerm and MeZinc. Br J Dermatol 1990;123(6):787–92.
155. Bennett LL, Rosenblum RS, Perlov C, et al. An in vivo comparison of topical agents on wound repair. Plast Reconstr Surg 2001;108(3):675–87.
156. Bergin SM, Wraight P. Silver based wound dressings and topical agents for treating diabetic foot ulcers. Cochrane Database Syst Rev 2006;(1):CD005082.
157. Armstrong DG, Salas P, Short B, et al. Maggot therapy in "lower-extremity hospice" wound care: fewer amputations and more antibiotic-free days. J Am Podiatr Med Assoc 2005;95(3):254–7.

158. Jaklic D, Lapanje A, Zupancic K, et al. Selective antimicrobial activity of maggots against pathogenic bacteria. J Med Microbiol 2008;57:617–25.
159. van der Plas MJ, Jukema GN, Wai SW, et al. Maggot excretions/secretions are differentially effective against biofilms of *Staphylococcus aureus* and *Pseudomonas aeruginosa*. J Antimicrob Chemother 2008;61(1):117–22.
160. Berendt AR, Peters EJ, Bakker K, et al. Diabetic foot osteomyelitis: a progress report on diagnosis and a systematic review of treatment. Diabetes Metab Res Rev 2008;24(Suppl 1):S145–61.
161. Gibbons GW. Lower extremity bypass in patients with diabetic foot ulcers. Surg Clin North Am 2003;83(3):659–69.
162. Bishop AJ, Mudge E. Diabetic foot ulcers treated with hyperbaric oxygen therapy: a review of the literature. Int Wound J 2012. [Epub ahead of print].
163. Barnes RC. Point: hyperbaric oxygen is beneficial for diabetic foot wounds. Clin Infect Dis 2006;43(2):188–92.
164. Berendt AR. Counterpoint: hyperbaric oxygen for diabetic foot wounds is not effective. Clin Infect Dis 2006;43(2):193–8.
165. Kranke P, Bennett MH, Martyn-St James M, et al. Hyperbaric oxygen therapy for chronic wounds. Cochrane Database Syst Rev 2012;(4):CD004123.
166. Abidia A, Laden G, Kuhan G, et al. The role of hyperbaric oxygen therapy in ischaemic diabetic lower extremity ulcers: a double-blind randomised-controlled trial. Eur J Vasc Endovasc Surg 2003;25(6):513–8.
167. Doctor N, Pandya S, Supe A. Hyperbaric oxygen therapy in diabetic foot. J Postgrad Med 1992;38(3):112–4, 111.
168. Faglia E, Favales F, Aldeghi A, et al. Adjunctive systemic hyperbaric oxygen therapy in treatment of severe prevalently ischemic diabetic foot ulcer. A randomized study. Diabetes Care 1996;19(12):1338–43.
169. Löndahl M, Katzman P, Nilsson A, et al. Hyperbaric oxygen therapy facilitates healing of chronic foot ulcers in patients with diabetes. Diabetes Care 2010;33(5):998–1003.
170. Ramsey SD, Newton K, Blough D, et al. Incidence, outcomes, and cost of foot ulcers in patients with diabetes. Diabetes Care 1999;22(3):382–7.
171. Newman LG, Waller J, Palestro CJ, et al. Unsuspected osteomyelitis in diabetic foot ulcers. Diagnosis and monitoring by leukocyte scanning with indium in 111 oxyquinoline. JAMA 1991;266(9):1246–51.
172. Lipsky BA. Osteomyelitis of the foot in diabetic patients. Clin Infect Dis 1997;25(6):1318–26.
173. Lavery LA, Sariaya M, Ashry H, et al. Microbiology of osteomyelitis in diabetic foot infections. J Foot Ankle Surg 1995;34(1):61–4.
174. Zimmerli W, Fluckiger U. Classification and microbiology of osteomyelitis. Orthopade 2004;33(3):267–72 [in German].
175. Game F, Jeffcoate W. MRSA and osteomyelitis of the foot in diabetes. Diabet Med 2004;21(Suppl 4):16–9.
176. Stewart PS. Mechanisms of antibiotic resistance in bacterial biofilms. Int J Med Microbiol 2002;292(2):107–13.
177. Gristina AG, Costerton JW. Bacterial adherence and the glycocalyx and their role in musculoskeletal infection. Orthop Clin North Am 1984;15(3):517–35.
178. Berendt T, Byren I. Bone and joint infection. Clin Med 2004;4(6):510–8.
179. Ciampolini J, Harding KG. Pathophysiology of chronic bacterial osteomyelitis. Why do antibiotics fail so often? Postgrad Med J 2000;76(898):479–83.
180. Donlan RM, Costerton JW. Biofilms: survival mechanisms of clinically relevant microorganisms. Clin Microbiol Rev 2002;15(2):167–93.

181. Whitchurch CB, Tolker-Nielsen T, Ragas PC, et al. Extracellular DNA required for bacterial biofilm formation. Science 2002;295(5559):1487.
182. Donlan RM. Role of biofilms in antimicrobial resistance. ASAIO J 2000;46(6): S47–52.
183. Patel R. Biofilms and antimicrobial resistance. Clin Orthop Relat Res 2005;(437): 41–7.
184. Weigel LM, Donlan RM, Shin DH, et al. High-level vancomycin-resistant *Staphylococcus aureus* isolates associated with a polymicrobial biofilm. Antimicrob Agents Chemother 2007;51(1):231–8.
185. Dinh MT, Abad CL, Safdar N. Diagnostic accuracy of the physical examination and imaging tests for osteomyelitis underlying diabetic foot ulcers: meta-analysis. Clin Infect Dis 2008;47(4):519–27.
186. Enderle MD, Coerper S, Schweizer HP, et al. Correlation of imaging techniques to histopathology in patients with diabetic foot syndrome and clinical suspicion of chronic osteomyelitis. The role of high-resolution ultrasound. Diabetes Care 1999;22(2):294–9.
187. Vesco L, Boulahdour H, Hamissa S, et al. The value of combined radionuclide and magnetic resonance imaging in the diagnosis and conservative management of minimal or localized osteomyelitis of the foot in diabetic patients. Metabolism 1999;48(7):922–7.
188. Armstrong DG, Lavery LA, Sariaya M, et al. Leukocytosis is a poor indicator of acute osteomyelitis of the foot in diabetes mellitus. J Foot Ankle Surg 1996; 35(4):280–3.
189. Grayson ML, Gibbons GW, Balogh K, et al. Probing to bone in infected pedal ulcers. A clinical sign of underlying osteomyelitis in diabetic patients. JAMA 1995;273(9):721–3.
190. Shone A, Burnside J, Chipchase S, et al. Probing the validity of the probe-to-bone test in the diagnosis of osteomyelitis of the foot in diabetes. Diabetes Care 2006;29(4):945.
191. Lavery LA, Armstrong DG, Peters EJ, et al. Probe-to-bone test for diagnosing diabetic foot osteomyelitis: reliable or relic? Diabetes Care 2007; 30(2):270–4.
192. Aragón-Sánchez J, Lipsky BA, Lázaro-Martínez JL. Diagnosing diabetic foot osteomyelitis: is the combination of probe-to-bone test and plain radiography sufficient for high-risk inpatients? Diabet Med 2011;28(2):191–4.
193. Mutluoglu M, Uzun G, Sildiroglu O, et al. Performance of the probe-to-bone test in a population suspected of having osteomyelitis of the foot in diabetes. J Am Podiatr Med Assoc 2012;102(5):369–73.
194. Morales Lozano R, Gonzalez Fernandez ML, Martinez Hernandez D, et al. Validating the probe-to-bone test and other tests for diagnosing chronic osteomyelitis in the diabetic foot. Diabetes Care 2010;33(10):2140–5.
195. Kaleta JL, Fleischli JW, Reilly CH. The diagnosis of osteomyelitis in diabetes using erythrocyte sedimentation rate: a pilot study. J Am Podiatr Med Assoc 2001; 91(9):445–50.
196. Butalia S, Palda VA, Sargeant RJ, et al. Does this patient with diabetes have osteomyelitis of the lower extremity? JAMA 2008;299(7):806–13.
197. DeStefano F, Newman J. Comparison of coronary heart disease mortality risk between black and white people with diabetes. Ethn Dis 1993;3(2):145–51.
198. Weinstein D, Wang A, Chambers R, et al. Evaluation of magnetic resonance imaging in the diagnosis of osteomyelitis in diabetic foot infections. Foot Ankle 1993;14(1):18–22.

199. Mettler MA. Essentials of radiology. Philadelphia: Elsevier Saunders; 2005.
200. Yuh WT, Corson JD, Baraniewski HM, et al. Osteomyelitis of the foot in diabetic patients: evaluation with plain film, 99mTc-MDP bone scintigraphy, and MR imaging. AJR Am J Roentgenol 1989;152(4):795–800.
201. Wang A, Weinstein D, Greenfield L, et al. MRI and diabetic foot infections. Magn Reson Imaging 1990;8(6):805–9.
202. Johnson JE, Kennedy EJ, Shereff MJ, et al. Prospective study of bone, indium-111-labeled white blood cell, and gallium-67 scanning for the evaluation of osteomyelitis in the diabetic foot. Foot Ankle Int 1996;17(1):10–6.
203. Lee SM, Lee RG, Wilinsky J, et al. Magnification radiography in osteomyelitis. Skeletal Radiol 1986;15(8):625–7.
204. Park HM, Wheat LJ, Siddiqui AR, et al. Scintigraphic evaluation of diabetic osteomyelitis: concise communication. J Nucl Med 1982;23(7):569–73.
205. Shults DW, Hunter GC, McIntyre KE, et al. Value of radiographs and bone scans in determining the need for therapy in diabetic patients with foot ulcers. Am J Surg 1989;158(6):525–9.
206. Croll SD, Nicholas GG, Osborne MA, et al. Role of magnetic resonance imaging in the diagnosis of osteomyelitis in diabetic foot infections. J Vasc Surg 1996;24(2):266–70.
207. Keenan AM, Tindel NL, Alavi A. Diagnosis of pedal osteomyelitis in diabetic patients using current scintigraphic techniques. Arch Intern Med 1989;149(10):2262–6.
208. Larcos G, Brown ML, Sutton RT. Diagnosis of osteomyelitis of the foot in diabetic patients: value of 111In-leukocyte scintigraphy. AJR Am J Roentgenol 1991;157(3):527–31.
209. Seldin DW, Heiken JP, Feldman F, et al. Effect of soft-tissue pathology on detection of pedal osteomyelitis in diabetics. J Nucl Med 1985;26(9):988–93.
210. Levine SE, Neagle CE, Esterhai JL, et al. Magnetic resonance imaging for the diagnosis of osteomyelitis in the diabetic patient with a foot ulcer. Foot Ankle Int 1994;15(3):151–6.
211. Oyen WJ, Netten PM, Lemmens JA, et al. Evaluation of infectious diabetic foot complications with indium-111-labeled human nonspecific immunoglobulin G. J Nucl Med 1992;33(7):1330–6.
212. Harwood SJ, Valdivia S, Hung GL, et al. Use of Sulesomab, a radiolabeled antibody fragment, to detect osteomyelitis in diabetic patients with foot ulcers by leukoscintigraphy. Clin Infect Dis 1999;28(6):1200–5.
213. Blume PA, Dey HM, Daley LJ, et al. Diagnosis of pedal osteomyelitis with Tc-99m HMPAO labeled leukocytes. J Foot Ankle Surg 1997;36(2):120–6.
214. Ertugrul MB, Baktiroglu S, Salman S, et al. The diagnosis of osteomyelitis of the foot in diabetes: microbiological examination vs. magnetic resonance imaging and labelled leucocyte scanning. Diabet Med 2006;23(6):649–53.
215. Newman LG, Waller J, Palestro CJ, et al. Leukocyte scanning with 111In is superior to magnetic resonance imaging in diagnosis of clinically unsuspected osteomyelitis in diabetic foot ulcers. Diabetes Care 1992;15(11):1527–30.
216. Craig JG, Amin MB, Wu K, et al. Osteomyelitis of the diabetic foot: MR imaging-pathologic correlation. Radiology 1997;203(3):849–55.
217. Horowitz JD, Durham JR, Nease DB, et al. Prospective evaluation of magnetic resonance imaging in the management of acute diabetic foot infections. Ann Vasc Surg 1993;7(1):44–50.
218. Kearney T, Pointin K, Cunningham D, et al. The detection of pedal osteomyelitis in diabetic patients. Practical Diabetes International 1999;16:98–100.

219. Ledermann HP, Schweitzer ME, Morrison WB. Nonenhancing tissue on MR imaging of pedal infection: characterization of necrotic tissue and associated limitations for diagnosis of osteomyelitis and abscess. AJR Am J Roentgenol 2002;178(1):215–22.

220. Lipman BT, Collier BD, Carrera GF, et al. Detection of osteomyelitis in the neuropathic foot: nuclear medicine, MRI and conventional radiography. Clin Nucl Med 1998;23(2):77–82.

221. Maas M, Slim EJ, Hoeksma AF, et al. MR imaging of neuropathic feet in leprosy patients with suspected osteomyelitis. Int J Lepr Other Mycobact Dis 2002; 70(2):97–103.

222. Morrison WB, Schweitzer ME, Batte WG, et al. Osteomyelitis of the foot: relative importance of primary and secondary MR imaging signs. Radiology 1998; 207(3):625–32.

223. Nigro ND, Bartynski WS, Grossman SJ, et al. Clinical impact of magnetic resonance imaging in foot osteomyelitis. J Am Podiatr Med Assoc 1992;82(12): 603–15.

224. Remedios D, Valabhji J, Oelbaum R, et al. 99mTc-nanocolloid scintigraphy for assessing osteomyelitis in diabetic neuropathic feet. Clin Radiol 1998;53(2): 120–5.

225. Kapoor A, Page S, Lavalley M, et al. Magnetic resonance imaging for diagnosing foot osteomyelitis: a meta-analysis. Arch Intern Med 2007;167(2): 125–32.

226. Karchevsky M, Schweitzer ME, Morrison WB, et al. MRI findings of septic arthritis and associated osteomyelitis in adults. AJR Am J Roentgenol 2004; 182(1):119–22.

227. Capriotti G, Chianelli M, Signore A. Nuclear medicine imaging of diabetic foot infection: results of meta-analysis. Nucl Med Commun 2006;27(10):757–64.

228. Devillers A, Moisan A, Hennion F, et al. Contribution of technetium-99m hexamethylpropylene amine oxime labelled leucocyte scintigraphy to the diagnosis of diabetic foot infection. Eur J Nucl Med 1998;25(2):132–8.

229. Harvey J, Cohen MM. Technetium-99-labeled leukocytes in diagnosing diabetic osteomyelitis in the foot. J Foot Ankle Surg 1997;36(3):209–14.

230. Unal SN, Birinci H, Baktiroglu S, et al. Comparison of Tc-99m methylene diphosphonate, Tc-99m human immune globulin, and Tc-99m-labeled white blood cell scintigraphy in the diabetic foot. Clin Nucl Med 2001;26(12):1016–21.

231. Zhuang H, Duarte PS, Pourdehand M, et al. Exclusion of chronic osteomyelitis with F-18 fluorodeoxyglucose positron emission tomographic imaging. Clin Nucl Med 2000;25(4):281–4.

232. Kalicke T, Schmitz A, Risse JH, et al. Fluorine-18 fluorodeoxyglucose PET in infectious bone diseases: results of histologically confirmed cases. Eur J Nucl Med 2000;27(5):524–8.

233. Meller J, Koster G, Liersch T, et al. Chronic bacterial osteomyelitis: prospective comparison of (18)F-FDG imaging with a dual-head coincidence camera and (111)In-labelled autologous leucocyte scintigraphy. Eur J Nucl Med Mol Imaging 2002;29(1):53–60.

234. Guhlmann A, Brecht-Krauss D, Suger G, et al. Chronic osteomyelitis: detection with FDG PET and correlation with histopathologic findings. Radiology 1998; 206(3):749–54.

235. Guhlmann A, Brecht-Krauss D, Suger G, et al. Fluorine-18-FDG PET and technetium-99m antigranulocyte antibody scintigraphy in chronic osteomyelitis. J Nucl Med 1998;39(12):2145–52.

236. Hartmann A, Eid K, Dora C, et al. Diagnostic value of 18F-FDG PET/CT in trauma patients with suspected chronic osteomyelitis. Eur J Nucl Med Mol Imaging 2007;34(5):704–14.

237. Basu S, Chryssikos T, Houseni M, et al. Potential role of FDG PET in the setting of diabetic neuro-osteoarthropathy: can it differentiate uncomplicated Charcot's neuroarthropathy from osteomyelitis and soft-tissue infection? Nucl Med Commun 2007;28(6):465–72.

238. Keidar Z, Militianu D, Melamed E, et al. The diabetic foot: initial experience with 18F-FDG PET/CT. J Nucl Med 2005;46(3):444–9.

239. Schwegler B, Stumpe KD, Weishaupt D, et al. Unsuspected osteomyelitis is frequent in persistent diabetic foot ulcer and better diagnosed by MRI than by 18F-FDG PET or 99mTc-MOAB. J Intern Med 2008;263(1):99–106.

240. Kagna O, Srour S, Melamed E, et al. FDG PET/CT imaging in the diagnosis of osteomyelitis in the diabetic foot. Eur J Nucl Med Mol Imaging 2012;39(10): 1545–50.

241. Nawaz A, Torigian DA, Siegelman ES, et al. Diagnostic performance of FDG-PET, MRI, and plain film radiography (PFR) for the diagnosis of osteomyelitis in the diabetic foot. Mol Imaging Biol 2010;12(3):335–42.

242. Senneville E, Morant H, Descamps D, et al. Needle puncture and transcutaneous bone biopsy cultures are inconsistent in patients with diabetes and suspected osteomyelitis of the foot. Clin Infect Dis 2009;48(7):888–93.

243. Slater RA, Lazarovitch T, Boldur I, et al. Swab cultures accurately identify bacterial pathogens in diabetic foot wounds not involving bone. Diabet Med 2004; 21(7):705–9.

244. Kessler L, Piemont Y, Ortega F, et al. Comparison of microbiological results of needle puncture vs. superficial swab in infected diabetic foot ulcer with osteomyelitis. Diabet Med 2006;23(1):99–102.

245. Jeffcoate WJ, Lipsky BA. Controversies in diagnosing and managing osteomyelitis of the foot in diabetes. Clin Infect Dis 2004;39(Suppl 2):S115–22.

246. Tan JS, Friedman NM, Hazelton-Miller C, et al. Can aggressive treatment of diabetic foot infections reduce the need for above-ankle amputation? Clin Infect Dis 1996;23(2):286–91.

247. Ha Van G, Siney H, Danan JP, et al. Treatment of osteomyelitis in the diabetic foot. Contribution of conservative surgery. Diabetes Care 1996;19(11):1257–60.

248. Pittet D, Wyssa B, Herter-Clavel C, et al. Outcome of diabetic foot infections treated conservatively: a retrospective cohort study with long-term follow-up. Arch Intern Med 1999;159(8):851–6.

249. Simpson AH, Deakin M, Latham JM. Chronic osteomyelitis. The effect of the extent of surgical resection on infection-free survival. J Bone Joint Surg Br 2001;83(3):403–7.

250. Henke PK, Blackburn SA, Wainess RW, et al. Osteomyelitis of the foot and toe in adults is a surgical disease: conservative management worsens lower extremity salvage. Ann Surg 2005;241(6):885–92.

251. Venkatesan P, Lawn S, Macfarlane RM, et al. Conservative management of osteomyelitis in the feet of diabetic patients. Diabet Med 1997;14(6):487–90.

252. Senneville E, Yazdanpanah Y, Cazaubiel M, et al. Rifampicin-ofloxacin oral regimen for the treatment of mild to moderate diabetic foot osteomyelitis. J Antimicrob Chemother 2001;48(6):927–30.

253. Yamaguchi Y, Yoshida S, Sumikawa Y, et al. Rapid healing of intractable diabetic foot ulcers with exposed bones following a novel therapy of exposing bone marrow cells and then grafting epidermal sheets. Br J Dermatol 2004;151(5):1019–28.

254. Kumagi SG, Mahoney CR, Fitzgibbons TC, et al. Treatment of diabetic (neuropathic) foot ulcers with two-stage debridement and closure. Foot Ankle Int 1998;19(3):160–5.
255. Kerstein MD. Osteomyelitis associated with vascular insufficiency. Curr Ther Res Clin Exp 1974;16(4):306–10.
256. Cohen M, Roman A, Malcolm WG. Panmetatarsal head resection and transmetatarsal amputation versus solitary partial ray resection in the neuropathic foot. J Foot Surg 1991;30(1):29–33.
257. Faglia E, Clerici G, Caminiti M, et al. The role of early surgical debridement and revascularization in patients with diabetes and deep foot space abscess: retrospective review of 106 patients with diabetes. J Foot Ankle Surg 2006;45(4): 220–6.
258. Murdoch DP, Armstrong DG, Dacus JB, et al. The natural history of great toe amputations. J Foot Ankle Surg 1997;36(3):204–8.
259. Quebedeaux TL, Lavery LA, Lavery DC. The development of foot deformities and ulcers after great toe amputation in diabetes. Diabetes Care 1996;19(2): 165–7.
260. Lavery LA, Lavery DC, Quebedeax-Farnham TL. Increased foot pressures after great toe amputation in diabetes. Diabetes Care 1995;18(11):1460–2.
261. Peters EJ, Lavery LA. Effectiveness of the diabetic foot risk classification system of the International Working Group on the Diabetic Foot. Diabetes Care 2001; 24(8):1442–7.
262. Hosch J, Quiroga C, Bosma J, et al. Outcomes of transmetatarsal amputations in patients with diabetes mellitus. J Foot Ankle Surg 1997;36(6):430–4.
263. Lazzarini L, Lipsky BA, Mader JT. Antibiotic treatment of osteomyelitis: what have we learned from 30 years of clinical trials? Int J Infect Dis 2005;9(3):127–38.
264. Saltoglu N, Dalkiran A, Tetiker T, et al. Piperacillin/tazobactam versus imipenem/ cilastatin for severe diabetic foot infections: a prospective, randomized clinical trial in a university hospital. Clin Microbiol Infect 2010;16(8):1252–7.
265. Erstad BL, McIntyre J. Prospective, randomized comparison of ampicillin/ sulbactam and cefoxitin for diabetic foot infections. Vasc Surg 1997;31(4): 419–26.
266. Spellberg B, Lipsky BA. Systemic antibiotic therapy for chronic osteomyelitis in adults. Clin Infect Dis 2012;54(3):393–407.
267. Walenkamp GH, Kleijn LL, de Leeuw M. Osteomyelitis treated with gentamicin-PMMA beads: 100 patients followed for 1-12 years. Acta Orthop Scand 1998; 69(5):518–22.
268. Klemm K. Gentamicin-PMMA-beads in treating bone and soft tissue infections (author's transl). Zentralbl Chir 1979;104(14):934–42 [in German].
269. Blaha JD, Calhoun JH, Nelson CL, et al. Comparison of the clinical efficacy and tolerance of gentamicin PMMA beads on surgical wire versus combined and systemic therapy for osteomyelitis. Clin Orthop Relat Res 1993;(295):8–12.
270. Jerosch J, Lindner N, Fuchs S. Results of long-term therapy of chronic, post-traumatic osteomyelitis with gentamycin PMMA chains. Unfallchirurg 1995; 98(6):338–43 [in German].
271. Barth RE, Vogely HC, Hoepelman AI, et al. To bead or not to bead? Treatment of osteomyelitis and prosthetic joint associated infections with gentamicin bead chains. Int J Antimicrob Agents 2011;38(5):371–5 (manuscript number: IJAA-D-11-00202).
272. Byren I, Peters EJ, Hoey C, et al. Pharmacotherapy of diabetic foot osteomyelitis. Expert Opin Pharmacother 2009;10(18):3033–47.

273. Norden CW. Lessons learned from animal models of osteomyelitis. Rev Infect Dis 1988;10(1):103–10.

274. Andros G, Armstrong DG, Attinger CE, et al. Consensus statement on negative pressure wound therapy (V.A.C. Therapy) for the management of diabetic foot wounds. Ostomy Wound Manage 2006;(Suppl):1–32.

Osteomyelitis in the Diabetic Foot
Diagnosis and Management

Frances L. Game, FRCP

KEYWORDS

- Diabetic foot • Osteomyelitis • Antibiotic therapy • Amputation

KEY POINTS

- Osteomyelitis of the foot in diabetes is common and frequently undiagnosed.
- Diagnosis should be clinical in the first instance and based on signs of infection, the size of the lesion, and the visibility of bone. but supported by the results of radiologic examination.
- The gold standard for diagnosis is the histologic and microbiological examination of bone, but this may not be possible or necessary in all patients. The possibility of sampling error must be taken into account.
- There is no clear consensus as to whether management should be primarily medical (antibiotics) or surgical; the pros and cons of each approach must be taken into account on an individual basis and after discussion with patients.

INTRODUCTION

Infection of the bone is a common complication of foot ulceration in diabetes and, depending on the study quoted, may complicate between 20% and 60% of the patients presenting with ulcers to a specialist clinic. Despite the existence of published guidelines,[1,2] there is little robust evidence on which much of the guidance is based and, as a result, approaches to management may vary widely. Professionals working in different countries and health care systems may hold differing views on diagnosis, the choice of antibiotics and their route and duration of administration, and the place of surgery.

PATHOLOGY

In general, the spread of infection into the bone of the foot of a patient with diabetes results from the contiguous spread of any infection of adjacent soft tissue, which may be complicating an ulcer. Bacteria enter through the cortex before spreading to the marrow. The bones affected, therefore, are those adjacent to areas where ulcers

Conflict of Interest: Nil.
Department of Diabetes and Endocrinology, Derby Hospitals NHS Trust, Uttoxeter Road, Derby DE22 3NE, UK
E-mail address: frances.game@nhs.net

Med Clin N Am 97 (2013) 947–956
http://dx.doi.org/10.1016/j.mcna.2013.03.010
0025-7125/13/$ – see front matter © 2013 Elsevier Inc. All rights reserved.

are most common—phalanges, metatarsal heads, and calcaneus. Because the spread of organisms is contiguous from the ulcers, causative organisms are similar to those isolated from complicated soft tissue infections (see the article by Peters and Lipsky elsewhere in this issue).

DIAGNOSIS
Histology and Culture of Bone

The gold standard of diagnosis of bone infection in the foot of patients with diabetes is said to be sampling of bone, which is then subjected to both histopathologic and microbiological examination.[2] This is usually done at the time of surgery or with fluoroscopic or CT guidance when surgery is not planned. In an insensate foot, a bone biopsy can be done with little or no anesthesia and the complication rate is low.[3] Histologic signs of osteomyelitis include bony necrosis and fragmentation with associated inflammatory infiltration, including leukocytes,[4] although there is currently a lack of standardized definition, which may lead to disagreement between pathologists as to the diagnosis.[5]

A condition from which it is sometimes difficult to distinguish bone infection (and may coexist) is the acute Charcot foot. Unfortunately, there are few descriptions in the literature of the histology of the acute Charcot foot to enable a histopathologist to confidently distinguish between the two. La Fontaine and colleagues[6] published the histology of a small series of 8 patients with Charcot foot in diabetes and described an inflammatory infiltrate in association with a disordered trabecular pattern. The inflammatory infiltrate was described as mainly lymphocytic in this small number of patients.

The microbiological definition of osteomyelitis relies on the culture of organisms from the bone. Care should be taken to avoid contamination, and hence, a false-positive result of the biopsy specimen, by taking a sample through skin uninvolved by ulceration. A falsely negative sample may occur from sampling error (biopsy taken from uninvolved bone) or previous treatment by antibiotics. The advantage of taking samples of bone for culture, however, is not only for diagnosis but also so that the organisms involved in the pathogenic process can be identified and targeted with appropriate and narrow-spectrum antimicrobial therapy. Unfortunately, culture of samples taken by swabbing the surface of wound has shown a less than 50% concordance with culture from bone.[7] Taking a deep tissue aspirate by needle aspiration close to bone is more accurate than surface swabs but still does not provide perfect concordance with organisms grown from bone.[8]

Although described as the gold standard, bone sampling is not performed in all patients in many specialist centers. There may be clinical reasons for this—patients are on anticoagulants, have severe ischemia, or have involvement of a very small bone, for example—but for some patients, it may be that there are doubts about whether it is a procedure that would provide an improvement in clinical outcome. A retrospective, non-randomised study from France[3] compared the outcome of patients whose management was based on biopsy-proved osteomyelitis (microbiology) versus those that were not and found an improvement in outcome in those patients who had had a biopsy (remission rates 81% vs 50%). There were other important clinical differences however, which may have affected the outcome of patients, including a higher use of Rifampicin in the centres performing bone biopsy. In addition, the outcomes of the patients who had biopsies were similar, however, to those in other reported series where no biopsies were routinely performed.[9] A further report from the same French group followed-up patients with negative biopsies for 2 years and found that 1 in 4 developed osteomyelitis after the original biopsy.[10]

Given these considerations, it is currently the recommendation of the Infectious Diseases Society of America[2] that bone biopsy be considered only in the following circumstances: (1) uncertainty regarding the diagnosis of osteomyelitis despite clinical and imaging evaluations; (2) an absence (or confusing mix) of culture data from soft tissue specimens; (3) failure of a patient to respond to empiric antibiotic therapy; and (4) a desire to use antibiotic agents that may be especially effective for osteomyelitis but have a high potential for selecting resistant organisms.

Clinical

Diagnosis is, in the first instance therefore, usually clinical and should be considered in any nonhealing wound of the foot in patients with diabetes when there is adequate perfusion and offloading has been optimized. There are various clinical features of a wound, however, that may be helpful in predicting the presence of bone infection. Of these, the depth and size of the ulcer has been considered predictive although the evidence to support this is weak. In a study where the prevalence of histology-proved osteomyelitis was 68%, the presence of exposed bone at the base of the ulcer had a sensitivity of only 32% but a specificity of 100% and an ulcer size greater than 2 cm had a sensitivity of only 52% but a specificity of 92%.[11]

Perhaps the most widely debated clinical sign is the probe-to-bone test. In one of the earliest studies,[12] a series of 76 infected ulcers were examined. Bone biopsy was not done to confirm the diagnosis in this study, but with a diagnosis on clinical criteria and in this population with a prevalence of osteomyelitis of 68%, a positive probe-to-bone test had a sensitivity of 66% and specificity of 87%, giving a positive predictive value of 89% and a negative predictive value of 56% for the diagnosis of osteomyelitis.

A subsequent UK study,[13] in a series of 81 consecutive outpatients with a total of 104 foot ulcers, both infected and noninfected, found a sensitivity of 38%, specificity of 91%, negative predictive value of 85%, and positive predictive value of only 53% for positive probe-to-bone tests to diagnose osteomyelitis (diagnosed radiologically, not by bone biopsy). The overall prevalence of osteomyelitis in this population was, however, only 23%. A further US study[14] evaluated the performance of the probe-to-bone test using the reference test of bone culture post-biopsy (not histology). In this series of 247 consecutive cases with only 12% prevalence of osteomyelitis, a positive probe-to-bone test had a sensitivity of 87%, specificity of 91%, negative predictive value of 96%, and positive predictive value of, again, only 57%. In this series, however, because only patients with a high clinical suspicion of osteomyelitis went on to have a bone biopsy and because it is uncertain whether treatment with antibiotics was started before bone culture, the prevalence of bone infection may have been higher than stated.

The only study to evaluate the probe-to-bone test in patients whose osteomyelitis was diagnosed on both bone histology and culture was performed in a series of 356 episodes of foot infections in 338 patients.[15] Almost all had surgery and biopsies were taken at the time of surgery. The prevalence of osteomyelitis was high, at 72.5%, and the sensitivity, specificity, and positive and negative predictive values for a positive probe-to-bone test for the diagnosis of osteomyelitis were 95%, 93%, 97%, and 83%, respectively.

What is clear is that the performance of the probe-to-bone test seems to vary with the prevalence of osteomyelitis in the population in which it is studied, with better positive predictive values demonstrated in populations with the highest prevalence. What is probably more important than prevalence is the pretest probability of osteomyelitis. The 2 centers with the highest prevalence of osteomyelitis were tertiary referral centers with a population of ulcers that were infected and not responding to standard therapies. Thus, the pretest probability of osteomyelitis was high. An analysis of the available data by Wrobel and Connolly[16] suggests that at the extremes of pretest probability (ie, <20% or >80%) the probe-to-bone test makes little difference to post-test probability. When the pretest probability is approximately 50%, however, then a positive or negative probe-to-bone test could possibly improve the post-test probability to approximately 80% (positive test) or to 30% (negative test), a performance similar to plain radiographs.

The situation is complicated by none of these studies having systematically assessed all patients, whether suspected or not clinically of having bone infection, with a bone biopsy, and perhaps it is unethical to do so. It is also of concern, however, that in the only published study to investigate the interobserver variability of the probe-to-bone test between professionals there seems to be only moderate to fair concordance.[17]

Blood Tests

Unfortunately the data to support the use of blood tests to definitively diagnose osteomyelitis in the foot of patients have been disappointing. In particular, an elevated white cell count was shown in 1 retrospective study to be absent in approximately half of patients presenting with bone infection.[18] Other markers of inflammation (eg, C-reactive protein [CRP] and erythrocyte sedimentation rate [ESR]) have also been investigated. Although 2 studies have shown that an ESR greater than 70 mm/h had 100% sensitivity for the diagnosis of osteomyelitis, the specificity of this was between 28% and 50%.[11,19]

Combination Tests

A recent prospective cohort study looked at combining the ulcer depth and CRP or ESR in a cohort of 54 patients with histology-proved osteomyelitis.[20] Combing the clinical and laboratory findings (ulcer depth >3 mm or CRP >30 mmol/L, ulcer depth >3 mm or ESR >60 mm/h) improved the sensitivity of the diagnosis of osteomyelitis to 100% with a specificity of 55%.

Imaging

There have been several reviews published of the utility of imaging for the diagnosis of osteomyelitis.[21–23] A recent meta-analysis found few studies, however, that compared the use of these investigations with diagnosis by bone histology and/or microbiology.[24]

Plain Radiograph

The sensitivity of plain radiographs is poor, particularly early in the disease process, because a loss of 30% to 50% of bone mineral content is required to produce noticeable changes. The first changes in bone on radiograph may be subtle and usually indicate that the infectious process has been present for at least 2 to 3 weeks. They include periosteal thickening, lytic lesions, osteopenia, loss of trabecular architecture, and new bone apposition.[25] Observational studies have demonstrated sensitivities of between 22% and 75% and specificities of 17% and 94% for the diagnosis of osteomyelitis.[26] The lack of specificity largely results from the difficulty in differentiating infection from Charcot neuro-osteoarthropathy in patients with bony destruction.

Despite the poor predictive value of a normal radiograph, however, it is recommended[2] that a plain radiograph be taken in all patients presenting with foot ulcers, because it could also indicate the presence of foreign bodies, bony deformities, or arterial calcification.

Radionucleotide Bone Scans

There are several published studies comparing the use of technetium Tc 99m phosphate bone scans with bone pathology for the diagnosis of osteomyelitis of the foot in diabetes. A meta-analysis[24] calculated the combined sensitivity of these studies as 81%, which is better than plain radiographs in the early diagnosis of the disease, but the calculated combined specificity was only 28%. Poor specificity generally relates to the inability of technetium bone scans to distinguish osteomyelitis from any other inflammatory process in the foot, in particular, again, an acute Charcot foot or even resolving osteomyelitis.[27] In addition, it is difficult to delineate the exact anatomic location or extent of the infection.

Other radionucleotide labeling techniques, which seem more specific for infection, such as indium In 111–labeled white cell, antigranulocyte Fab' fragment antibody, or technetium Tc 99m –labeled monoclonal antigranulocyte antibody scans, should, in theory, help distinguish between an acute Charcot foot and osteomyelitis.

In 1 meta-analysis, the pooled sensitivity of indium In 111–labeled white cell scans was 74% and the pooled specificity 68%.[24] Other labeled scans have been evaluated in small studies with no real improvement in sensitivity or specificity. The downside of labeled white cell scans includes the time taken to label cells, the need to handle blood and scan at 2 time points—4 and 24 hours, and the lack of anatomic definition.[28] The sensitivity may be reduced further in an ischemic foot.[4] Combining tests, such as labeled white cell or antigranulocyte Fab' fragment antibody with technetium-labeled bone scans, should, in theory, improve specificity. Studies to prove this have been small, however, and generally of poor quality.[26] Equally, combining single-photon emission (SPECT) CT/CT with bone and leukocyte scanning should, in theory, improve the spatial location of bone infection but suffers from all the other drawbacks of labeled white cell scans. Again, early studies are small and more evidence of utility and cost-effectiveness is required.[29,30]

MRI

MRI scans have the advantage over radionucleotide bone scans of being able to accurately define the anatomic location and extent of inflammatory change in the foot as well as any soft tissue infection, including sinus tracts, deep tissue necrosis, or abscesses. In a meta-analysis of 4 studies comparing the performance of MRI scans to bone pathology for the diagnosis of osteomyelitis, the combined sensitivity was 90% and the pooled specificity 79%.[24] The lower specificity in diabetes is usually attributable to the difficulty of distinguishing osteomyelitis from other causes of bone edema, in particular, Charcot neuroarthropathy.[31]

Other Types of Scan

Preliminary data suggest a possible role for combined fluorodeoxyglucose F 18–positron emission tomography/CT. The studies, however, are small, and vary not only in patient population but also in how the images are analyzed and the absence of correlation with bone pathology in the majority.[28] Standard CT scanning is more sensitive than plain radiography (and in some cases MRI) in detecting cortical disruption, periosteal reaction, and sequestrae but has low specificity.[29]

There is no single test that absolutely confirms or refutes a diagnosis of osteomyelitis in the diabetic foot. In 2008, a consensus group of the International Working Group on the Diabetic Foot described a suggested algorithm for the diagnosis of osteomyelitis based on clinical examination imaging and bone sampling methods that stratified the diagnosis into unlikely (<10% probability), possible (10%–50%), probable

(51%–90%), and definite (>90%).[1] At present, however, there is no robust validation of this scheme.

MANAGEMENT CHOICES

Approaches to the management of osteomyelitis of the foot in diabetes vary widely from center to center and country to country. Clinicians differ on such fundamental management issues as the choice route and duration of antibiotics but perhaps most frequently on the place of surgery. Many specialists maintain that early surgical excision of all infected bone is essential[32,33] whereas others maintain that the majority of patients can be managed with antibiotics alone.[34] These debates will continue as long as the data to support clinical decision making are not particularly robust (as shown in the systematic reviews by the International Working Group on the Diabetic Foot[1] and the Infectious Diseases Society of America[2]).

Conservative (Primarily Nonsurgical) Treatment

In support of a conservative, that is, primarily nonsurgical, approach is the evidence from more than 500 reported cases in the literature, in which initial management was primarily with antibiotics and in which there was a mean rate of eradication of infection of greater than 60%.[4] These data are all, however, from uncontrolled observational series and may have been affected by case selection, in particular, the exclusion of those who may have required early limb salvage surgery. One series of 147 cases from a UK center did, however, study a consecutive series of patients presenting with osteomyelitis of the foot, including those who had immediate surgery.[9] In this series, 80% of those who had no initial surgery had apparent arrest of their infection with antimicrobial therapy alone, although this represented only 63% of the total series if those who had immediate limb saving surgery are counted. Overall, there was a 23% minor and 8.8% major amputation rate. These case series have been criticized by some investigators, however, as failing to specify a definition of osteomyelitis, how patients were selected, and how much nonoperative débridement of bone was performed.[2]

A further criticism of this approach is the perceived requirement for excessively prolonged antimicrobial treatment compared with those having surgical resection. In the single-center UK series above, the median length of antibiotic treatment was 61 days.[9] Other investigators have reported even more prolonged courses of antibiotic treatment, with more than 50% of patients requiring 6 months or more antibiotic treatment in a separate UK series[35] and a mean of 40 weeks' treatment in a series from Canada.[36] Using prolonged courses of broad-spectrum antibiotics in this way undoubtedly increases the risk of side-effects (including the development of *Clostridium difficile* diarrhea) and an increased risk of allowing the emergence of antibiotic-resistant bacteria, such as methicillin-resistant *Staphylococcus aureus*.

Antibiotic Choices

At present, there are few robust data to guide clinicians in the choice, duration, or route of antimicrobial therapy.[1] Because the pathogens involved are generally those involved in soft tissue infection, it makes sense that regimens should be derived from protocols for the management of this complication of foot ulceration (see the article by Peters and Lipsky elsewhere in this issue).

There has been some interest in the use of implanted antibiotic carriers (eg, polymethyl methacrylate beads or calcium sulfate pellets) in conjunction with surgery[2] but the advantages of their use have yet to be confirmed in properly designed randomized trials.[37]

Primarily Surgical Treatment

There are few published data to support the view that surgical intervention is imperative in all cases in the management of osteomyelitis of the diabetic foot. The International Working Group on the Diabetic Foot systematic review[1] found only a few small case series and no randomized studies that directly compared primarily surgical and primarily nonsurgical management. A single-center retrospective analysis[38] of 112 patients (65 with osteomyelitis) admitted for management of infection of the foot in diabetes found that those in whom surgery was delayed by 3 days or more had a worse outcome. Details on the baseline characteristics of the patients, in particular, the clinical reasons why surgery may have been delayed, are not, however, explained in the article. In a larger retrospective series of 224 patients with osteomyelitis,[33] there seemed again to be an increased risk of eventual major amputation in those who had had surgery delayed compared with those who had immediate minor amputation of the affected area. The overall major amputation rate of the cohort was, however, high, at 25%. Another study[39] looked at 32 patients with diabetic forefoot osteomyelitis who had limited débridement of the infected area (ulcerectomy plus limited débridement of the underlying phalanx or metatarsal), with an eventual healing rate of 78%. There was, however, a mean duration of antibiotic therapy of 111 days in this series.

A more recent study[40] examined 185 sequential cases of diabetic foot osteomyelitis that were treated in a single center. After initial broad-spectrum intravenous antibiotics, limited conservative surgery was performed on the majority, although 71 had initial minor and 3 major amputations. The overall major amputation rate was only 8.1%, with a minor amputation rate of 48%. This published series gives no data on antibiotic usage, but in a subsequent series from the same center,[41] the median use of antibiotics was 36 days.

One of the consistent features of the published surgical series is the number of patients reported who, despite apparent débridement of infected bone, whether conservative or minor, had recurrence of the infection, requiring further surgical intervention. In the 2 most recent series,[40,41] this is reported as 18% and 25%, respectively. A possible explanation for this observation comes from 2 small studies,[42,43] both of which examined the histology of bone specimens taken at the osteotomy site at the time of minor amputation of the diabetic foot. In both there was histologic evidence of osteomyelitis at the osteotomy site, in 60% of 54 minor amputations and 35% of 111 patients, respectively. It is possible, therefore, that the difficulty of clinically distinguishing infected from noninfected bone at the time of operation is one explanation for the finding that the surgical series with the lowest postoperative risk of amputation have included antibiotics either preoperatively or postoperatively. Although it seems from a single published surgical series[41] as if the duration of antibiotic could potentially be shorter in those having surgery compared with the published series of primarily medical management, no direct comparisons have been made.

Another identified complication of surgical solutions to osteomyelitis is that the potential alteration of foot architecture may cause transfer ulceration, that is, skin breakdown at a new high-pressure site. In a single published study, the risk of transfer ulcers postsurgery was 41% but varied depending on the site of surgery; the highest risk of ulceration followed surgery to the first metatarsal head (28%) and the lowest the 5th metatarsal head (8%).[44]

Primarily Conservative Versus Primarily Surgical Approach?

The superiority of either approach, primarily nonsurgical or early conservative surgery, is currently unclear and clinicians need to weigh the risks of prolonged antibiotics with those of repeated surgery and possible transfer ulcers. Only future well-designed controlled trials will answer this question and in which situations either approach may be clearly superior. From published series, however, those centers with the lowest major amputation rates (even allowing for the question of baseline characteristics of the patients) are those that offer a combined approach to the patient. Either initial antibiotic treatment with surgical débridement after a period of observation or conservative surgery initially with antibiotic treatment postoperatively. Thus, as in all areas of management of the diabetic foot, it is apparent that a multidisciplinary approach is imperative, with surgeons, physicians, and specialists in infectious diseases and microbiology all involved in a holistic approach to patients but with the patients' own views at the heart of the decision making.

SUMMARY

Although osteomyelitis of the foot in diabetes remains common in specialist foot clinics across the world, the quality of published work to guide clinicians in the diagnosis and management is generally poor. Diagnosis should be based primarily on clinical signs supported by results of pathologic and radiologic investigations. Although the gold standard comes from the histologic and microbiological examination of bone, clinicians should be aware of the problems of sampling error. This lack of standardization of diagnostic criteria and of consensus on the choice of outcome measures poses further difficulties when seeking evidence to support management decisions. Experts have traditionally recommended surgical removal of infected bone but available evidence suggests that in many cases (excepting those in whom immediate surgery is required to save life or limb) a nonsurgical approach to management of osteomyelitis may be effective for many, if not most, patients with osteomyelitis of the diabetic foot. The benefits and limitations of both approaches need, however, to be established in prospective trials so that appropriate therapy can be offered to appropriate patients at the appropriate time, with the patients' views taken fully into account.

REFERENCES

1. Berendt AR, Peters EJ, Bakker K, et al. Diabetic foot osteomyelitis: a progress report on diagnosis and a systematic review of treatment. Diabetes Metab Res Rev 2008;24(Suppl 1):S145–61.
2. Lipsky BA, Berendt AR, Cornia PB, et al. 2012 Infectious Diseases Society of America clinical practice guideline for the diagnosis and treatment of diabetic foot infections. Clin Infect Dis 2012;54(12):132–73.
3. Senneville E, Lombart A, Beltrand E, et al. Outcome of diabetic foot osteomyelitis treated non-surgically: a retrospective cohort study. Diabetes Care 2008;31: 637–42.
4. Jeffcoate WJ, Lipsky BA. Controversies in diagnosing and managing osteomyelitis of the foot in diabetes. Clin Infect Dis 2004;39(Suppl 2):S115–22.
5. Meyr AJ, Singh S, Zhang X, et al. Statistical reliability of bone biopsy for the diagnosis of diabetic foot osteomyelitis. J Foot Ankle Surg 2011;50(6):663–7.
6. La Fontaine J, Shibuya N, Sampson HW, et al. Trabecular quality and cellular characteristics of normal, diabetic, and charcot bone. J Foot Ankle Surg 2011; 50(6):648–53.
7. Elamurugan TP, Jagdish S, Kate V, et al. Role of bone biopsy specimen culture in the management of diabetic foot osteomyelitis. Int J Surg 2011;9:214–6.

8. Kessler L, Piemont Y, Ortega F, et al. Comparison of microbiological results of needle puncture vs. superficial swab in infected diabetic foot ulcer with osteomyelitis. Diabet Med 2006;23:99–102.

9. Game FL, Jeffcoate WJ. Primarily non-surgical management of osteomyelitis of the foot in diabetes. Diabetologia 2008;51:962–7.

10. Senneville E, Gaworowska D, Topolinski H, et al. Outcome of patients with diabetes with negative percutaneous bone biopsy performed for suspicion of osteomyelitis of the foot. Diabet Med 2012;29:56–61.

11. Newman LG, Waller J, Palestro CJ, et al. Unsuspected osteomyelitis in diabetic foot ulcers: diagnosis and monitoring by leukocyte scanning with indium in 111 oxyquinoline. JAMA 1991;266:1246–51.

12. Grayson ML, Gibbons GW, Balogh K, et al. Probing to bone in infected pedal ulcers: a clinical sign of underlying osteomyelitis in diabetic patients. JAMA 1995; 273:721–3.

13. Shone A, Burnside J, Chipchase S, et al. Probing the validity of the probe-to-bone test in the diagnosis of osteomyelitis of the foot in diabetes. Diabetes Care 2006; 29:945.

14. Lavery LA, Armstrong DG, Peters EJ, et al. Probe-to-bone test for diagnosing diabetic foot osteomyelitis: reliable or relic? Diabetes Care 2007;30:270–4.

15. Aragón-Sánchez J, Lipsky BA, Lázaro-Martínez JL. Diagnosing diabetic foot osteomyelitis: is the combination of probe-to-bone test and plain radiography sufficient for high-risk inpatients? Diabet Med 2011;28(2):191–4.

16. Wrobel JS, Connolly JE. Making the diagnosis of osteomyelitis. The role of prevalence. J Am Podiatr Med Assoc 1998;88(7):337–43.

17. Garcia Morales E, Lazaro-Martinez JL, Aragon-Sanchez FJ, et al. Inter-observer reproducibility of probing to bone in the diagnosis of diabetic foot osteomyelitis. Diabet Med 2011;28:1238–40.

18. Armstrong DG, Lavery LA, Sariaya M, et al. Leukocytosis is a poor indicator of acute osteomyelitis of the foot in diabetes mellitus. J Foot Ankle Surg 1996;35: 280–3.

19. Eneroth M, Larsson J, Apelqvist J. Deep foot infections in patients with diabetes and foot ulcer: an entity with different characteristics, treatments, and prognosis. J Diabet Complications 1999;13:254–63.

20. Fleischer AE, Didyk AA, Woods JB, et al. Combined clinical and laboratory testing improves diagnostic accuracy for osteomyelitis in the diabetic foot. J Foot Ankle Surg 2009;48(1):39–46.

21. Becker W. Imaging osteomyelitis and the diabetic foot. Q J Nucl Med 1999;43: 9–20.

22. Eckman MH, Greenfield S, Mackey WC, et al. Foot infections in diabetic patients. Decision and cost-effectiveness analyses. JAMA 1995;273:712–20.

23. Tomas MB, Patel M, Marwin SE, et al. The diabetic foot. Br J Radiol 2000;73: 443–50.

24. Dinh MT, Abad CL, Safdar N. Diagnostic accuracy of the physical examination and imaging tests for osteomyelitis underlying diabetic foot ulcers: meta-analysis. Clin Infect Dis 2008;47:519–27.

25. Pineda C, Espinosa R, Pena A. Radiographic imaging in osteomyelitis: the role of plain radiography, computed tomography, ultrasonography, magnetic resonance imaging, and scintigraphy. Semin Plast Surg 2009;23(2):80–9.

26. National Institute for Health and Clinical Excellence. Diabetic foot problems Inpatient management of diabetic foot problems. 2011. Available at: http://www.nice.org.uk/nicemedia/live/13416/57943/57943.pdf. Accessed January 12, 2013.

27. Sella EJ. Current concepts review: diagnostic imaging of the diabetic foot. Foot Ankle Int 2009;30:568–76.
28. Gnanasegaran G, Vijayanathan S, Fogelman I. Diagnosis of infection in the diabetic foot using 18F-FDG PET/CT: a sweet alternative? Eur J Nucl Med Mol Imaging 2012;39:1525–7.
29. Erdman WA, Buethe J, Bhore R, et al. Indexing severity of diabetic foot infection with 99mTc-WBC SPECT/CT hybrid imaging. Diabetes Care 2012;35(9):1826–31.
30. Heiba SI, Kolker D, Mocherla B. The optimized evaluation of diabetic foot infection by dual isotope SPECT/CT imaging protocol. J Foot Ankle Surg 2010;49: 529–36.
31. Craig JG, Amin MB, Wu K, et al. Osteomyelitis of the diabetic foot: MR imaging-pathologic correlation. Radiology 1997;203:849–55.
32. Lipsky BA, Berendt AR. Principles and practice of antibiotic therapy of diabetic foot infections. Diabetes Metab Res Rev 2000;16(Suppl 1):S42–6.
33. Henke PK, Blackburn SA, Wainess RW, et al. Osteomyelitis of the foot and toe in adults is a surgical disease: conservative management worsens lower extremity salvage. Ann Surg 2005;241(6):885–94.
34. Game F. Management of osteomyelitis of the foot in diabetes mellitus. Nat Rev Endocrinol 2010;6:43–7.
35. Valabhji J, Oliver N, Samarasinghe D, et al. Conservative management of diabetic forefoot ulceration complicated by underlying osteomyelitis: the benefits of magnetic resonance imaging. Diabet Med 2009;26(11):1127–34.
36. Embil JM, Rose G, Trepman E, et al. Oral antimicrobial therapy for diabetic foot osteomyelitis. Foot Ankle Int 2006;27(10):771–9.
37. Barth RE, Vogely HC, Hoepelman AI, et al. 'To bead or not to bead?' Treatment of osteomyelitis and prosthetic joint-associated infections with gentamicin bead chains. Int J Antimicrob Agents 2011;38(5):371–5.
38. Tan JS, Friedman NM, Hazelton-Miller C, et al. Can aggressive treatment of diabetic foot infections reduce the need for above-ankle amputation? Clin Infect Dis 1996;23:286–91.
39. Ha Van G, Siney H, Danan JP, et al. Treatment of osteomyelitis in the diabetic foot. Contribution of conservative surgery. Diabetes Care 1996;19:1257–60.
40. Aragón-Sánchez FJ, Cabrera-Galván JJ, Quintana-Marrero Y, et al. Outcomes of surgical treatment of diabetic foot osteomyelitis: a series of 185 patients with histopathological confirmation of bone involvement. Diabetologia 2008;51(11): 1962–70.
41. Aragón-Sánchez J, Lázaro-Martínez JL, Hernández-Herrero C, et al. Does osteomyelitis in the feet of patients with diabetes really recur after surgical treatment? Natural history of a surgical series. Diabet Med 2012;29(6):813–8.
42. Hachmöller A. Outcome of minor amputations at the diabetic foot in relation to bone histopathology: a clinical audit. Zentralbl Chir 2007;132:491–6.
43. Kowalski TJ, Matsuda M, Sorenson MD, et al. The effect of residual osteomyelitis at the resection margin in patients with surgically treated diabetic foot infection. J Foot Ankle Surg 2011;50(2):171–5.
44. Molines-Barroso RJ, Lázaro-Martínez JL, Aragón-Sánchez FJ, et al. Analysis of transfer lesions in patients who underwent surgery for diabetic foot ulcers located on the plantar aspect of the metatarsal heads. Diabet Med 2013.

Hyperbaric Oxygen Therapy as Adjunctive Treatment of Diabetic Foot Ulcers

Magnus Löndahl, MD, PhD[a,b,*]

KEYWORDS

- Diabetes • Foot ulcers • Hyperbaric oxygen therapy • Hyperbaric oxygen • Healing
- Amputation

KEY POINTS

- Hyperbaric oxygen therapy (HBO) is a short-term, high-dose oxygen inhalation and diffusion therapy, delivered systemically through airways and blood under high pressure, using hyperbaric chambers.
- HBO therapy stimulates angiogenesis, reduces edema, augments granulation tissue formation by enhancing fibroblasts, and improves leukocyte function by elevating the partial pressure of oxygen in tissue.
- The widespread use of HBO as an adjunctive treatment of diabetic foot ulcers has been founded on weak scientific evidence, but the consistency in positive outcomes in trials evaluating HBO for ulcer healing is noteworthy.

INTRODUCTION

In clinical practice, all aspects of the multifactorial etiology of diabetic foot ulcers must be considered. Therefore, treatment of diabetic foot ulcers requires a multifactorial approach and must at least include regular minor debridement, off-loading of areas with high pressures, optimizing control of metabolism and concomitant diseases, foot care, education of foot care, and provision of protective shoes. Further important aspects include revascularization to restore adequate blood flow, aggressive control of infection by use of local and systemic antibiotics as well as regular debridement, and extensive surgical debridement and amputations as needed. Treatment is best offered by multidisciplinary clinics.[1,2] Most patients will heal if these treatment

This work was supported by the Faculty of Medicine (ALF), Lund University, Lund, Sweden. The author has nothing to disclose.

[a] Department of Clinical Sciences, Lund University, Lund S-221 85, Sweden; [b] Department of Endocrinology, Skane University Hospital, Hudhuset, Lund S-221 85, Sweden
* Department of Endocrinology, Skane University Hospital, Hudhuset, Lund S-221 85, Sweden.
E-mail address: magnus.londahl@med.lu.se

strategies are applied.[3] Failure to heal, despite applying all conventional treatment methods, should imply consideration of adjunctive therapies such as topical growth factors, bioengineered biological coverings, systemically applied colony-stimulating growth factors, and hyperbaric oxygen therapy (HBO).[4–6]

HYPERBARIC OXYGEN THERAPY

HBO has been used in the armamentarium of diabetic foot therapy for more than 4 decades, but its utility has been controversial, not least because evidence has been scarce, but also because charlatans have unscrupulously promoted HBO as a cure of almost any disease.[7] In fact, although evidence supporting the usefulness of HBO in the healing of diabetic foot ulcers has been limited, it has not been inferior to that of many other more commonly used treatment modalities for diabetic feet.[8] More recently, 2 double-blind, randomized controlled trials have shown beneficial effects of HBO in terms of improved ulcer healing and improved health-related quality of life.[9–11]

In this article the indications, contraindications, and complications, as well as basic and clinical evidence of HBO therapy for diabetic foot ulcers, are discussed.

DEFINITION OF HBO

HBO can be described as a short-term, high-dose oxygen inhalation and diffusion therapy, delivered systemically through airways and blood, achieved by having the patient breathing concentrated oxygen at a pressure higher than 1 absolute atmosphere (ATA).[12] In clinical practice, hyperbaric chambers are used to achieve this, and in the diabetic foot pressures between 2.0 and 2.5 ATA are usually endorsed.

Breathing high-dose concentrations of oxygen at surface levels or topical exposure of limbs to high-dose concentrations of oxygen are not included in this definition of HBO.

PHYSIOLOGIC EFFECTS OF HBO

HBO is all about gases and bubbles, and might to be considered as a treatment modality when there is a need for increased oxygen delivery to tissues or when gas bubbles are present in tissues or vessels. The effects of HBO are founded on pure physics, and common gas laws explain the theoretical framework as well as usual clinical experiences of HBO treatment.

Boyle's law states that during constant temperature, a volume of a gas is inversely proportional to its pressure. For example, the volume of gas-containing cavities in a body will alter if HBO is applied. A clinical illustration is the squeeze phenomenon, taking place when compression of the Eustachian tube prevents equalization of gas pressure between the middle ear and surrounding air. According to the same physical law, trapped gas expands during decompression and can thereby cause severe tissue damage.

According to Charles' law, there is a relationship between absolute pressure and temperature as long as the volume is constant, which explains the increasing temperature in a hyperbaric chamber during compression and decreasing temperature during decompression.

At sea level the air above the ground (the atmosphere) exerts a total pressure of 760 mm Hg on the earth's surface, which rationally corresponds to the pressure of 1 absolute atmosphere (ATA). According to Dalton's law (of partial pressures), the total pressure exerted by a gaseous mixture is equal to the sum of the partial pressures of each individual component in the gas mixture. As the atmosphere constitutes 20.94 volume-% oxygen, 78.08 volume-% nitrogen, 0.04 volume-% CO_2, and traces of several other gases, the partial pressure of oxygen (Po_2) in air is approximately 160 mm Hg (760 mm Hg $\times$ 21% = 160 mm Hg). The partial pressure a gas is exerting on its environment will increase if the pressure increases or the gas concentration in the gas mixture increases.

As stated by Henry's law, the concentration of a specific gas in a solution, such as water or body fluids, is determined by its partial pressure and by its solubility coefficient. Under ordinary perfusion conditions, resting tissues extract about 50 mL of oxygen per liter of blood, most of which is delivered by hemoglobin. During air breathing at normobaric pressure, hemoglobin is saturated to about 97% when leaving the pulmonary circulation, and only a small fraction of oxygen is dissolved in blood, about 3 mL of oxygen per liter of blood. If 100% oxygen is administered, the volume of dissolved oxygen increases to 15 mL per liter of blood, and during HBO at 2.5 ATA almost 60 mL of oxygen is dissolved in each liter.[13] This phenomenon is graphically illustrated in **Fig. 1**. This state is sufficient to support resting tissues without any contribution of oxygen bound to hemoglobin.[13] In fact, in 1960 Boerema and colleagues[14] showed that life can be maintained in pigs in the absence of erythrocytes using HBO. Furthermore, in solution oxygen can more easily reach physically obstructed areas where red cells cannot pass or diffusion distances are long. However, the microcirculation is also enhanced by increased erythrocyte flexibility caused by HBO.[15]

In summary, by increasing pressure and oxygen concentration, HBO treatment increases Po_2, and thereby additional oxygen molecules are dissolved in the patient's blood. **Table 1** shows the ideal alveolar and arterial partial pressures of oxygen at different pressure levels in patients during air and oxygen breathing.

After transportation to the capillary bed, oxygen depends on diffusion to reach cells and intracellular spaces. The rate of oxygen delivery is inversely proportional to the square distance and directly proportional to Po_2 at the initial point at the capillary.[16]

Intercapillary distances vary between different types of tissue. A major denominator of capillary density is metabolic rate; that is, distances between capillaries are short in muscle and other highly oxygen-consuming tissues but are considerably longer in slow-healing tissues with lower metabolic rates, such as tendon, fascia, and subcutis.

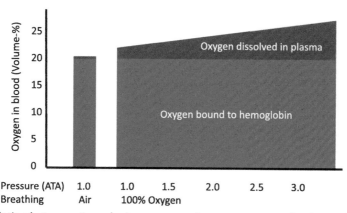

Fig. 1. Relation between atmospheric pressure and oxygen concentration in arterial blood. The volume bound to hemoglobin is almost constant around 20 volume-%, whereas the dissolved volume is increasing with pressure, according to Henry's law. ATA, absolute atmosphere.

Table 1
Ideal alveolar and arterial Po₂ during air and oxygen breathing

	Breathing Air		Breathing 100% Oxygen	
	Po_2	Po_2	Po_2	Po_2
	Alveolar (mm Hg)	Arterial (mm Hg)	Alveolar (mm Hg)	Arterial (mm Hg)
1.0 ATA	102	0.32	673	2.09
2.0 ATA	262	0.81	1433	4.44
2.5 ATA	342	1.06	1813	5.62
3.0 ATA	422	1.31	2193	6.80

Abbreviations: ATA, absolute atmosphere; Po₂, partial pressure of oxygen.

In diabetic microvascular disease, capillary function is declined and distances between capillaries are increased. To avoid hypoxia in the presence of microvascular disease, oxygen needs to diffuse longer distances, thus requiring higher Po₂ levels at the edge of the capillaries. The increase in Po₂ at therapeutic hyperbaric conditions generates a potential 3-fold augmentation in diffusion distance.[17] The importance of this feature is outlined in **Fig. 2**.

Several other effects of HBO and hyperoxygenation on the human body have been described, the most important of which are summarized in **Table 2**. These effects may vary according to several factors, among which patients' health states, pressures used, and exposition time to HBO are the most important. For example, in general HBO treatment is followed by peripheral vessel constriction, whereas the opposite, vasodilation, seems to appear in ischemic tissues.[18] Moreover, effects are more pronounced at higher pressures; that is, clinically notable effects of reduced cerebral blood flow on the central nervous systems are seldom seen at pressures below 2.0 ATA, whereas the risk of oxygen convulsions significantly increases when pressures exceed 3.0 ATA. However, the clinical relevance of many of these effects is as yet unknown.

CLINICAL SETTING OF HBO

There are 2 different kinds of hyperbaric chambers: monoplace and multiplace chambers. The size, shape, and construction of chambers vary considerably, but the

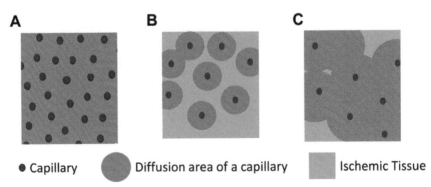

● Capillary   ● Diffusion area of a capillary   ▇ Ischemic Tissue

Fig. 2. Clinical implications of change in diffusion distances at different pressures according to Krogh. (*Panel A*) Non-ischemic tissue with an adequate number of capillaries with normal capillary function. (*Panel B*) Ischemic tissue in a diabetic patient caused by loss of capillaries and capillary function due to microvascular disease. (*Panel C*) Restoration of ischemia as the diffusion distance from each capillary increases as pressures increases during an HBO session.

Table 2	
Important effects of exposure of HBO treatment to a healthy human body	
Cardiovascular system	Bradycardia
	Decreased cardiac output
	Decreased cerebral blood flow
	Increased risk of cardiac arrhythmias
	Increased systolic blood pressure
	Decreased diastolic blood pressure
Respiratory system	Depressed ventilation caused by suppression of aortic and carotid bodies
	Washout of N_2 with subsequent increased risk of pulmonary collapse
Peripheral vessels	Increased peripheral resistance
	Vasoconstriction
Blood/coagulation	Stimulated fibrinolytic activity hours after exposure
	Reduced platelet aggregation
	Increased elasticity of erythrocytes
Metabolism	Changed cerebral glucose metabolism
Oxygen metabolism	Decreased importance of hemoglobin as oxygen transporter

common denominator is that the construction is built to withstand pressurization. **Fig. 3** shows different models of hyperbaric chambers.

Monoplace chambers are the most commonly used. These chambers are easily moveable and require less patient compliance but, in contrast to multiplace chambers, direct patient access is very restricted. A monoplace hyperbaric chamber is generally made of acrylic material and permits direct patient observation. The cylinder is either pressurized entirely with oxygen or air, having the patients breathing oxygen via a mask.

Multiplace chambers are typically steel constructions in which 2 or more patients are pressurized. For safety reasons (fire hazards) the chamber is pressurized with air, and patients breathe oxygen via tightly fitted hoods or masks. Multiplace chambers usually have an anteroom that can be used as a fast passage, admitting personnel going into or patients going out of the pressurized chamber.

Robust evidence is lacking for a selection of treatment regimens leading to optimal therapeutic benefit, such as hyperbaric pressure level, duration of treatment sessions, number of HBO sessions, and, not least, best timing of treatment initiation. In clinical practice, HBO in the management of patients with diabetic foot ulcers are usually accomplished with daily treatment sessions at pressures of 2.0 to 2.5 ATA.[19] During a treatment session, patients usually breathe oxygen for 80 to 90 minutes. Another 5 to 10 minutes per session is generally required for compression and decompression. To minimize the risk of oxygen toxicity, a rare but severe complication of HBO, the treatment period of oxygen breathing may be interrupted by 1 or 2 5-minute intervals of air breathing. A typical treatment protocol consists of 30 to 40 treatment sessions.[19]

Differences between monoplace and multiplace hyperbaric chambers are listed in **Table 3**.

INDICATIONS FOR HBO IN THE DIABETIC FOOT

The rational for HBO is in counteracting hypoxia, edema, and infection. It has been used in clinical practice for a long time, but evidence has been limited, as discussed later in this article.

No worldwide consensus for plausible indications of HBO in the diabetic foot is present today. The Underwater and Hyperbaric Medical Society suggests HBO as

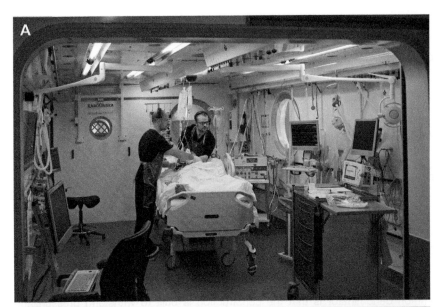

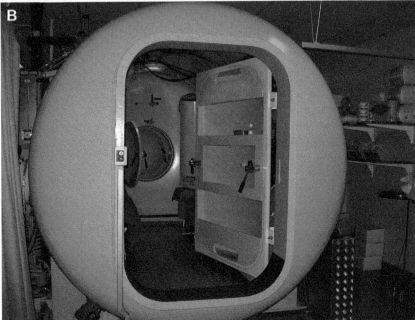

Fig. 3. Three different models of hyperbaric chamber. (*A*) Modern stationary multiplace chamber at Karolinska Hospital, Sweden. (*B*) An older movable multiplace chamber at Helsingborg Hospital, Sweden. (*C*) A mobile monoplace chamber. ([*A, C*] *Courtesy of* Dr Folke Lind, Karolinska Hospital, Solna, Sweden; photography by Folke Lind [*A*], Magnus Löndahl [*B*], and Per Eliasson [*C*].)

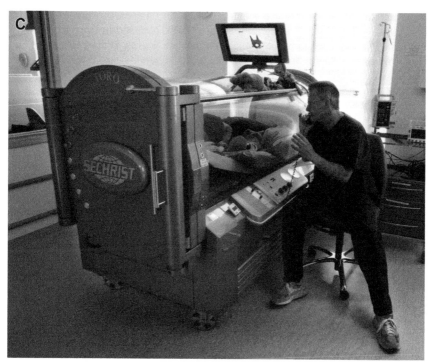

Fig. 3. (*continued*)

Table 3		
Comparison between monoplace and multiplace hyperbaric chambers		
	Monoplace Chamber	**Multiplace Chamber**
Environment	Claustrophobic	More space
Accessibility	Limited access to the patient	Health care personnel can be in or enter the chamber to deal with acute clinical situations Physical/medical/surgical therapy can be performed inside the chamber Intensive care treatment possible
Number of patients	One Newer devices may admit 2 patients	From a few to 20
Risk of fire	Increased if chamber is pressurized with oxygen	Less, as chamber is pressurized with air
Masks/hoods	Not needed if pressurized with oxygen, otherwise yes	Tight-fitting masks or hoods are required
Infection	Less risk as patients are treated individually	Risk for cross infection if more than 1 patient is treated at the same time
Cost	Lower investment cost	Lower cost per treated patient
Portable	Yes	No
Pressure	Usually 3 ATA	Up to 6 ATA

an adjuvant treatment of refractory osteomyelitis and selected problem wounds in patients with arterial insufficiency. The issue is not discussed in a recent Cochrane report. The National Institute of Clinical Excellence in the United Kingdom does not recommend HBO for treating diabetic foot ulcer, whereas the US Food and Drug Administration approve HBO for the treatment of diabetic problem foot wounds.[20]

The International Working Group on the Diabetic Foot concludes in their most recent guideline on ulcer healing that the scientific evidence for use of HBO as an adjunctive therapy for nonhealing diabetic foot ulcers is firmer than before.[8] Several investigators in are supporting this opinion, and the inclusion criteria in the studies with the highest Jadad scores have been suggested as a clinical selection standard.[19,21–23] Such a standard might include the following selection criteria:

- Diabetic full-skin foot ulcers, not healing despite best available care in a multidisciplinary diabetic foot clinic setting for at least 3 months (Löndahl and colleagues[9]) or 6 weeks (Abidia and colleagues[11])
- No need for or no ability of vascular surgical intervention in the affected lower limb
- Capacity and ability to complete an HBO session series
- Absence of contraindications for HBO

Several large case series, as well as data from some randomized clinical trials, are suggesting that patients with very low transcutaneous oxygen pressure (TcPo$_2$) levels in the affected foot, without substantial response to pure oxygen breathing, have less beneficial effect from HBO. However, reported positive predictive values of these measurements as predictors for nonhealing after HBO are low.[24] In a large cohort study by Fife and colleagues,[24] in-chamber wound-area TcPo$_2$ levels less than 200 mm Hg during HBO treatment predicted nonhealing with 74% reliability.

CONTRAINDICATIONS

Absolute contraindications for HBO include untreated pneumothorax and concomitant use of certain chemotherapeutics, such as doxorubicin or cisplatin. Concomitant treatment with disulfiram is also a contraindication, as this drug inhibits production of superoxide dismutase, a protective antioxidant.

Relative contraindications include sinusitis, severe chronic obstructive pulmonary disease, history of pneumothorax or thoracic surgery, uncontrolled high fever, claustrophobia, upper respiratory infection, and inability to equalize pressure in the middle ear. Many of these contraindications are related to known complications of HBO, such as barotrauma, which can be exacerbated by emphysema or inability to equalize middle ear pressure, and seizures for which an uncontrolled fever can be a predisposing factor. Congenital spherocytosis is also a relative contraindication, as these patients have fragile erythrocytes, and high O$_2$ partial pressures may cause severe hemolysis in these patients.

Animal studies have shown an increased incidence of congenital malformations during early pregnancy after exposure to HBO. Although human cases series with women from all trimesters have mitigated this risk, pregnancy is considered as a contraindication unless vast gain is anticipated.

As HBO increases tissue Po$_2$ levels and stimulates activation of stem progenitor cells, concerns about tumor growth have been raised. In 1967 Johnson and Lauchlan[25] reported on a plausible tumor-stimulatory effect of HBO by demonstrating increased metastatic burden in HBO-treated patients with cervical cancer. Twenty years later Eltorai and colleagues[26] presented 3 cases with occult carcinoma becoming clinically evident after HBO, and suggested that presence of known malignancy should be a contraindication of HBO. These findings have been verified neither in animal studies nor in other clinical studies.[27–30] In fact, HBO has been suggested as an adjunctive treatment in cancer therapy, as facilitated oxygenation of hypoxic regions could enhance tumor destruction by mechanisms of increased intratumor levels of reactive oxygen species and decreased hypoxic stimulation of angiogenesis, and may cause the cells to enter a proliferative stage and thus sensitize them for chemotherapy or radiotherapy.[31,32]

COMPLICATIONS

Although HBO has several potential side effects, in comparison with many other medical therapies it may be considered as reasonably safe.[33] Barotrauma is among the most prevalent complications. It may occur at any tissue and gas interface within the body, but in clinical practice middle-ear barotrauma is the most common. Of 94 randomized patients in a Swedish study, 1 endured barotraumatic otitis and another 4 required myringotomy with tube placement, owing to pain caused by the inability to equilibrate air pressure through the eustachian tube.[9] In a case series of 11,376 treatment sessions, 17% of all patients reported ear pain or discomfort during compression.[34] However, persistent injuries visible on ear microscopy are less common, with reported incidences between 0.5% and 3.8%.[9,34,35] Nevertheless, as barotrauma might lead to persistent hear loss or vertigo, tympanostomy with tube placement ought to be considered when patients have problems in equalizing pressures. Dental barotrauma may occur if cavities are present in a tooth, such as after an inappropriate filling.

Pulmonary barotrauma is a rare but potentially life-threatening complication. The intrapulmonary gas volume increases during decompression, and if this additional gas volume cannot be exhaled this overpressure might cause pulmonary tears, leading to pneumothorax, emphysema, or, in a worst-case scenario, air emboli. The incidence of pulmonary barotrauma is about 1 in 50,000 to 60,000 treatments.[33,36]

Reversible myopia is a common side effect affecting up to every fifth patient.[37] Cataract is not a clinical problem during normal treatment series, but seems to be persistent and highly frequent after prolonged treatment series (>150 treatment sessions).[38] Such exposures are therefore no longer recommended. Prolonged exposures to oxygen may cause pneumonitis and alveolitis, but these consequences of pulmonary oxygen toxicity are not a problem in the clinical use of HBO.

Oxygen seizure is a rare and self-limiting complication without any long-term implications.[34]

Diabetic patients, especially those on insulin therapy, are at increased risk of hypoglycemia, usually occurring within 2 to 6 hours of the HBO session.[9,39] In the trial by Löndahl and colleagues[9] (3225 treatment sessions and 94 patients), 6 incidents with hypoglycemia (symptoms and blood glucose $\leq$54 mg/dL [$\leq$3.0 mmol/L]) within 6 hours after treatment were reported.

Some data indicate that HBO treatment may improve peripheral insulin sensitivity.[40] The mechanism is still unknown, but the effect seems to be acute and sustainable for at least a period of 30 treatment sessions.[40]

The most common fatal complication is associated with fire in the chamber. At least 88 human fatalities in 36 separate hyperbaric chamber fires have been reported.[41] Increased fire risk applies especially to chambers pressurized with oxygen.

RATIONALE OF HBO IN ULCER HEALING

HBO has been shown to stimulate angiogenesis, reduce edema, augment the formation of granulation tissue by enhancing fibroblasts, and improve leukocyte function by elevating tissue P_{O_2}.[42–45]

Neovascularization emerges by 2 mechanisms: angiogenesis and vasculogenesis. Regional factors stimulate the former, and recruitment and differentiation of circulating stem/progenitor cells (SPC) the latter.[46,47] HBO enhances these processes by increasing production of growth factors such as vascular endothelial growth factor, the most specific growth factor for neovascularization.[48,49] Oxidative stress at sites of neovascularization stimulates growth-factor synthesis by augmenting synthesis and stabilization of hypoxia-inducible factor 1, a process further enhanced by HBO.[50–54] HBO also enhances extracellular matrix formation, an O_2-dependent process closely linked to neovascularization.[55,56]

Activity of nitric oxide synthase (NOS)-3 is required for SPC mobilization from the bone marrow, a process that is impaired in patients with diabetes, probably because of reduced NOS activity caused by hyperglycemia and insulin resistance.[57,58] HBO mobilizes SPC in people with and without diabetes by stimulating nitric oxide synthesis in bone marrow.[51,59]

HBO reduces tissue edema by mechanisms of vasoconstriction in nonischemic tissue.[45]

Throughout reperfusion, leukocytes cause pathologic vasoconstriction and tissue damage by releasing proteases and free radicals after adhering to ischemic tissues. HBO treatment has been shown to reduce postischemic leukocyte adherence and vasoconstriction in ischemic rat tissue.[60]

High lactate concentrations, as present in wounds, stimulate procollagen synthesis.[43] The enzymatic steps whereby procollagen is converted to collagen, and cross-linked to collagen matrix, are oxygen dependent.[60] In animal experiments, collagen deposition in a hyperoxic environment has been shown to increase 3-fold compared with deposition in a hypoxic environment. Correction of both vasoconstriction and hypoxemia might increase collagen deposition as much as 10-fold.[61] Furthermore, fibroblast replication is most optimal at tissue P_{O_2} of 40 to 60 mm Hg.[16] Epithelialization is promoted by oxygen exposure, and seems also to be enhanced by HBO.[62,63]

The single most bactericidal mechanism in wounds is oxidant production by leukocytes, and P_{O_2} has a far higher impact on bactericidal production in human leukocytes than blood glucose concentration, pH, and temperature.[64] HBO facilitates the oxygen-dependent peroxidase system in leukocytes, increases the generation of oxygen free radicals, and thereby enhances oxidation of proteins and membrane lipids while inhibiting bacterial metabolic function.[65,66] In ischemic tissue, restoration of tissue P_{O_2} reestablishes the phagocytic function of macrophages.[67,68] HBO augments oxygen-dependent transport of certain antibiotics across bacterial cell walls.[69,70] Moreover, with increasing tissue P_{O_2} hypoxic environments become less suitable for anaerobic bacteria.

CLINICAL EVIDENCE OF HBO

The first outcome of HBO treatment in patients with diabetic foot ulcers was reported in 1979 by Hart and Strauss.[71] In this small retrospective study of patients with chronic, nonhealing ulcers, 10 of 11 participants healed after HBO. Since then numerous retrospective studies have been published. The study characteristics and outcomes of some of these are given in **Table 4**. Even if these studies have different

Table 4
Characteristics and outcomes of retrospective studies/case series evaluating the effect of HBO in patients with diabetes foot ulcers

Authors,[Ref.] Year	Wound Description	No. of Patients	Outcome and Comments
Hart and Strauss,[71] 1979	Chronic nonhealing diabetic foot ulcers	11	Healing rate 10/11 (91%)
Matos,[111] 1983	Nonhealing diabetic foot ulcers Ischemia, infection, or neuropathy present	70	Healing or significant improvement seen in 60% of all patients
Perrins and Barr,[112] 1986	Unknown	26	Healing rate 67% Amputation avoided in 18%
Davis,[113] 1987	Wagner grade 3 and 4 Daily HBO for 30–60 d	168	Healing rate 70% Treatment failures seen in older patents with peripheral arterial disease and absent pedal pulses
Wattel et al,[105] 1990	Ulcers; 11 diabetic and 9 arteriosclerotic HBO 2.5 ATA Two sessions of 90 min/d Median 46 (15–108) sessions	20	Healing seen in 15 patients Transcutaneous oxygen pressure a predictive factor for ulcer healing
Cianci et al,[114] 1991	Wagner grade 4 Limb-threatening infection in 97% Revascularization in 55%	41	Limbs salvaged in 78%
Weisz et al,[115] 1993	Ulcer duration >3 mo All palpable foot pulses HBO, 2.5 ATA Median 56 ± 10 sessions	14	Healing seen in 11 patients
Lee et al,[116] 1997	Infected foot ulcers HBO Mean 35 ± 22 sessions	31	Major amputation 6 Healing 25
Ciaravino et al,[72] 1996	Nonhealing wounds Diabetes 17/54 patients HBO Mean 30 sessions	54	Some improvement 11% No improvement 80% Inconclusive 9% Complications in 63% (barotraumas 43%)
Kaya et al,[117] 2009	Prospective HBO, 2.4 ATA, 120 min, mean 39 sessions	184	At 1 y follow-up 115 (62.5%) patients healed
Bishop and Mudge,[104] 2012	Retrospective Mean 40 sessions of HBO	30	Index ulcer healing rate 3 mo after completion of HBO: 26.7% Amputation rate 3.9%

patient selection criteria and design, all (with one exception) suggest a beneficial effect of HBO on ulcer healing.[72]

The first prospective controlled study was performed by Baroni and colleagues[73] and was published in 1987. Eighteen hospitalized patients with diabetic foot ulcers of Wagner grades were treated with HBO. Outcome was compared with that of a control group matched for duration, lesion size, depth, and severity of diabetes. Attending surgeons taking decisions about amputations were blinded as to which group a patient belonged. Sixteen patients healed and 2 underwent amputation in the HBO group, compared with 1 healed and 4 amputated patients in the control group. The investigators concluded that HBO was beneficial to patients with diabetic ulcers of Wagner grade 3 and 4 below the ankle. This study was followed by several nonrandomized controlled studies as listed in **Table 5**. In the nonrandomized controlled study by Kalani and colleagues,[74] 38 patients with neuropathy, local ischemia, and foot ulcer with a duration of at least 2 months were followed for 3 years. Healing rates at the 3-year follow-up visit were 76%, compared with 48% in the HBO and control groups, respectively. Two of 17 patients (12%) had been amputated above the ankle in the HBO group and 7 of 21 (33%) in the control group. There were no differences in arterial toe blood pressure or basal $TcPo_2$ levels between healed or amputated patients, whereas $TcPo_2$ levels during oxygen breathing were higher in healers.[74]

Earlier this year Margolis and colleagues[75] published a large cohort trial using longitudinal data from the National Healing Corporation (2005–2011) to compare diabetic foot ulcer healing and amputation rates at 16 weeks in 793 patients receiving HBO therapy with 5466 patients not receiving HBO. The results in this study are in contrast to those in the earlier nonrandomized controlled trials, as ulcer healing rates were lower and amputation rates higher in the group of HBO-treated patients. These results persist also after adjustment for plausible registered selection biases. The conclusion of the investigators is that the usefulness of HBO in the treatment of diabetic foot ulcers needs to be reevaluated. This wording may be incisive and, as applies to every study, this one also needs to be discussed and evaluated in detail. Such a discussion is beyond the scope of this review, but some concerns are stressed here. The ulcer duration at inclusion was 1 month, which might be considered as short for ulcers that are difficult to heal. As shown in **Table 5**, frequencies of Wagner grade 3 ulcers differed between groups, and deeper ulcers were more common in those patients selected for HBO. The median HBO series included 29 treatment sessions, and all patients receiving at least 8 treatment sessions were included in the intention-to-treat analysis. The length of the follow-up period is an important issue; 16 weeks might be too short to identify the full effects of HBO, as indicated by the 16 weeks' ulcer-healing rate of less than 15% in the HBO group in the randomized, placebo-controlled, double-blind HODFU study.[9] In the author's opinion, the major importance of this study is its assessment of HBO usage in everyday clinical practice in the United States, although the follow-up time might be too short to fully do so. The randomized clinical trial is still considered to be the best available method to reduce selection and other biases, especially those difficult to identify.

Outcomes from 8 randomized clinical trials evaluating the effect of HBO as an adjunctive therapy in the management of chronic diabetic foot ulcers have been reported.[9,11,76–81] One of these trials, comparing effects of HBO and hyperbaric air on Tco_2 levels in 29 diabetic patients, has been presented only as an abstract and not as a peer-reviewed article.[78] In an open-label, randomized trial shockwave therapy healed more ulcers than treatment with 20 HBO sessions at 2.5 ATA. This trial has been considered to be at high risk of both performance bias and attrition bias, as participants who withdrew were excluded from the analysis; it is therefore not included in the further discussion.[20]

In the first randomized controlled trial (RCT) evaluating the effect of HBO as an adjunctive therapy in the management of diabetic foot ulcers by Doctor and colleagues,[76] amputations were significantly fewer in patients receiving 4 HBO sessions

Table 5
Characteristics and outcomes of prospective nonrandomized studies evaluating the effect of HBO in patients with diabetes foot ulcers

Authors,[Ref.] Year	Study Design and Ulcer Characteristics	No. of Patients	Outcome and Comments
Baroni et al,[73] 1987	Wagner grade 3 and 4 Matched control group Surgeons blinded	I: 18 C: 16	Healing: I 16/18; C 1/16 Amputation: I 2/18; C 4/16 Amputation rates at the center 40%
Faglia et al, 1987[a]	Wagner grade 3 and 4 Matched control group Surgeons blinded Follow-up (group-extension?) of Baroni study	I: 26 C: 20	Healing: I 24/26; C 2/20 Amputation: I 2/26; C 8/20
Oriani et al,[84] 1990	Controls were selected for, but refused, HBO Group-extension of Baroni study?	I: 62 C: 18	Healing: I 66%; C 33%
Zamboni et al,[85] 1997	HBO, 2.0 ATA, 30 sessions	I: 5 C: 5	Healing at 4–6 mo follow-up: I 80%; C 20%
Kalani et al,[74] 2002	Basal $TcPo_2$ <40 mm Hg and >100 mm Hg breathing O_2. HBO, 2.5 ATA, 40–60 sessions	I: 17 C: 21	Three-year follow-up: Healing: I 76%; C 48% Amputation: I 12%; C 33%
Lyon,[118] 2008	Retrospective Standard care (a) vs HBO (b) vs platelet-derived growth factors (PDGF) (c) vs PDGF + HBO (d). Larger wounds in group d		Healing rates at 8 wk follow-up: a. 15% (n = 25) b. 30% (n = 13) c. 82% (n = 26) d. 72% (n = 25)
Chen et al,[119] 2010	Prospective <10 HBO sessions (a) vs ≥10 sessions (b)	42	Healing rates: a. 33.3% b. 76.2%
Margolis et al,[75] 2013	Longitudinal data from NHC (2005–2011) 16 wk follow-up Inclusion criteria: <40% ulcer area reduction during 28 d Plantar ulcer Adequate arterial flow in the leg Ulcer duration at inclusion: 1 mo Wagner grade ≥3: I 45.7%; C 18.4%		

Abbreviations: C, control group; I, intervention group; NHC, National Healing Corporation; $TcPo_2$, transcutaneous oxygen pressure.
[a] The original paper could not be identified; data from fourth ECHM Consensus Conference.[120]

(3.0 ATA) over 4 weeks, compared with those given standard care alone. Double-blind sham therapy with compressed air was used in 2 of the remaining 5 studies, and these 2 scored 5 out of 5 points on the Jadad scale.[9,11] Study settings, inclusion criteria, and outcomes in these RCTs are given in **Tables 6** and **7**. Although all these prospective,

Table 6
Characteristics of clinical randomized studies evaluating the effect of HBO in patients with diabetes foot ulcers

Authors,[Ref.] Year	Wound Description	No. of Patients	Treatment Control vs Intervention
Doctor et al,[76] 1992	Chronic ulcers, not further specified. Randomization after necessary debridement and 3 d of antibiotic treatment in hospital	I: 15 C: 15	Multidisciplinary wound care only vs Multidisciplinary wound care HBO, 3.0 ATA, 45 min/session 4 sessions over 4 wk
Faglia et al,[79] 1996	Wagner grade 2–4 Duration >3 mo	I: 36 C: 34	Multidisciplinary wound care only vs Multidisciplinary wound care HBO, 2.2–2.5 ATA, 90 min/session 38 ± 8 sessions Follow-up time approximately 7 wk
Kessler et al,[80] 2003	Wagner grade 1–3 Duration >3 mo Neuropathy present	I: 14 C: 13	Multidisciplinary wound care only vs Multidisciplinary wound care HBO, 2.5 ATA, 90 min/session 20 sessions in 10 d Follow-up time 4 wk
Abidia et al,[11] 2003	Ulcer duration $\geq$6 wk Diameter 1–10 cm^2 ABI <0.8 or TBI <0.7 HbA_{1c} <8.5%	I: 9 C: 9	Double-blinded design Multidisciplinary wound care Hyperbaric air (sham) therapy vs Multidisciplinary wound care HBO, 2.4 ATA, 90 min/session 30 sessions Follow-up time 1 y
Duzgun et al,[77] 2008	Ulcer duration $\geq$4 wk	I: 50 C: 50	Multidisciplinary wound care only vs Multidisciplinary wound care HBO, 2.5 ATA, 90 min/session 30–45 sessions Mean follow-up time 92 ± 12 wk
Löndahl et al,[9] 2010	Ulcer duration >3 mo At least 2 mo treatment in a diabetic foot clinic Need for or ability of vascular surgical intervention ruled out	I: 49 C: 45	Multidisciplinary wound care and hyperbaric air treatment 2.5 ATA, 90 min/session, 40 sessions vs Multidisciplinary wound care HBO, 2.5 ATA, 90 min/session 40 sessions Follow-up time 40 wk

Abbreviations: ABI, ankle-brachial index; C, control; HbA_{1c}, hemoglobin A_{1c}; I, intervention; TBI, toe-brachial index.

Table 7
Outcomes of clinical randomized studies evaluating the effect of HBO in patients with diabetes foot ulcers

	Follow-Up Period	No. of Patients I/C Groups	Major Amputation[a] I/C Groups	Minor Amputation[b] I/C Groups	Ulcer Healing[c] I/C Groups
Doctor et al,[76] 1992	Until discharge	15/15	13%/47% (2/7)	27%/13% (4/2)	
Faglia et al,[79] 1996	±49 d	35/33	9%/33% (3/11)	60%/36% (21/12)	
Abidia et al,[11] 2003	1 y	8/8	13%/13% (1/1)	13%/0% (1/0)	63%/0% (5/0)
Duzgun et al,[77] 2008	92 ± 12 wk	50/50	0%/34% (0/17)	8%/48% (4/24)	82%/66% (41/33)
Löndahl et al,[9] 2010, ITT - analysis	1 y	49/45	7%/2% (3/1)	8%/9% (4/4)	52%/29% (25/12)
Löndahl et al,[9] 2010, per-protocol analysis	1 y	38/37	3%/3% (1/1)	11%/8% (4/3)	61%/27% (23/10)

Abbreviations: C, control; I, intervention.
[a] In the study by Duzgun et al, proximal of metatarsophalangeal joints in all other studies above ankle.
[b] In the study by Duzgun et al, distal of metatarsophalangeal joints in all other studies below ankle.
[c] Censored for deaths during the follow-up period (I = 1 and C = 3).

randomized trials demonstrate outcomes in favor of HBO, results should be interpreted cautiously, as study methodologies have been criticized.[15,82] Detailed information of randomization procedures or concomitant therapies are lacking in some of the studies. Patient-selection procedures are not always easy to follow, and withdrawals are not always reported. Furthermore, investigators and outcomes assessors may unintentionally lend bias to study outcomes in the open-labeled trials.

Other interventions during follow-up periods might bias the study outcomes, particularly in nonblinded trials. The impact of vascular surgery interventions during follow-up times is such an issue in HBO trials. In the trial by Faglia and colleagues,[79] vascular surgical intervention was performed in 38% of all patients during the follow-up period after HBO, and the implications of the outcome of these interventions have been debated.[7,79,83] Although more than 50% of the patients had had at least one previous vascular intervention at the time of randomization, and the need for (or possibility of) vascular surgical intervention had been excluded at time of inclusion in the Löndahl trial,[9] percutaneous transluminal angioplasty (PTA) was performed in 10 patients (11%) within 1 year of randomization. However, these interventions cannot explain the higher rate of ulcer healing in the HBO group, as only 3 ulcers, of which 1 was in the placebo group, healed following PTA.

As there are possibilities of both clinical and study-related heterogeneities between these RCTs, owing to differential wound severity and size across studies at time of inclusion as well as variability in inclusion criteria and the nature and timing of outcome assessments, it might be most proper to let every study stand for itself, and avoid data pooling; thus, pooled data analyses should be interpreted with caution.

Ulcer Healing

Long-term ulcer healing is reported in 3 studies.[9,11,77] Löndahl and colleagues[9] and Abidia and colleagues[11] report healing at 1 year of follow-up. During the follow-up time of 92 ± 12 weeks, 91% of all patients either healed or underwent an amputation in the trial conducted by Duzgun and colleagues.[77] The primary end point in this study was healing without surgical intervention in an operating theater. According to this definition 66% of the patients in the HBO group healed, compared with none in the control group. However, 18% healed after debridement in the operating room, and are considered as healers in the following analysis so as to be in accordance with the trials by Abida and Löndahl.

Altogether 210 patients have been included in RCTs reporting long-term follow-up (at least 1 year), 107 being randomized to HBO and 103 to placebo or control groups. Sixty-three (59%) of the HBO-treated patients healed compared with 21 (20%) patients randomized to non-HBO in the control groups.

Published nonrandomized controlled studies, with follow-up times between 3 and 36 months, reported outcome in 128 HBO-treated and 80 non–HBO-treated patients. Healing rates were significantly higher in patients treated with HBO (77% vs 25%).[73,74,84,85]

Major Amputation

Frequencies of major amputation are reported in 5 RCTs, but the definition of major amputation differs in Duzgun's trial,[77] and it is accordingly separately discussed. Two hundred eight patients were included in the other 4 trials (107 HBO and 101 non-HBO). Twenty (19%) major amputations were performed in patients randomized to no HBO treatment, compared with 9 (8%) in HBO-treated patients. However, amputation rates in the control groups were considerably higher in the earlier nonblinded RCTs in comparison with the more recent double-blinded RCTs (36% vs 4%). In the hospitalized study population of patients with infected Wagner grade 3 and 4 patients in the trial by Faglia and colleagues,[79] significantly fewer (8.6 vs 33.3%) above-ankle amputations were done in those randomized to HBO, compared with best care without HBO. Doctor and colleagues[76] report a similar outcome. Only 6 patients, of whom 4 were in control groups, underwent above-ankle amputations in the 2 double-blind RCTs.[9,11] This finding may be explained by different study populations, but might also mirror a change in indications for major amputation, as nonhealing of a chronic ulcer could be an indication for major amputation in the setting of the earlier studies by Doctor and colleagues[76] and Faglia and colleagues,[79] but not in the later studies by Abidia and colleagues[11] and Löndahl and colleagues.[9] In the open-labeled randomized trial by Duzgun and colleagues,[77] 24 (48%) patients in the standard treatment group were amputated proximal to the metatarsophalangeal joint, compared with 4 (8%) in the HBO group.

Health-Related Quality Of Life

Diabetic foot ulceration is a source of severe disability, and reported health-related quality of life (HRQoL) in these patients is as low as in patients treated for breast cancer.[10,86–92] Ulcer healing is associated with improved HRQoL.[88,93]

HBO has been shown to improve HRQoL in patients with diabetes and chronic foot ulcers. In a small study by Lin and colleagues[94] evaluating HRQoL in 15 patients with foot ulcers (11 diabetic patients), overall quality of life was enhanced after HBO therapy. HRQoL was also evaluated in the 2 double-blind RCTs. In the trial by Abidia and colleagues,[11] SF-36 domains General Health and Vitality improved in patients randomized to HBO. The SF-36 domains Role Limitations Due to Physical and Emotional Health and Mental Health Summary Score were significantly higher after 1 year compared with baseline in HBO-treated patients in the study by Löndahl and colleagues.[10] No improvements occurred in the placebo group. This study was the first to identify improvement in mental health summary score after healing of a diabetic foot ulcer, which might be attributable to longer follow-up time and more severe baseline ulcer conditions. Furthermore, focus-group interviews with 19 study participants identified development of positive contacts and social relations with other patients as a main advantage of HBO treatment.[95] Patients perceived HBO as unproblematic and pleasant, although time consuming and tiring.[95] The social interaction accomplished by treatment in a multiplace hyperbaric chamber during an 8-week-long treatment period might thus improve long-term well-being by increased social interaction, improved self-confidence, and reduced depression.

Other Effects

Patients with diabetes and a history of chronic foot ulcer are at a high risk for cardiovascular morbidity and mortality. Some data indicate that HBO treatment may reduce this risk level. Some small, nonrandomized studies indicate beneficial effects, at least in the short term, on diastolic dysfunction, heart rate, and blood pressure.[96,97] HBO treatment may also decrease QT dispersion, thereby reducing the risk of lethal arrhythmias.[98] Three-year follow-up data from the double-blind randomized HODFU study suggest that HBO treatment may improve survival (Löndahl M, Hammarlund C, and Katzman P, personal communication, 2013).

Health Economics

Cost-effectiveness is a central issue in modern health care. The cost of a full course of HBO treatment for diabetic foot ulcers varies from one place to another and depends on several factors, such as setup costs, ongoing costs, reimbursement systems, and number of patients treated per center. Charges between US$200 and $1250 per treatment session have been reported from reimbursed health care units.[11,99,100] These figures do not include accompanying expenses such as travel and hotel costs. Of more importance than the actual cost is outcome from a full health-economic evaluation of the treatment. Some health-economic analyses evaluating the cost-effectiveness of HBO as adjunctive therapy for diabetic foot ulcers have been published, but are limited by deficient primary clinical data and should be interpreted with caution.[11,101,102] Nevertheless they suggest a potential cost-effectiveness of HBO. A crude analysis of the small but high-quality double-blind RCT by Abidia and colleagues,[11] taking only HBO and dressing costs into account, suggests a saving of £2960 per patient during the first year of follow-up. However, the cost-effectiveness of HBO cannot be considered as established as long as robust health-economic evaluations based on large placebo-controlled RCTs evaluating the effect of HBO as adjunctive treatment are lacking.

Selection of Patients

HBO is a time-consuming and expensive treatment modality; therefore, being able to predict who will benefit from therapy would indeed be valuable. In the study by Löndahl and colleagues,[10] neither ankle-brachial index nor toe blood pressure could be used as predictors for ulcer healing. In the prospective study by Kalani and colleagues,[74] toe blood pressure could not be used as predictor for healing or amputation after HBO. Likewise, ankle-brachial index was not reported as a factor influencing outcome in a retrospective study including 1006 patients with diabetic foot ulcers from 5 hyperbaric facilities in the United States.[103] Patients without the presence of peripheral arterial disease (PAD) achieved a better outcome after HBO than those with PAD in a small recent case series by Bishop and Mudge.[104]

TcPo$_2$ seems to be associated with healing after HBO. In a case series including 20 patients (11 diabetic patients and 9 patients with arterial insufficiency but without diabetes) given adjunctive treatment with HBO, Wattel and colleagues[105] reported higher basal TcPo$_2$ levels in healers than in nonhealers (32 mm Hg and 12 mm Hg, respectively). Similarly, in a retrospective study of 35 patients who received 16 to 20 sessions of HBO after partial foot amputation, healing was achieved in all patients with a TcPo$_2$ higher than 29 mm Hg.[106] Oubre and colleagues[107] performed a retrospective analysis of 73 HBO-treated patients (37 with diabetes) with 85 chronic lower extremity ulcers. Robust healing was achieved in 33 ulcers, minimal healing in 31, and no healing in 21. Basal mean TcPo$_2$ in each of these groups was 57 mm Hg, 44 mm Hg, and 38 mm Hg, respectively. In the randomized double-blind trial by Löndahl and colleagues,[108] TcPo$_2$ before the first treatment session was significantly related to ulcer healing after HBO. In this study, no complete epithelialization occurred in patients with TcPo$_2$ levels lower than 25 mm Hg, and all ulcers healed at TcPo$_2$ levels greater than 75 mm Hg. In patients with TcPo$_2$ between 26 to 50 mm Hg and 51 to 75 mm Hg, healing rates were 50% and 73%, respectively.[108] In addition, more than 70% of all HBO-treated patients with a TcPo$_2$ level higher than 100 mm Hg during 100% oxygen breathing healed, compared with only one-fifth of the patients with a level lower than 100 mm Hg. No ulcer healed if TcPo$_2$ during oxygen breathing was lower than 50 mm Hg. However, stimulated TcPo$_2$ was strongly correlated to basal TcPo$_2$, and in a regression analysis stimulated TcPo$_2$ was not superior to basal TcPo$_2$ in predicting ulcer healing.[108] A similar outcome, indicating less probability of healing after HBO if TcPo$_2$ at baseline was lower than 25 mm Hg breathing air or lower than 50 mm Hg breathing oxygen, has been reported by Fife and colleagues.[24] These conclusions were based on a multicenter follow-up study including 629 patients. However, when various potential cutoff scores were evaluated, the positive predictive values of these analyses were all less than 50%. The investigators recommend TcPo$_2$ measurement under hyperbaric conditions as the best way to predict healing after HBO therapy in diabetic patients with chronic foot ulcers, with a cutoff level of 200 mm Hg,[109] but of course this is not practical in diabetic foot clinics without hyperbaric chambers.

SUMMARY

The widespread use of HBO as an adjunctive treatment of diabetic foot ulcers has been founded on weak scientific evidence, but the consistency in positive outcomes in trials evaluating HBO on ulcer healing is noteworthy, not least as these results are in concert with data from in vitro and physiologic studies supporting the theoretical framework of HBO reversing hypoxia-induced abnormality. The long-term ulcer-healing rates of the nonrandomized controlled studies before the recent study by Margolis and colleagues,[75] 77% with HBO versus 25% with standard treatment, are in concert with 1-year follow-up data from the 2 double-blind RCTs, 54% versus 25%. These 2 trials have put the use of HBO on firmer ground, but several issues, including health economics, developing robust selection criteria for treatment, optimizing treatment protocols, and identifying standards for when to start and stop treatment, remain to be elucidated.[100] Not least, outcomes from further high-quality studies are needed.

At present, HBO may be used as an adjunctive therapy in a select group of patients with diabetic foot ulcers that are difficult to heal.[21,100,110]

REFERENCES

1. Hunt D. Foot ulcers and amputations in diabetes. Clin Evid 2005;14:455–62.
2. Boulton AJ. The diabetic foot: grand overview, epidemiology and pathogenesis. Diabetes Metab Res Rev 2008;24(Suppl 1):S3–6.
3. Barnes R. Point: hyperbaric oxygen is beneficial for diabetic foot ulcers. Clin Infect Dis 2006;43:188–92.
4. Boulton AJ, Armstrong DG, Albert SF, et al. Comprehensive foot examination and risk assessment: a report of the task force of the foot care interest group of the American Diabetes Association, with endorsement by the American Association of Clinical Endocrinologists. Diabetes care 2008;31: 1679–85.
5. Jeffcoate WJ, Lipsky BA, Berendt AR, et al. Unresolved issues in the management of ulcers of the foot in diabetes. Diabet Med 2008;25:1380–9.
6. Jeffcoate WJ, Price P, Harding KG. Wound healing and treatments for people with diabetic foot ulcers. Diabetes Metab Res Rev 2004;20(Suppl 1): S78–89.
7. Berendt AR. Counterpoint: hyperbaric oxygen for diabetic foot wounds is not effective. Clin Infect Dis 2006;43:193–8.
8. Game FL, Hinchliffe RJ, Apelqvist J, et al. A systematic review of interventions to enhance the healing of chronic ulcers of the foot in diabetes. Diabetes Metab Res Rev 2012;28(Suppl 1):119–41.
9. Löndahl M, Katzman P, Nilsson A, et al. Hyperbaric oxygen therapy facilitates healing of chronic foot ulcers in patients with diabetes. Diabetes care 2010; 33:998–1003.
10. Löndahl M, Landin-Olsson M, Katzman P. Hyperbaric oxygen therapy improves health-related quality of life in patients with diabetes and chronic foot ulcer. Diabet Med 2011;28:186–90.
11. Abidia A, Laden G, Kuhan G, et al. The role of hyperbaric oxygen therapy in ischaemic diabetic lower extremity ulcers: a double-blind randomised-controlled trial. Eur J Vasc Endovasc Surg 2003;25:513–8.
12. Hammarlund C. Hyperbaric oxygenation and wound repair in man. Lund (Sweden): Anesthesiology and Intensive Care; 1995.
13. Tibbles PM, Edelsberg JS. Hyperbaric-oxygen therapy. N Engl J Med 1996;334: 1642–8.
14. Boerema I, Meyne NG, Brummelkamp WH, et al. Life without blood. Ned Tijdschr Geneeskd 1960;104:949–54 [in Dutch].
15. Bakker DJ. Hyperbaric oxygen therapy and the diabetic foot. Diabetes Metab Res Rev 2000;16(Suppl 1):S55–8.
16. Hunt TK, Hopf HW. Wound healing and wound infection. What surgeons and anesthesiologists can do. Surg Clin North Am 1997;77:587–606.
17. Krogh A. The number and distribution of capillaries in muscles with calculations of the oxygen pressure head necessary for supplying the tissue. J Physiol 1919; 52:409–15.
18. Hammarlund C, Sundberg T. Hyperbaric oxygen reduced size of chronic leg ulcers: a randomized double-blind study. Plast Reconstr Surg 1994;93:829–33 [discussion: 834].
19. Löndahl M, Fagher K, Katzman P. What is the role of hyperbaric oxygen in the management of diabetic foot disease? Curr Diab Rep 2011;11:285–93.
20. Kranke P, Bennett MH, Martyn-St James M, et al. Hyperbaric oxygen therapy for chronic wounds. Cochrane Database Syst Rev 2012;(4):CD004123.

21. Boulton AJ. Hyperbaric oxygen in the management of chronic diabetic foot ulcers. Curr Diab Rep 2010;10:255–6.

22. Lind F, Eriksson B, Frostell C, et al. How we work with hyperbaric oxygen therapy. Lakartidningen 2011;108:1914–5 [in Swedish].

23. Wu SC, Marston W, Armstrong DG. Wound care: the role of advanced wound-healing technologies. J Am Podiatr Med Assoc 2010;100:385–94.

24. Fife CE, Buyukcakir C, Otto GH, et al. The predictive value of transcutaneous oxygen tension measurement in diabetic lower extremity ulcers treated with hyperbaric oxygen therapy: a retrospective analysis of 1,144 patients. Wound Repair Regen 2002;10:198–207.

25. Johnson R, Lauchlan SC. Epidermoid carcinoma of cervix treated by ^{60}Co therapy and hyperbaric oxygen. In: Proceedings Int Cong of Hyperb Med 1966: 648–652.

26. Eltorai I, Hart GB, Strauss MB, et al. Does hyperbaric oxygen provoke an occult carcinoma in man? In: Kindwall EP, editor. Proceedings of the eighth international congress on hyperbaric medicine. San Pedro: Best Publishing; 1987. p. 18–29.

27. Shewell J, Thompson SC. The effect of hyperbaric oxygen treatment on pulmonary metastasis in the C3H mouse. Eur J Cancer 1980;16:253–9.

28. McMillan T, Calhoun KH, Mader JT, et al. The effect of hyperbaric oxygen therapy of oral mucosal carcinoma. Laryngoscope 1989;99:241–4.

29. Lian QL, Hang RC, Yan HF, et al. Effects of hyperbaric oxygen on S-180 sarcoma in mice. Undersea Hyperb Med 1995;22:153–60.

30. Feldmeier JJ, Heimbach RD, Davolt DA, et al. Does hyperbaric oxygen have a cancer-causing or -promoting effect? A review of the pertinent literature. Undersea Hyperb Med 1994;21:467–75.

31. Sealy R, Cridland S, Barry L, et al. Irradiation with misonidazole and hyperbaric oxygen: final report on a randomized trial in advanced head and neck cancer. Int J Radiat Oncol Biol Phys 1986;12:1343–6.

32. Daruwalla J, Christophi C. The effect of hyperbaric oxygen therapy on tumour growth in a mouse model of colorectal cancer liver metastases. Eur J Cancer 2006;42:3304–11.

33. Trytko BE, Bennett M. Hyperbaric oxygen therapy. Complication rates are much lower than author suggest. BMJ 1999;318:1077–8.

34. Plafki C, Peters P, Almeling M, et al. Complications and side effects of hyperbaric oxygen therapy. Aviat Space Environ Med 2000;71:119–24.

35. Sheffield PJ, Smith PS. Physiological and pharmacological basis of hyperbaric oxygen therapy. In: Bakker DJ, Cramer FS, editors. Hyperbaric Surgery Perioperative Care. Flagstaff (AZ): Best Publishing Company; 2002. p. 63–110.

36. Murphy DG, Sloan EP, Hart RG, et al. Tension pneumothorax associated with hyperbaric oxygen therapy. Am J Emerg Med 1991;9:176–9.

37. Heyneman CA, Lawless-Liday C. Using hyperbaric oxygen to treat diabetic foot ulcers: safety and effectiveness. Crit Care Nurse 2002;22:52–60.

38. Palmquist BM, Philipson B, Barr PO. Nuclear cataract and myopia during hyperbaric oxygen therapy. Br J Ophthalmol 1984;68:113–7.

39. Broussard CL. Hyperbaric oxygenation and wound healing. J Vasc Nurs 2004; 22:42–8.

40. Wilkinson D, Chapman IM, Heilbronn LK. Hyperbaric oxygen therapy improves peripheral insulin sensitivity in humans. Diabet Med 2012;29:986–9.

41. Sheffield PJ, Desautels DA. Hyperbaric and hypobaric chamber fires: a 73-year analysis. Undersea Hyperb Med 1997;24:153–64.

42. Knighton DR, Silver IA, Hunt TK. Regulation of wound-healing angiogenesis—effect of oxygen gradients and inspired oxygen concentration. Surgery 1981; 90:262–70.

43. Hunt TK, Pai MP. The effect of varying ambient oxygen tensions on wound metabolism and collagen synthesis. Surg Gynecol Obstet 1972;135:561–7.

44. Hunt TK, Linsey M, Grislis H, et al. The effect of differing ambient oxygen tensions on wound infection. Ann Surg 1975;181:35–9.

45. Wattel F, Mathieu D, Neviere R, et al. Acute peripheral ischaemia and compartment syndromes: a role for hyperbaric oxygenation. Anaesthesia 1998;53(Suppl 2): 63–5.

46. Carmeliet P. Mechanisms of angiogenesis and arteriogenesis. Nat Med 2000;6: 389–95.

47. Hattori K, Dias S, Heissig B, et al. Vascular endothelial growth factor and angiopoietin-1 stimulate postnatal hematopoiesis by recruitment of vasculogenic and hematopoietic stem cells. J Exp Med 2001;193:1005–14.

48. Sheikh AY, Rollins MD, Hopf HW, et al. Hyperoxia improves microvascular perfusion in a murine wound model. Wound Repair Regen 2005;13(3):303–8.

49. Sheikh AY, Gibson JJ, Rollins MD, et al. Effect of hyperoxia on vascular endothelial growth factor levels in a wound model. Arch Surg 2000;135(11): 1293–7.

50. Gallagher KA, Goldstein LJ, Thom SR, et al. Hyperbaric oxygen and bone marrow-derived endothelial progenitor cells in diabetic wound healing. Vascular 2006;14:328–37.

51. Milovanova TN, Bhopale VM, Sorokina EM, et al. Hyperbaric oxygen stimulates vasculogenic stem cell growth and differentiation in vivo. J Appl Physiol 2009; 106:711–28.

52. Hunt TK, Aslam RS, Beckert S, et al. Aerobically derived lactate stimulates revascularization and tissue repair via redox mechanisms. Antioxid Redox Signal 2007;9:1115–24.

53. Thom SR. Oxidative stress is fundamental to hyperbaric oxygen therapy. J Appl Physiol 2009;106:988–95.

54. Milovanova TN, Bhopale VM, Sorokina EM, et al. Lactate stimulates vasculogenic stem cells via the thioredoxin system and engages an autocrine activation loop involving hypoxia-inducible factor 1. Mol Cell Biol 2008;28: 6248–61.

55. Dinar S, Agir H, Sen C, et al. Effects of hyperbaric oxygen therapy on fibrovascular ingrowth in porous polyethylene blocks implanted under burn scar tissue: an experimental study. Burns 2008;34:467–73.

56. Hopf HW, Gibson JJ, Angeles AP, et al. Hyperoxia and angiogenesis. Wound Repair Regen 2005;13:558–64.

57. Du X, Edelstein D, Obici S, et al. Insulin resistance reduces arterial prostacyclin synthase and eNOS activities by increasing endothelial fatty acid oxidation. J Clin Invest 2006;116:1071–80.

58. Bucci M, Roviezzo F, Brancaleone V, et al. Diabetic mouse angiopathy is linked to progressive sympathetic receptor deletion coupled to an enhanced caveolin-1 expression. Arterioscler Thromb Vasc Biol 2004;24:721–6.

59. Thom SR, Bhopale VM, Velazquez OC, et al. Stem cell mobilization by hyperbaric oxygen. Am J Physiol Heart Circ Physiol 2006;290:1378–86.

60. Hussain MZ, Ghani QP, Hunt TK. Inhibition of prolyl hydroxylase by poly(ADP-ribose) and phosphoribosyl-AMP. Possible role of ADP-ribosylation in intracellular prolyl hydroxylase regulation. J Biol Chem 1989;264:7850–5.

61. Hartmann M, Jonsson K, Zederfeldt B. Effect of tissue perfusion and oxygenation on accumulation of collagen in healing wounds. Randomized study in patients after major abdominal operations. Eur J Surg 1992;158:521-6.

62. Medawar PB. The cultivation of adult mammalian skin epithelium in vitro. Q J Microsc Sci 1948;89:187-96.

63. Uhl E, Sirsjo A, Haapaniemi T, et al. Hyperbaric oxygen improves wound healing in normal and ischemic skin tissue. Plast Reconstr Surg 1994;93: 835-41.

64. Allen DB, Maguire JJ, Mahdavian M, et al. Wound hypoxia and acidosis limit neutrophil bacterial killing mechanisms. Arch Surg 1997;132:991-6.

65. Knighton DR, Halliday B, Hunt TK. Oxygen as an antibiotic. A comparison of the effects of inspired oxygen concentration and antibiotic administration on in vivo bacterial clearance. Arch Surg 1986;121:191-5.

66. Mandell GL. Bactericidal activity of aerobic and anaerobic polymorphonuclear neutrophils. Infect Immun 1974;9:337-41.

67. Mader JT, Brown GL, Guckian JC, et al. A mechanism for the amelioration by hyperbaric oxygen of experimental staphylococcal osteomyelitis in rabbits. J Infect Dis 1980;142:915-22.

68. Babior BM. Oxygen-dependent microbial killing by phagocytes (second of two parts). N Engl J Med 1978;298:721-5.

69. Hind J, Attwell RW. The effect of antibiotics on bacteria under hyperbaric conditions. J Antimicrob Chemother 1996;37:253-63.

70. Kent TA, Sheftel TG, Sutton TE, et al. Effect of hyperbaric oxygen on the blood: cerebrospinal fluid transfer of tobramycin. Aviat Space Environ Med 1986;57: 664-6.

71. Hart GB, Strauss M. Response of ischemic ulcerative conditions to OHP. In: Smith G, editor. Proceedings of the Sixth International Congress on Hyperbaric Medicine. Aberdeen: Aberdeen University Press; 1997. p. 312-4.

72. Ciaravino ME, Friedell ML, Kammerlocher TC. Is hyperbaric oxygen a useful adjunct in the management of problem lower extremity wounds? Ann Vasc Surg 1996;10:558-62.

73. Baroni G, Porro T, Faglia E, et al. Hyperbaric oxygen in diabetic gangrene treatment. Diabetes Care 1987;10:81-6.

74. Kalani M, Jorneskog G, Naderi N, et al. Hyperbaric oxygen (HBO) therapy in treatment of diabetic foot ulcers. Long-term follow-up. J Diabet Complications 2002;16:153-8.

75. Margolis DJ, Gupta J, Hoffstad O, et al. Lack of effectiveness of hyperbaric oxygen therapy for the treatment of diabetic foot ulcer and the prevention of amputation: a cohort study. Diabetes care 2013;36:1961-6.

76. Doctor N, Pandya S, Supe A. Hyperbaric oxygen therapy in diabetic foot. J Postgrad Med 1992;38:112-4, 111.

77. Duzgun AP, Satir HZ, Ozozan O, et al. Effect of hyperbaric oxygen therapy on healing of diabetic foot ulcers. J Foot Ankle Surg 2008;47:515-9.

78. Lin TF, Chen S, Niu K. The vascular effects of hyperbaric oxygen therapy in treatment of early diabetic foot. Undersea Hyperb Med 2001;28:63.

79. Faglia E, Favales F, Aldeghi A, et al. Adjunctive systemic hyperbaric oxygen therapy in treatment of severe prevalently ischemic diabetic foot ulcer. A randomized study. Diabetes care 1996;19:1338-43.

80. Kessler L, Bilbault P, Ortega F, et al. Hyperbaric oxygenation accelerates the healing rate of nonischemic chronic diabetic foot ulcers: a prospective randomized study. Diabetes care 2003;26:2378-82.

81. Wang CJ, Wu RW, Yang YJ. Treatment of diabetic foot ulcers: a comparative study of extracorporeal shockwave therapy and hyperbaric oxygen therapy. Diabetes Res Clin Pract 2011;92:187–93.

82. Roeckl-Wiedmann I, Bennett M, Kranke P. Systematic review of hyperbaric oxygen in the management of chronic wounds. Br J Surg 2005;92:24–32.

83. Hinchliffe RJ, Valk GD, Apelqvist J, et al. A systematic review of the effectiveness of interventions to enhance the healing of chronic ulcers of the foot in diabetes. Diabetes Metab Res Rev 2008;24(Suppl 1):S119–44.

84. Oriani G, Meazza D, Favales F. Hyperbaric oxygen therapy in diabetic gangrene. J Hyperb Med 1990;5(3):171–5.

85. Zamboni WA, Wong HP, Stephenson LL, et al. Evaluation of hyperbaric oxygen for diabetic wounds: a prospective study. Undersea Hyperb Med 1997;24:175–9.

86. Wilson RW, Hutson LM, Vanstry D. Comparison of 2 quality-of-life questionnaires in women treated for breast cancer: the RAND 36-Item Health Survey and the Functional Living Index-Cancer. Phys Ther 2005;85:851–60.

87. Muller-Nordhorn J, Nolte CH, Rossnagel K, et al. The use of the 12-item short-form health status instrument in a longitudinal study of patients with stroke and transient ischaemic attack. Neuroepidemiology 2005;24:196–202.

88. Armstrong DG, Lavery LA, Wrobel JS, et al. Quality of life in healing diabetic wounds: does the end justify the means? J Foot Ankle Surg 2008;47:278–82.

89. Meijer JW, Trip J, Jaegers SM, et al. Quality of life in patients with diabetic foot ulcers. Disabil Rehabil 2001;23:336–40.

90. Vileikyte L. Diabetic foot ulcers: a quality of life issue. Diabetes Metab Res Rev 2001;17:246–9.

91. Willrich A, Pinzur M, McNeil M, et al. Health related quality of life, cognitive function, and depression in diabetic patients with foot ulcer or amputation. A preliminary study. Foot Ankle Int 2005;26:128–34.

92. Nabuurs-Franssen MH, Huijberts MS, Nieuwenhuijzen Kruseman AC, et al. Health-related quality of life of diabetic foot ulcer patients and their caregivers. Diabetologia 2005;48:1906–10.

93. Ragnarson Tennvall G, Apelqvist J. Health-related quality of life in patients with diabetes mellitus and foot ulcers. J Diabet Complications 2000;14:235–41.

94. Lin LC, Yau G, Lin TF, et al. The efficacy of hyperbaric oxygen therapy in improving the quality of life in patients with problem wounds. J Nurs Res 2006;14:219–27.

95. Hjelm K, Löndahl M, Katzman P, et al. Diabetic persons with foot ulcers and their perceptions of hyperbaric oxygen chamber therapy. J Clin Nurs 2009;18:1975–85.

96. Al-Waili NS, Butler GJ. Effects of hyperbaric oxygen on inflammatory response to wound and trauma: possible mechanism of action. ScientificWorldJournal 2006;6:425–41.

97. Karadurmus N, Sahin M, Tasci C, et al. Potential benefits of hyperbaric oxygen therapy on atherosclerosis and glycaemic control in patients with diabetic foot. Endokrynol Pol 2010;61:275–9.

98. Kardesoglu E, Aparci M, Uzun G, et al. Hyperbaric oxygen therapy decreases QT dispersion in diabetic patients. Tohoku J Exp Med 2008;215:113–7.

99. van der Staal SR, Ubbink DT, Lubbers MJ. Comment on: Lipsky and Berendt. Hyperbaric oxygen therapy for diabetic foot wounds: has hope hurdled hype? Diabetes Care 2010;33:1143–5 Diabetes care 2011;34:e110; [author reply: e111].

100. Lipsky BA, Berendt AR. Hyperbaric oxygen therapy for diabetic foot wounds: has hope hurdled hype? Diabetes care 2010;33:1143–5.

101. Chow I, Lemos EV, Einarson TR. Management and prevention of diabetic foot ulcers and infections: a health economic review. Pharmacoeconomics 2008; 26:1019–35.

102. Chuck AW, Hailey D, Jacobs P, et al. Cost-effectiveness and budget impact of adjunctive hyperbaric oxygen therapy for diabetic foot ulcers. Int J Technol Assess Health Care 2008;24:178–83.

103. Fife CE, Buyukcakir C, Otto G, et al. Factors influencing the outcome of lower-extremity diabetic ulcers treated with hyperbaric oxygen therapy. Wound Repair Regen 2007;15:322–31.

104. Bishop AJ, Mudge E. A retrospective study of diabetic foot ulcers treated with hyperbaric oxygen therapy. Int Wound J 2012;9:665–76.

105. Wattel F, Mathieu D, Coget JM, et al. Hyperbaric oxygen therapy in chronic vascular wound management. Angiology 1990;41:59–65.

106. Zgonis T, Garbalosa JC, Burns P, et al. A retrospective study of patients with diabetes mellitus after partial foot amputation and hyperbaric oxygen treatment. J Foot Ankle Surg 2005;44:276–80.

107. Oubre CM, Roy A, Toner C, et al. Retrospective study of factors affecting non-healing of wounds during hyperbaric oxygen therapy. J Wound Care 2007;16: 245–50.

108. Löndahl M, Katzman P, Hammarlund C, et al. Relationship between ulcer healing after hyperbaric oxygen therapy and transcutaneous oximetry, toe blood pressure and ankle-brachial index in patients with diabetes and chronic foot ulcers. Diabetologia 2011;54:65–8.

109. Fife CE, Smart DR, Sheffield PJ, et al. Transcutaneous oximetry in clinical practice: consensus statements from an expert panel based on evidence. Undersea Hyperb Med 2009;36:43–53.

110. Tiaka EK, Papanas N, Manolakis AC, et al. The role of hyperbaric oxygen in the treatment of diabetic foot ulcers. Angiology 2012;63:302–14.

111. Matos L. Preliminary report of the use of hyperbarics as adjunctive therapy in diabetics with chronic non-healing wounds. HBO Review 1983;4:88–9.

112. Perrins JD, Barr PO. HBO and wound healing. In: Schmutz J, editor. Proceedings of the First Swiss Symposium of Hyperbaric Oxygenation; September 18–20, 1985; Basel: Foundation for Hyperbaric Medicine, 1986: 119–32

113. Davis JC. The use of adjuvant hyperbaric oxygen in treatment of the diabetic foot. Clin Podiatr Med Surg 1987;4:429–37.

114. Cianci P, Petrone G, Green B. Adjunctive hyperbaric oxygen in salvage of the diabetic foot. Undersea Biomed Res 1991;18:108.

115. Weisz G, Ramon Y, Melamed T. Treatment of the diabetic foot by hyperbaric oxygen. Harefuah 1993;124:678–81.

116. Lee S, Chen C, Chan YW, et al. Hyperbaric oxygen in the treatment of diabetic foot infection. Changgeng Yi Xue Za Zhi 1997;20:17–22.

117. Kaya A, Aydin F, Altay T, et al. Can major amputation rates be decreased in diabetic foot ulcers with hyperbaric oxygen therapy? Int Orthop 2009;33:441–6.

118. Lyon KC. The case for evidence in wound care: investigating advanced treatment modalities in healing chronic diabetic lower extremity wounds. J Wound Ostomy Continence Nurs 2008;35:585–90.

119. Chen CE, Ko JY, Fong CY, et al. Treatment of diabetic foot infection with hyperbaric oxygen therapy. Foot Ankle Surg 2010;16:91–5.

120. Fourth ECHM Consensus Conference. In: Medicine ECfH. December 4–5, 1998 London, 1999.

Index

Note: Page numbers of article titles are in **boldface** type.

A

Achilles tendon pathology, surgical correction of, 815
Adalimumab, for Charcot foot, 866–867
Advanced glycation end products, in Charcot foot, 860
Age factors, in ulceration, 780
Alendronate, for Charcot foot, 864–865
Allogenic bilayered human skin equivalent, 886, 891
American Diabetes Association, consensus report on Charcot neuropathy, 867
Aminobisphosphonates, for Charcot foot, 864
Amoxicillin/clavulanate, 918, 922
Ampicillin-sulbactam, 918, 921
Amputation, **791–805**
    counting methods for, 792–794
    for Charcot foot, 878
    for osteomyelitis, 930, 953–954
    frequency of, hyperbaric oxygen therapy effects on, 972
    pathway to, 782–783
    variation in observed incidence of, 794–798
    versus revascularization, 796, 798, 801
Anaerobic infections, 917, 919, 922
Anakinra, for Charcot foot, 867
Angiogenesis, in hyperbaric oxygen therapy, 966
Angiography, therapeutic, 841–842
Angioplasty, for revascularization, 827, 830, 839, 842–843
Angiosome theory, 840, 842
Ankle brachial index, 777, 824
Ankle equinus deformity, in Charcot foot, 860
Ankle joint, Charcot foot involvement of, 861
Ankle-foot orthosis, for Charcot foot, 863
Apoptosis, in Charcot foot, 858–859
Arthrodesis, for Charcot foot, 877–878
Arthroplasty, for ulceration prevention, 816
Autologous platelet-rich plasma, 887, 892–893
Autonomic neuropathy
    in Charcot foot, 859–860
    sympathetic, 779–780
    ulceration in, 779–780
Aztreonam, 919

B

Balloon angioplasty, for peripheral vascular disease, 842–843
Barotrauma, in hyperbaric oxygen therapy, 965

Med Clin N Am 97 (2013) 981–992
http://dx.doi.org/10.1016/S0025-7125(13)00109-0
0025-7125/13/$ – see front matter © 2013 Elsevier Inc. All rights reserved.

medical.theclinics.com

Printed and bound by CPI Group (UK) Ltd, Croydon, CR0 4YY

03/10/2024

01040439-0006